OSCE Stations for Medical Finals Book 1

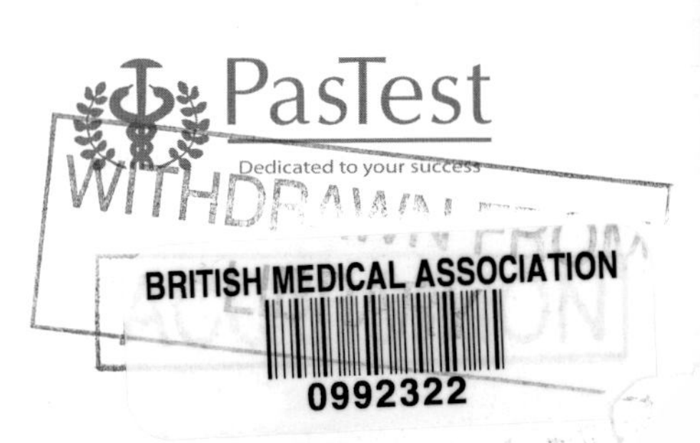

OSCE Stations for Medical Finals Book 1

Adam Feather FRCP
Senior Lecturer in Medical Education,
St. Bartholomew's and The London Medical School,
Consultant Geriatrician
Newham University Hospital NHS Trust

Ashling Lillis BA (Cantab) MB BS MRCP(UK)
Acute Medicine Registrar,
King George Hospital,
Essex

Tony Joy MBChB MRCS(Eng) DCH
'Darzi' Fellow in Clinical Leadership
Registrar in Emergency Medicine
North East Thames Rotation
London

John S P Lumley MS FRCS
Emeritus Professor of Vascular Surgery,
St Bartholomew's and the Royal London
School of Medicine and Dentistry

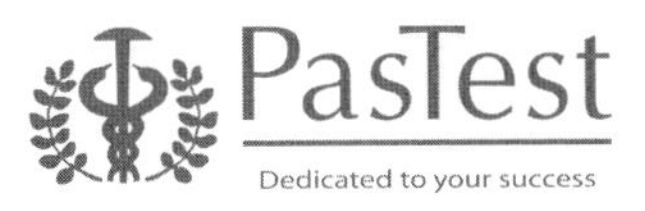

Egerton Court

Parkgate Estate
Knutsford
Cheshire
WA16 8DX

Telephone: 01565 752000

First Published 2012

ISBN: 978 1905 635 795
A catalogue record for this book is available from the British Library.

Text prepared by Carnegie Book Production, Lancaster
Printed and bound in the UK by Page Bros, Norwich

Contents

About the Authors *vi*
Preface *vii*
Acknowledgements *viii*
How to Use This Book *ix*
Introductory Chapter *xi*

SCENARIOS

1. What a wheeze 1
2. Heartache 19
3. Tummy pain 39
4. Party girl 55
5. Diarrhoea and vomiting 72
6. Washed out and totally drained 98
7. Breathless patient 115
8. Cold feet 132
9. Feeling awful 149
10. Tingle in my fingers 163
11. Confused young man 179
12. Out of breath 203
13. Funny turns 219
14. Fallen Community leader 239
15. Off legs 262
16. All of a sudden 286
17. Couldn't get up 304
18. Heart's a flutter 318
19. Don't sweat it 338
20. Unsteady on my feet 353

Blank Charts *368*
Station Index *374*
Subject Index *376*

About the Authors

Dr Ashling Lillis BA (Cantab) MB BS MRCP(UK)
Ashling is a trainee in Acute Internal Medicine in North East London. Having completed medical school and foundation training in Cambridge and then the East End of London she left for sunnier climbs with a year of medical practice in New Zealand. She returned to the East End to complete acute care core training at the Royal London Hospital, Whitechapel, at which time she became a clinical skills tutor at Bart's and the London School of Medicine and Dentistry. She is now starting out on dual training in Acute Internal and General Medicine.

Dr Tony Joy MBChB MRCS(Eng) DCH
Tony is a Registrar in Emergency Medicine on the Northeast Thames Rotation in London. He is currently working as a 'Darzi' Fellow in Clinical Leadership at Newham University Hospital. Having qualified from the University of Sheffield in 2004, he worked briefly in Sri Lanka following the Boxing Day tsunami. After moving to London in 2005 he became interested in trauma and emergency medicine when working at the Royal London Hospital. He aims to become an Emergency Medicine Consultant, with particular interests in pre-hospital care, medical education and clinical leadership. In 2011 he married Amanda, and they are currently awaiting the imminent arrival of their first child.

Dr Adam Feather FRCP
Adam Feather is a Geriatrician at Newham University Hospital Trust and a Senior Lecturer in Medical Education at Barts and The London Medical School. He is the Lead for Clinical Skills and the Head of Final Year, and as such has responsibilities in supporting and preparing final year students in their transition to qualified doctors. He has been involved with the finals assessment both as a major contributor and lead for the past ten years. He is passionate about undergraduate medical education and has diverse interests including assessment, student support and curriculum design. He is perhaps best known for being the father of the soon to be famous Jack Barney Feather.

John S P Lumley MS FRCS
John Lumley was formerly Honorary Consultant Surgeon to St Bartholomew's Hospital, The National Hospital for Neurology and Neurosurgery, Queen Square and the Hospital for Sick Children, Great Ormond Street, London. He has been World President of the International College of Surgeons, and Council Member, Journal Editor and Chairman of the Primary Fellowship Examiners of the Royal College of Surgeons. He has authored/edited over 50 texts, including one on conducting, having founded and conducted the Barts Academic Festival Choir and Orchestra (BAFCO) for over 40 years.

Preface

OSCEs for Finals are based on clinical cases, each assessing you on the sequential management of a clinical problem. This form of scenario-based assessment is more akin to your future clinical practice than the more common independent OSCE format. We also give emphasis to the critical thinking, diagnostic reasoning and other aspects of professionalism that are essential for a practicing doctor: these features are highlighted by icons and summary boxes throughout the text. Case-based assessment is widely used in postgraduate examinations, and is increasingly being introduced into the undergraduate curriculum and into finals.

The first two volumes of the series cover general medicine and surgery. The third volume is devoted to the specialities commonly included in the foundation programmes. Each clinical problem assesses history taking, examination, communication and data interpretation, and where appropriate, procedural and prescribing skills. The three volumes cover all of the procedures required by Tomorrow's Doctors (2009) and the Foundation Programme Application System (FPAS), and are the first set of books covering the skills and knowledge to be assessed in the new national prescribing skills assessment (PSA).

If successive tasks (stations) provide unwanted clues, they are placed on separate pages, as are the answers and patient prompts. Possible navigation difficulties are overcome by clear numbering, and the use of icons. Uniform timing of stations can be a problem in a clinical examination; a text has no such limitations, and appropriate times are given for each question.

We advise working through the scenarios in student pairs, one of you being the examinee and the other the 'patient' and examiner (or a third member can take on one of these tasks): the separation of the patient history, examination and investigations of each scenario facilitates this approach. Marking is against a defined protocol, with grades from A-E: involvement in clinical practice and discussions with your teachers will indicate the required level of competence at each stage of your training. As you approach finals, your professional competence should be A or B, even if there are still gaps in your knowledge of specific diseases.

The texts are intended to refine your diagnostic approach, but they can also serve to revise the clinical features and investigation of specific conditions – this is facilitated by the refection and consolidation sections that bring together the salient features of each problem. Use the index to find the condition, and the icons in each scenario to locate individual stations for abnormal symptoms, signs and investigations. Consider how these abnormalities relate to the severity of the problem and how you would treat the patient at each stage of their disease.

Most stations refer to the reader as an FY1 doctor, rather than a medical student: this emphasises that the qualifying examination is to ensure that you are well trained and safe to progress to this level. The final's examiner expects fluency of your diagnostic approach, a reasoned differential diagnosis, and a caring and complete understanding of patient management.

Acknowledgements

Thanks to Rebecca Spendiff, Consultant Radiologist at Colchester General Hospital

How to Use This Book

The OSCEs in this text are based on 20 clinical problems (Scenarios), and follow their management through diagnosis and treatment: thus reflecting the typical process used in clinical practice. In this case-based format, you need information for each station, but it must not give clues that could pre-empt subsequent questions and answers. To facilitate this, you are advised to work in pairs, one acting as a candidate and the other as the examiner – if you are the examiner, use the grey shaded patient instructions to respond to the candidate's questions, and then use the examiner's questions to assess and mark the candidate's performance. The patient/carer scripts state what information should be volunteered and areas that should be left for the candidate to actively explore. A third member can act as the patient for the **History** and **Examination** stations. Rotate the roles so that you all experience the various components of the OSCE format.

Each scenario is made up of a number of stations: the questions for these are sequential, followed by the answer section. The type of station content is indicated by a specific icon, so that they can be quickly identified in the question and answer sections. Cases do not necessarily have all types of station, but each begins with a **History**, followed by an **Examination** station. The **History** station starts with an instruction to the candidate, specifying their role and what is expected of them, eg whether you should take a full history or concentrate on a specific aspect – **read all OSCE instructions very carefully**. If not specified, take a full history of the presenting complaint and question the patient's past – drug use, allergies, social and family history – and undertake a systemic enquiry (by finals this should be a rapid review, and it is the examiner's job to ensure that you do not miss important information, as this could be detrimental in your subsequent clinical practice).

As you approach finals, you are expected to be competent in patient management, particularly in taking a history and examining a patient. You will probably have revised the factual content of clinical problems, but this series also gives prominence to the professionalism, the diagnostic process, your **Clinical communication skills** and the diagnostic reasoning that must underpin your answers. All participants must read the paragraphs on each history page to understand the meaning of the previous sentence. Icons are used to both emphasise these features in the examiner's assessment and to avoid writing them out again in full.

When assessing the history taking and presentation, the examiner gives a mark for content, professionalism, the diagnostic process, communication skills and, when questioned, the candidate's diagnostic reasoning, followed by a global mark for the whole – be aware that the examiner is taking into account all these elements of your history taking.

Marking is not further discussed in this chapter, but for more information on the subject go to page xxii. Similarly go to page xv for discussion on timing – examination circuits have to run to a schedule, and the time allowed for a station is usually more than adequate for a fair assessment. Be aware of the suggested times in the text, but you can be fluid in their use, as between you, you should cover and discuss all aspects of each station.

Your examination can be carried out, and assessed, on a model or a mannequin. Although abnormal signs are absent, with your partners, you can talk through the clinical features you are looking for and the techniques you are using, as you would in an observed examination station in finals. One of you acting as the model, or the examiner, can indicate the abnormal findings present as the examination proceeds. Again read the instructions with icons on the initial examination sheet and make sure they are taken into account in your presentation and assessment. An alternative approach is also given – the examination findings are provided, to be read and then presented. Take enough time to take in this material, but be aware that a time may be suggested in finals. (The difficulty of avoiding pre-emptive clues in a text has already been mentioned – **avoid reading these pages before examining a model**.)

Clinical communication skills are essential in clinical practice and a number of these stations have been included to assess your approach to difficult explanations, such as surgical consent and terminal illness. Read the instructions thoroughly, including the additional icon linked material: be aware that, as with the **History** and **Examination** stations, the examiner is assessing your skills and training in all these areas.

Data interpretation is a key domain in your final assessment. Normal values are usually embedded in the question, but commit normal values of common investigations to memory. The questions in some of these stations are extended beyond the single case of the scenario, to expand their educational and assessment value.

The assessment of **Prescribing skills** is a mandatory part of finals (page xxi): as the NHS does not have a standard prescription chart, use either that of your local trust, or photocopy the chart(s) at the back of this book. In view of the potential harmful effect on patient safety, you must spend time to ensure competency in this area: marking must be stringent. Compare your answers with those in the text to ensure their accuracy in every detail.

Procedural skills cannot be assessed on patients in finals, but models or mannequins may be appropriate, or the candidate's understanding of the relevant apparatus can be tested. The text follows the same pattern and covers the competencies that are expected of a qualifying doctor (page xxi).

The **Consolidation and Reflection** section summarises the case and its components, and can serve as a reminder of these facts on completion of the scenario or at a later date. This information can be expanded and reinforced by use of the **Further reading** section.

Introductory Chapter

Diagnostic Medical Graduates

Professor Sir George Paget introduced clinical assessments into the graduating finals at Cambridge University in the 1840s. Some may suggest that little changed until Harden and Gleason introduced the Objective Structured Clinical Examination (OSCE) in 1975. OSCEs, a derivation from the traditional approach of clinical short cases, and the 'bell day' or 'steeplechase' used in many anatomy examinations, introduced and reinforced several educationally important concepts. Perhaps most importantly, each student taking a formal clinical examination underwent a similar, objective and structured assessment. Their performance was observed by multiple examiners who marked the candidates' performance against a validated set of criteria, recorded on an itemised checklist.

Despite their 'educational excellence' it was not until the 1990s that they were fully embraced and developed further by the UK Medical Schools. However, like the 'Pagetoid' Final Examinations of the 19th and 20th century, over the last 10 years (both nationally and internationally) OSCEs have largely stagnated, and their reliability and defensibility, so important in an era of increasing litigation, have come to totally dominate other psychometric aspects, in particular face and content validity.

OSCEs are made up of a circuit of 'stations', each station being a self contained area (a room or cubicle) in which the candidate is asked to perform a given clinical task. The tasks are largely independent of one another and the knowledge and skills utilised in one are neither required nor utilised in subsequent stations. The tasks may vary in duration but are often artificially remodelled and time limited by the practicalities of the examination.

As the candidate proceeds around the circuit they are asked to perform tasks in multiple and varying contexts and roles, each task observed by a different assessor. Whilst these multiple clinical 'biopsies' are the strength of the OSCE, this format poorly reflects the reality of working in the clinical environment, and students move from task to task with little or no testing of the linked diagnostic process required when seeing a single, 'real' patient.

In the earlier phases of the course, ie until such time as a student can demonstrate minimal competence, students and the assessments rightly concentrate on the content and to a far lesser extent the process, of the tasks. Sadly the 'what' (content), rather than the 'how' (process) has become the priority for the majority of students and has resulted in the modern phenomenon of the 'OSCE performance'; students enacting a performance to gain the necessary pass marks. This is sadly repeated in all station-based examinations, including final MB graduating examinations, and latterly has been creeping into the PACES assessment of the MRCP.

At graduation candidates should be expected to function at a more sophisticated level, being challenged and assessed around the 'how, when and why' and not simply the 'what'. In short our assessments need to encourage and test the **clinical diagnostic process and reasoning.**

Clinical Diagnostic Process

In its simplest form the diagnostic process consists of taking a history from a patient, examining them, formulating a diagnosis, and then planning appropriate investigation and the subsequent therapeutic interventions. This involves a complex interaction between knowledge and skills, and is difficult to define, teach and perhaps most importantly, learn and assess.

Diagnostic History + Diagnostic Examination = Diagnostic Clinical Assessment

Imagine you are a clinician in the middle of nowhere, for example on an arctic expedition, on board a 747 mid Pacific, or in the outback of Australia or rural Africa. There are no triage teams, no monitoring machines or near patient testing, and CRP is the local beer. Given the limited clinical resources you may have at your disposal you must formulate an action plan based on the severity of the presentation. In the 'middle of nowhere' this may mean asking a plane with 400 fellow passengers on board to land, calling in the flying doctor service, rescue vessels or even an extraction team, so you had better be right! Now one begins to understand the potential importance of a diagnostic clinical assessment. By taking a history and performing a full, appropriate examination, one derives a working diagnosis and differentials. From these arise the management plan, including investigations and therapeutic interventions

The history should be well structured, appropriate to the severity of the presentation, and should include all important and relevant information. This process can only be achieved if supported by the necessary background knowledge. One must also be able to present this history in a logical, coherent and appropriate manner so that others can assist and intervene as required.

The subsequent ***clinical examination*** should confirm or refute the initial list of differentials from the history, and include such things as supporting evidence, eg associated risk factors. Thus the history and examination are intimately related and together form the ***'clinical assessment'***. This assessment needs to acknowledge the '**severity of the presentation**', and should be used to target / focus the ***'action plan'***, ie the subsequent investigations and management, including procedures and other therapeutic interventions: but above all, this assessment must lead to a working diagnosis. Whether one is learning the process as a novice or taking a history as a senior clinician, the focus must be diagnostic. This diagnostic focus is perhaps the thing that separates doctors from many other clinicians.

How do we teach and learn these processes, knowledge and skills? There is a definite pathway of maturation from the competent FY1 to the experienced senior clinician. However, the way a working FY1 assesses a patient and formulates an action plan, increasingly bears less resemblance to that of our graduating finalists, and is almost unrecognisable in our novice clinical students. It is difficult to identify where this disjunction arose. Some may say it has ever been thus, but if so, it may reflect our over-reliance and underdevelopment of the OSCE: our over-dependence on this single clinical assessment format has reinforced and even exaggerated these differences. It is time for our teaching, the clinical learning environment we create, and the assessments we use, to promote and recognise this maturation process, and reverse the trend away from simple 'performance' and back towards focussed, diagnostic assessment and management.

Back to the Future

Most undergraduate OSCE stations utilise detailed, itemised checklists. These checklists and the duration of stations, mean students have become 'performance' orientated. The format of the objective checklist encourages students to work their way through the items on the list, gaining the necessary marks to pass the task, but failing to think about the clinical meaning and importance of their findings. Rarely are students required to act upon the clinical information they have gathered. Unchallenged and untested decisions and conclusions have no impact on the care of simulated patients and manikins.

Scenario (case/patient)-Based Assessment

This series of books promotes a new approach to the OSCE, developing a scenario-based assessment for the 21st century. Circuits consist of a series of clinical cases or scenarios. We suggest three or four cases be used in a major summative assessment, reflecting realistic and deliverable circuits, but the number may vary with cohort numbers and available resources. Each case / scenario is subdivided into a number of sequential, interdependent tasks (typically 5 or 6), always starting with a history taking station and progressing through stations on the relevant examination, data interpretation, procedures and clinical therapeutics. **Linking** the tasks together promotes clinical diagnostic reasoning, and the application and utilisation of knowledge and skills, requiring candidates to think and act on the clinical information they have gathered in previous stations. As the stations and tasks are linked, the candidate must start at station 1, and move through each of the subsequent stations in the given order. In real life, each task is performed with or on the same patient and their carers. But to retain the OSCEs' strength of multiple reviews by multiple people each task is performed at a separate station, observed by a different person.

Domain based checklists

We have also promoted a more clinical approach to the tasks by removing the detailed itemised lists. Each station is subdivided into **DOMAINS**, and these are marked globally from Grade A (Excellent) to Grade E (Clear Fail). The items within each of the generic domains are considered below, and repeated (both boxed and unique **icons**) at the start of the history and examination stations. The CONTENT ('what you did') domain differs between cases and is retained full.

We hope through use of these domain based prompts you will think about what you are doing and the relevance of the clinical findings, rather than simply your 'performance'. In the following paragraphs we have indicated the typical percentage of the total marks that each domain represents within a given station. This reinforces their relative importance, not only in each station but in the examination overall – reflecting the significant contribution these areas make to the care of patients, their carers and to effective team working.

We have re-introduced a number of important generic tasks that need reinforcement at an undergraduate level. These include assessment of (a) clinical diagnostic reasoning through a structured viva voce at the end of most stations, and (b) presentation skills – including presenting diagnostic summaries and interpretation of histories and examination findings. The 'ideal' presentation of history and examination can be found at the end of each case, along with web-links and further reading.

Mixing observed and unobserved stations – purists may suggest that many of the unobserved stations we have included are simply written assessments, and argue that these have no place in an OSCE. However, they assesses contextualised knowledge, that occurs in real life – interpreting clinical data, challenging knowledge around differentials, therapeutics and completing relevant forms, eg a death certificate. With the increasing sophistication and utilisation of computer based assessment, the often arbitrary division 'written' and 'clinical' assessment will probably blur and even merge in the near future.

OSCEs for Finals

The OSCEs for Finals Series aims to prepare you for finals with common case-based scenarios that provide you with a broad cover of the curriculum. Early in your course you can work slowly through these cases, learning how to approach a clinical problem, while later you can use the cases to manage problems that you are likely to encounter in finals, and under examination conditions.

The following paragraphs consider the design of the scenario-based OSCE, the domains we have chosen and the scoring system: these are of interest to both teachers and students. If, however, you are already conversant with these aspects of the assessment and just want to get on with it, go to 'How to use this book' on page ix, and proceed.

Scenarios

This text contains 20 clinical scenarios; each is subdivided into five or six tasks, starting with taking a history from a patient or relative / carer, and progressing to the relevant diagnostic examination, data interpretation, procedures, therapeutic interventions and explanation stations. Unlike traditional OSCE circuits, students must all begin at a history station at the start of a given scenario, and thus the subsequent stations remain empty until such time as each student has passed through their starting history station and moved on sequentially through the tasks.

In the book we have tried to make all stations ten minutes in duration, but some are divided into two or three tasks: these timings are guestimates and you may find them too short or too long, depending on your year and level of skills. In a real examination this needs careful consideration and matching. We have also largely ignored the resources (especially trained examiners) required to run such examinations, but feel assessment teams may mix and match stations and scenarios to take account of such important issues.

You should work your way sequentially through each scenario before attempting a second. This allows the instructions of each station within a given scenario to give confirmatory findings regarding the preceding station, eg after completing the history, the examination instructions may confirm the working diagnosis and ask you to examine for additional diagnostic evidence. The data interpretation and therapeutic stations may give further confirmatory information, allowing all students to start the stations on equal footing, regardless of how they performed and the conclusions they reached in the preceding station. Although this 'double jeopardy' is true of real life working, ie if you get the diagnosis wrong all your subsequent actions, including investigations and interventions, are likewise wrong (double jeopardy), in an assessment where one is interested in the task as much as the correct answer, this needs to be avoided.

The answer section of each scenario is made up of several key elements:

(a) **Patient, relative/carer scripts** (with shaded background) – these are paired with the appropriate histories and clinical communication stations. They facilitate a student role play of the various characters involved in the scenario

(b) **Content** – this contains the icons of the three or four **constituent domains** within the larger itemised contents box. This content box is principally for the benefit of student- learning and revision. In summative OSCEs, appropriately trained clinicians act as examiners, and as with other domains, in an examination, this box is simply presented as an icon or space. The repetition of the icons should prompt you to think about important clinical issues such as professionalism, diagnostic reasoning, process, presentation and communication skills.

(c) The succinct '**presentation'** to colleagues of key, diagnostic findings is an essential skill that is rarely taught, and poorly learnt in the busy clinical areas of today's NHS. In each of the examination question stations we have provided a list of 'key' clinical findings (with a specific balloon icon). Study these lists and present them to a colleague as if they are in the named clinical area.

Presentation is not an easy skill to master. However, as you approach graduation it is essential that you progress from merely being able to complete a history or examination in the correct order, as a novice clinician, to a more diagnostic appreciation and holistic approach. Through practice using these books with colleagues, and in the clinical areas to senior clinical colleagues, such presentations become second nature. Take note of how different clinical contexts allow for different presentations. Think how you might present cases to colleagues, on teaching rounds, business rounds, over the phone or written in the medical records or a referral letter. Each has its own skills and nuances and can only truly be learnt experientially within the clinical environment.

Keeping good medical notes is also an essential skill required of all graduating students, and although this is beyond the scope of these books, we recommend you think about how you would write up these cases in the medical notes.

(d) **Clinical Diagnostic Reasoning** – these boxes are set out as a structured viva voce; several questions are included towards the end of each station allowing assessment of diagnostic reasoning, data interpretation and therapeutic intervention.

(e) **Reflection and Consolidation** – At the end of each scenario there is a diagnostic summary box that should prompt you to reflect on your performance, knowledge and skills. The case presentations are examples of an A-grade requirement. They are also a rapid reference for consolidating knowledge in the lead up to exams.

(f) **Further reading and web links** – These direct you to key, up to date guidelines and other useful reading.

Domains

If one looks at a typical itemised checklist used in undergraduate OSCEs it contains several generic items that are common to many stations, eg hand cleaning, introduction, gaining consent, formal completion, demonstrating a caring and professional attitude and a logical approach. These can be grouped together under common themes, or domains. Each domain is similar whatever the focus of the station. By including the domains, rather than the individual items, we hope students who have mastered the basic knowledge and skills of a given task will refocus away from the 'tick box mentality' and back towards a more holistic and diagnostic approach.

The following section explains each of the domains contained in these volumes. They are an amalgamation of our own observations, and domains used in other formal clinical assessments, eg PACES (MRCP). The explanations include typical items that are included in these domains with the icons as they appear within the book. Within these explanations there is also an indication of the percentage of marks that each domain might represent in a given station, and this in turn should guide you as to the proportion such domains represent of the total exam marks. For examiners and students this potentially allows for more meaningful and focussed feedback. When viewed in such a strategic light, you will appreciate how these essential but often disregarded components, differentiate the excellent from the competent, and the competent from the failing student.

It remains almost impossible to define what makes a good doctor. The heterogeneity of the various specialities and the characteristics of their specialists exclude a simple, unifying answer. However, if you ask the general public what they want from their doctor, common, essential characteristics emerge, including professionalism, demonstrating a caring and empathetic manner, and being knowledgeable and skilful. These are reflected in the domains we and others include in our stations.

Domain – Professionalism

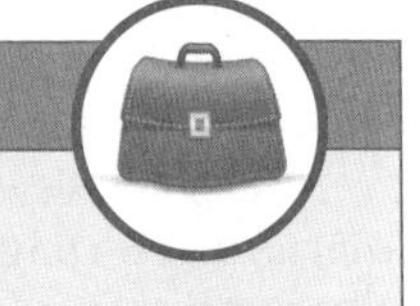

What is being assessed? These are the holistic skills and attributes that are implicit in being a good doctor. Individually they are easily defined and effects are often far more than their sum. In the clinical arena they include NHS or locally regulated dress code, cleanliness, punctuality, caritas, reliability, trustworthiness, honour and attitude. These are extremely difficult to measure in an OSCE situation and so we rely on such items as hygiene, appearance / dress code, and elements of communication and process (checking patient identity, explanation of role) as proxies of true professionalism. Despite this use of proxies in exams, all clinicians should think about how they present themselves to their patients and how they interact with them.

Typical percentage of a station 5 - 10%

Typical Items included from checklists

- Professional appearance (NHS dress code) – including general appearance, hair and jewellery
- Maintains patient and personal safety
- Polite introduction; identifies patient or interviewee correctly; confirms patient's date of birth from name band or other source
- Obtains informal consent; maintains patient's privacy
- Displays empathetic and caring attitudes and behaviours throughout

Domain – Process

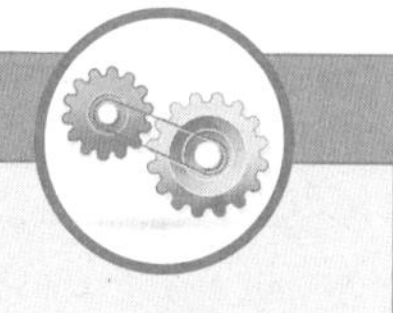

Typical percentage of a station 10 – 20%

What is being assessed? Process is 'how' one completes a task. Whilst the majority of undergraduates concentrate on the content items on the checklists, many are unaware or disregard the process, ie how they achieve the end result. At the novice stage this approach may be quite appropriate but as one clinically matures, process becomes increasingly important, ensuring clinical acceptability (as defined by patients' expectations, colleagues, guidelines and professional standards), and a clinically relevant, appropriate and functional outcome. Whilst simulation has an important role in learning and practising clinical skills, low fidelity manikins cannot tell a student they are hurting them, have poor technique or are uncaring. Students often define OSCE tasks by the title of the station, eg In a phlebotomy station, students regard the task as ending up with blood in a blood bottle regardless of ***how*** they obtain that blood. It may be suggested that in real life, the process is the part that keeps you and the patient safe, and defines defensible practise. Ignoring these important factors often increases the likelihood of complication and harm.

Typical Items included from checklists

In the History

- Good organisation and structure; appropriate use of open and closed questions
- Appropriate fluency / rhythm / pace to the interview – this may change depending on environment and acute nature of problem
- Allows appropriate time for patient to respond / reply to questions
- Appropriately acknowledges difficult or emotional areas of the patient's history

In the Examination

- Appropriate fluency / rhythm / pace to the examination – this may change depending on environment and acute nature of problem
- Organisation and structure of examination; sensitive and empathetic approach
- Uses appropriate clinical techniques throughout
- Maintains privacy and dignity throughout

Domain – Content

CARRIES THE ICON OF THE STATION

What is being assessed? This domain makes up the majority of marks within any given station, and has been largely left as an itemised checklist in these new volumes. Although this goes against our move towards a holistic / diagnostic focus it cannot be avoided if these volumes are to be useful aids to facilitate students' learning. In post-graduate examinations (eg PACES) and at medical schools where they are using domain based checklists, this domain, like all the others, is simply represented by a box with a grading system, and it is left to the 'expert' examiner to use their experience and judgement as to the coverage of the task by the candidate.

Students will focus on this domain for exam purposes, but we once again remind you that it is often their 'overall' performance that influences an examiner's global mark, and their 'excellence' of content may be downgraded by poor hygiene, communication, appearance and attitudes. Although these are rarely considered or practised by students they may lead to your downfall.

Typical percentage of a station 60 – 70%

Domain – Clinical Communication (in History and Examination stations)

What is being assessed? This incredibly important part of the doctor-patient interaction has become increasingly rewarded within procedure and clinical examination stations. It is now common for manikins to be 'molded' to a simulated patient to facilitate a more realistic interaction during a procedure or examination, eg DRE, Vaginal and Breast examination, and phlebotomy, arterial blood gas sampling and insertion of an intravenous cannula. Newly qualified clinicians quickly realise how essential these elements can be in calming, instilling confidence, and building rapport with acutely ill, frightened or emotional patients.

Typical percentage of a station 5 – 10%

Typical items included from checklists for clinical communication

In the History
- Demonstrates a caring and sympathetic attitude
- Asks open questions
- Invites patient to ask questions and answers them appropriately
- Addresses patient's ideas, concerns and expectations

In an examination or procedure
- Explains purpose of examination / procedure; explains examination / procedure as it proceeds
- Offers information in a clear, structured and fluent manner; avoiding jargon
- Listens to patient and responds appropriately
- Demonstrates appropriate body language

Domain – Clinical Diagnostic Reasoning (CDR)

What is being assessed? This domain assesses

- The quality of the information the student has gathered from their interaction with the patient, and
- How they are able to apply and utilise this information to the patient in front of them.

Typically you are asked to present your history or clinical findings to the examiner, and are expected to demonstrate how you arrived at your clinical diagnosis. Subsidiary questions are directed around the major differentials diagnoses, and the future management of the patient, including investigations and therapeutic interventions.

Unlike the novice clinician, the graduating student must develop a method of synthesising this information as they proceed through the history or examination process, and be ready to present and utilise it a short period after completing these tasks. It is a difficult skill to learn but one that is essential in the time pressured atmosphere of the 21st century NHS.

Typical percentage of a station 20 – 25%

OTHER STATIONS AND ICONS USED IN THESE BOOKS

Examination station

EXAMINATION STATIONS – These differ from traditional, formal examination stations, in that they cover all the elements of an appropriate, focussed and diagnostic clinical assessment, including all relevant clinical observations. By their inclusion we hope to progress students from simply reproducing a robotic, limited 'OSCE performance', to a complete assessment that they can apply in the real world. The two should be synonymous but sadly are often a long way apart, especially in the student's mind.

Clinical findings

CLINICAL FINDINGS – This icon is used when you are expected to read and present examination findings to a colleague. It is not included as a separate domain, but is assessed within clinical diagnostic reasoning. Read this information carefully, organising it into systems so that it is easily recalled. No time limit is given for this task, as it is more important for the information to fully understood, and the time needed varies between individuals; it reduces considerably with experience. We encourage you to listen to, read, and reflect upon the way clinical information is presented in different clinical contexts. Presentation of information, verbal (face to face), verbal (telephone), written in the medical records, via email or referral letter all have particular nuances and skills and we hope these volumes challenge you to reflect upon and improve your own abilities in these areas. **[NB If you have a model do not read this section]**

Data interpretation

DATA INTERPRETATION – These stations include interpretation of haematological, biochemical, microbiological, radiological and specialist investigation results. The majority of the data is directly relevant to the patient case (scenario) but we have used 'poetic license' to extend this to include data that is commonly assessed within final graduating examinations. Although it is common practice to allow candidates to use normal values embedded within the assessment, we encourage you to learn the normal ranges of common clinical data.

Communication skills

COMMUNICATION SKILLS – This is an important part of history taking, as considered above: independent communication stations focus on specific, difficult areas such as consent and giving important or difficult news to a patient or carer.

Prescribing

PRESCRIBING – These (and other) stations cover all aspects of prescribing and in particular ensure you are confident in the types of skills and knowledge being assessed in the new national Prescribing Skills Assessment (PSA). These include:

- Prescription review
- Adverse drug reactions
- Drug calculations
- Communication with patients
- Data interpretation
- Drug monitoring
- Planning therapeutic management
- Prescribing

We encourage you to use locally employed drug and fluid prescribing charts but have also provided copies that can be photocopied (page 368): use the Drug memo (page 373) to be sure you include all relevant data

Procedure stations

PROCEDURE STATIONS – The Foundation Programme Application System (FPAS) and Tomorrow's Doctors (2009) set out a series of 20 – 30 competencies that all graduating students must be proficient with before starting their FY1 employment. We have ensured that all of these competencies are fully covered through this series of books. We recommend that you are familiar with all the procedures included in these documents and are both competent and confident in your ability to perform them.
www.gmc-uk.org/static/documents/content/GMC_TD_09__1.11.11.pdf
www.foundationprogramme.nhs.uk/pages/home

Consolidation and reflection

CONSOLIDATION AND REFLECTION – This section, at the end of each scenario is to encourage you to reflect on your skills and knowledge in the key areas covered. You should find the section useful to direct your learning and examination preparation. The history and examination sections can be used as a guide to presenting the key diagnostic information in an appropriate manner for both clinical practice and graduating OSCEs.

Further reading and web links

FURTHER READING AND WEB LINKS – This concluding section contains useful web links and reading that we have used when writing the scenarios.

Setting the pass mark using domain based lists

The standard setting of the pass / fail cut off, ie the pass mark in high stakes summative assessments (like finals) has become increasingly sophisticated and important over the past twenty years. The general public, the GMC, clinical colleagues and peers wish to know that newly graduating doctors have passed a robust set of assessments that are able to differentiate the competent from the incompetent. Likewise, students want to be certain that their performance can be quantified as a pass or fail with a reasonable degree of certainty.

Most UK undergraduate OSCE assessments utilise two methods to pass and fail candidates. The first is an absolute score. Each item on the checklist is given a value according to its perceived importance and contribution to the overall task. These are then summed to give a total for each station.

Previously **norm referenced** methods were commonly used, whereby the distribution of examination marks were drawn out and a set percentage of the cohort passed or failed. This was an arbitrary division and did not take into account the variation in cohort performance. The same number would pass or fail regardless of the candidates' performance. Today **criterion referenced** methods are preferred. These measure the performance of the cohort against a given set of criteria, setting the pass mark prior to the examination. There is no set number of passing and failing students but such methods rely on large numbers of experienced examiners being involved in setting the scores.

The Global Score

A third variation has developed with the use of OSCEs. The **borderline group** method is an **'on the day'** criterion referenced method whereby candidates are graded against the expected performance and each other. Candidates are given a global grade at the end of the station based on the examiner's expert opinion. This does not contribute to the overall score but is used to define the pass mark of the station and the overall examination. Each student is graded as Competent, Borderline or Fail, or variations thereof. The 'borderline' students' checklist scores are added together and the mean of these scores is used to define the pass mark of each station. These mean scores are then added together, and this gives the pass mark for the whole examination. More recently the **borderline regression method** has become increasingly employed. This involves two borderline grades, borderline pass and borderline fail. These in turn are used to derive the pass mark.

In keeping with a borderline regression method we have chosen to have five grades, A – E for both our domains and our global scores. Whilst peers may not be expert enough to differentiate passing and failing performances, we hope teachers and students alike will appreciate the inclusion of these grades.

A – Excellent – This applies to a candidate who in the opinion of the assessor gives a near perfect or perfect performance. Such students often receive every available (or very nearly every available) mark within the station or the domain. Their technique, their interaction with the patient and their professionalism are all excellent, and are perhaps above the standard expected of a student at this level of training.

B – Good – This applies to a candidate who in the opinion of the assessor gives a good, but not perfect performance. This type of student often is awarded the majority of the available marks but their interaction, communication, clinical technique or fluency may not be quite as good as the excellent student.

C – Borderline Pass – This is a candidate who in the examiner's opinion was just competent and demonstrated techniques, knowledge and skills that perhaps raise a few concerns.

D – Borderline Fail – This is a candidate who in the examiner's opinion demonstrated techniques, knowledge and skills that raised a number of concerns, and is deemed just below the standard required to pass the examination.

E – Clear Fail – This is a candidate who in the opinion of the examiner has clearly failed the examination. They often have poor examination technique, poor knowledge and skills, and their interaction with the patient or examiner may be poor or dangerous.

In this series of books we have produced a hybrid checklist containing elements of an itemised checklist and domain based list. If a pure domain based list were to be used, each candidate would need to get a C (borderline pass) or above in all the domains and the global rating to pass the station. If it were needed to quantify the grades obtained, each element of each domain would need to be assigned a score by an expert set of judges / examiners. This is unnecessary in examinations where a pass or fail grade is awarded but may be necessary in examinations of excellence.

Glossary

AA	Alcoholics anonymous
ABGs	Arterial blood gases
ABE	Actual base excess
AC	Abdominal circumference
ACE inhibitors	Angiotensin converting enzyme
ACTH	Adrenocorticotrophic hormone
ACS	Acute coronary syndrome
ADH	Anti-diuretic hormone
ADL	Activity of daily living
AF	Atrial fibrilation
AFP	Alpha-fetoprotein
aGBM	Anti-glomerular basement membrane
AGT	Angiotensin
AHBe/c	Anti Hepatitis B envelope/core
AKI	Acute kidney injury
AIDS	Acquired immune deficiency syndrome
AKA	Also known as
Alb	Albumin
Alk phos	Alkaline phosphatase
ALT	Alanine amino-transferase
AMA	Anti-mitochondrial antibody
AMTS	Abridged mental test score
ANCA	Anti neutrophil cytoplasmic antibody
Anti dsDNA	Double stranded deoxyribonucleic acid
Anti-Jo	Specific antigen
Anti-La	Specific antigen
Anti-RNP	Ribonucleic protein
Anti-Ro	Specific antigen
Anti-SCL70	Specific antigen
Anti-TPO	Anti-thyroid peroxidase
Anti-TG	Anti-thyroglobulin
AP	Antero-posterior
APC gene	Adenomatosis polyposis coli
APTT	Activated partial thromboplastin time
APVU	Alert; Pain; Voice; Unresponsive
A2RB	Angiotensin 2 receptor blocker
ARDS	Adult respiratory distress syndrome
ARM	Artificial rupture of membranes
AS	Aortic stenosis
ASH	Action on smoking and health
ASMA	Anti-smooth muscle antibody
ASO(T)	Anti streptolysin-O-titre

AST	Aspartate amino-transferase
ATLS	Advanced trauma life support
AV	Arterio-venous
AV	Atrio-ventricular
aVF	Augmented voltage lead left lower leg
aVL	Augmented voltage lead left arm
aVR	Augmented voltage lead right arm
AVSD	Atrioventricular septal defect
AXR	Abdominal X-ray
AZT	Azidothymidine (generic name: Zidovudine)
BAL	Broncho-alveolar lavage
BBB	Bundle branch block
BCC	Basal cell carcinoma
BCG	Bacille Calmette-Guerin
Beta HCG	Beta human chorionic gonadotrophin
b.d.	Twice daily (bis die)
BE	Base excess
BHL	Bilateral hilar lymphadenopathy
BiPAP	Biphasic positive airway pressure
BMA	British Medical Association
BM stix	Blood monitoring
BM	Bone marrow
BMI	Body mass index
BMR	Basal metabolic rate
BNF	British national formulary
BP	Blood pressure
Bpm	Beats per minute
BRCA	Breast cancer susceptibility genes
BXS	Base excess
C	Cervical
Ca	Cancer
CA	Cyclic AMP
Ca^{++}	Calcium
CABG	Coronary bypass graft
CAGE questionnaire	Cut down Annoyed Guilty Eye-opener
CAPD	Chronic ambulatory peritoneal dialysis
CBD	Common bile duct
CBG	Capillary blood glucose
CCa^{++}	Corrected calcium
CD4	A surface antigen principally found on helper-inducer T-lymphocyte
CDR	Clinical diagnostic reasoning
CEX	Ckinical evaluation exercise
CK	Creatinine phosphokinase
Cl	Chloride
CLL	Chronic lymphocytic leukaemia

cm	Centimetre
CML	Chronic myeloid leukaemia
CMV	Cytomegalovirus
CNS	Central nervous system
CO	Complaining of
CO_2	Carbon dioxide
COCP	Combined oral contraceptive pill
COMT	Catechol *O*-methyl transferase
COPD	Chronic obstructive pulmonary disease
CPAP	Continuous positive airway pressure
CPN	Community psychiatric nurse
CPR	Cardio pulmonary resuscitation
Cr	Creatinine
CRP	C-reactive protein
CRT	Capillary refill time
CS	Caesarean section
CSF	Cerebro-spinal fluid
CSU	Catheter specimen of urine
CT	Computerised tomography
CTG	Cardiotocography
CTPA	CT-pulmonary angiogram
CVA	Cerebro-vascular accident
CVP	Central venous pressure
CVS	Chorionic villi sampling
CWD	Consistent with dates
CXR	Chest radiograph
DCCT	Diabetes control and complications trial
DDAVP	Desmopressin, synthetic vasopressin
DIC	Disseminated intravascular coagulopathy
DIP joints	Distal inter-phalangeal joints
DKA	Diabetic keto-acidosis
dl	Decilitres
DM	Diabetes mellitus
DMSA	Dimercaptosuccinic acid
DNA	Deoxyribonucleic acid
DNAR	Do not attempt resusitation
DOB	Date of birth
DOPS	Directly observed procedural skills
DRE	Digital rectal examination
DSN	Diabetic specialist nurse
DT	Delirium tremens
D&V	Diarrhoea and vomiting
DVT	Deep vein thrombosis
DVLA	Driving vehicle licensing authority
ECG	Electrocardiogram
ED	Emergency department

EDV	End diastolic department
EEG	Electroencephalogram
eGFR	Estimated glomerula filtration rate
EMQ	Extended matching question
ENT	Ear, nose and throat
ERCP	Endoscopic retrograde cholangiopancreatography
ESR	Erythrocyte sedimentation rate
ET	Exercise test
ETEC	Enterotoxigenic *Escherichia coli*
ETT	Exercise tolerance test
EUA	Examination under anaesthesia
FBC	Full blood count
FDP	Fibrin degredation products
FEV1	Forced expiratory volume in one second
FFP	Fresh frozen plasma
FH	Family history
FHx	Family history
5-FU	5-Fluoro-uracil
5HT	5-Hydroxy-tryptamine
fl	Femtolitres
F:M	Female:male (ratio)
FNA	Fine needle aspirate
FPIO	Family practice – prescription chart
FRIVII/R	Fixed rate intravenous insulin infusion/rate
FTA	Fluorescent treponemal antibody
fT4	Free thyroxine
FVC	Forced vital capacity
FY1/2	Foundation year 1/2
G	Gram
GABA	Gamma-amino butyric acid
GCS	Glasgow coma scale
gGT	Gama-elutamyl transferase
GFR	Glomerula filtration rate
GI	Gastrointestinal
GIT	Gastrointestinal tract
GP	General Practitioner
GRACE	Global registry of acute coronary events
G6PD	Glucosa 6 phosphate dehydrogenase
GTN	Glyceryl trinitrate
GU	Genito-urinary
HAV	Hepatitis A virus
Hb	Haemoglobin
HBA-1c	Haemoglobin A-1c
HBD	Hepatobiliary disease
HBe	Hepatitis Be
HC	Hepatitis C

HCO_3^-	Bicarbonate
HCV	Hepatitis C virus
HONK	Hyperosmolar-non-ketotic
HIB	*Haemophilus influenzae* type B (vaccine)
HIV	Human immunodeficiency virus
HLA	Human leucocyte antigen
HR	Heart rate
HS	Heart sound
ICP	Intra-cranial pressure
ICU	Intensive care unit
IDDM	Insulin dependent diabetes mellitus
Ig	Immunoglobulin
IgM	Immunoglobulin M
IGT	Impaired glucose tolerance
IHD	Ischaemic heart disease
Im	Intramuscular
INR	International ratio
ISMN	Iso-sorbide mono-nitrate
ITU	Intensive therapy unit
IU	International unit(s)
IVI	Intravenous infusion
IV	Intravenous
IVP	Intravenous pyelogram
IVU	Intravenous urogram
JVP	Jugulovenous pressure
K^+	Potassium
kg	Kilogram
kPa	Kilopascals
KUB	Kidneys/ureters/bladder
L	Litre
LAD	Left anterior descending
LBBB	Left bundle branch block
LDH	Lactate dehydrogenase
LDL	Low-density lipoprotein
LFT	Liver function tests
LKM-1	Liver, kidney, muscle
LMA	Laryngeal mask airway
LMN	Lower motor neurone
LMW	Low molecular weight
LMWH	Low molecular weight heparin
LOC	Loss of conciousness
LTOT	Long term oxygen therapy
LV	Left ventricle
LVEF	Left ventricular ejection fraction
LT	Light touch
m	Meter

MAOI	Mono-amine oxidase inhibitor
MAU	Medical admissions unit
MCH	Mean corpuscular haemoglobin
MC&S	Microscopy, culture and sensitivity
MCV	Mean corpuscular volume
Mg^{++}	Magnesium
mg	Milligram
MI	Myocardial infarction
mmol	Millimoles
MPTP	1-methyl 4-phenyl-1.2.3.6 tetrahydropyridine
MR	Mitral regurgitation
MRA	Magnetic resonance angiogram
MRI	Magnetic resonance imaging
MRSA	Methicillin resistant staphylococcus
MS	Multiple sclerosis or Mitral stenosis
MSU	Mid stream urine
Na^{+}	Sodium
NAD	No abnormality detected
NEC	Necrotising enterocolitis
Neut	Neutrophilis
NG(T)	Nasogastric (tube)
NIDDM	Non-insulin dependent diabetes mellitus
NIPPV	Noninvasive positive pressure ventilation
NIV	Noninvasive ventilation
NKDA	No known drug allergy
Non-STEMI	ST elevation myocardial infarction
NSAID	Non steroidal anti-inflammatory drug
O2	Oxygen
Obs	Observations
OCP	Oral contraceptive pill
Od	Omni die (once daily)
OGD	Oesophagogastroduodenoscopy
OSCE	Objective structured clinical examination
PA	Postero-anterior
$PaCO_2$	Arterial pressure of carbon dioxide
PaO_2	Arterial pressure of oxygen
PAN	Perinuclear anti-neutrophilic
PCA	Patient controlled analgesia
PCI	Percutaneous coronary intervension
PCR	Polymerase chain reaction
PCV	Packed cell volume
PD	Parkinson's disease
PDA	Patent ductus arteriosus
PE	Pulmonary embolism
PEA	Persistent electrical activity
PEFR	Peak expiratory flow rate

PERL(A)	Pupils equal reactive to light (and accommodation)
PET	Positron emission tomography
pH	Puissance d'Hydrogen = – log (H^+)
Plats	Platelets
PMH	Previous medical history
Pmol	Picomol
PND	Paroxysmal nocturnal dyspnoea
PNS	Peripheral nervous system
PO	Per oral
PO_4^-	Phosphate
PR	Per rectum
PQRST	ECG complex
PRN	As required (*pro re nata*)
PT	Prothrombin time
Q	ECG wave
QRST	ECG complex
Qds	Four times/day (quarter in die)
RBC	Red blood count
RCT	Randomised, controlled trial
Retics	Reticulocytes
ROM	Range of movement
SACD	Subacute combined degeneration of the spinal cord
SAH	Subarachnoid haemorrhage
SARS	Severe acute respiratory syndrome
Sats	Saturation
SDH	Subdural haemorrhage
SE	Side effects
SHx	Social history
SIADH	Syndrome inappropriate antidiuretic hormone secretion
SL	Sublingual
SLE	Systemic lupus erythematosus
SOA	Swelling of ankle
SOCRATES	Site/Onset/Character/Radiation/Association/Times/ Exacerbations/relieving factors/severity
SOL	Space occupying lesion
SpO2	Saturation percentage oxygen
SpR	Specialist registrar
SROM	Spontaneous rupture of membranes
SSRI	Selective serotonin reuptake inhibitors
ST	ECG interval
ST 1-4	Specialist trainee (years 1–4)
Stat	Statim (immediately)
STEMI	ST elevation MI
SVT	Supraventricular tachycardia
SXR	Skull X-ray
T	ECG wave/temperature

T3	Tri-iodo-thyronine
T4	Tetra-iodo-thyronine (thyroxine)
TB	Tuberculosis
TBil	Total bilirubin
T cholesterol	Total cholesterol
T2DM	Type 2 diabetes melitus
tds	Ter die sumendus – (to be taken three times daily)
TED	Thrombo-embolic
Temp	Temperature
TFTs	Thyroid function tests
TIA	Transient ischaemic attack
TOP	Termination of pregnancy
TPA	Tissue plasminogen activator
TSH	Thyroid stimulating hormone
TT	Thrombin time
TVF	Tactile vocal fremitus
U&Es	Urea and electrolytes
UGIB	Upper gastrointestinal bleed
UGT/UGIT	Upper gastrointestinal tract
UMN	Upper motor neurone
UO	Urine output
Ur	Urea
USS	Ultrasound scan
UTI	Urinary tract infection
UV	Ultraviolet
V 1-6	ECG chest leads
VDRL	Venereal disease research laboratory
VF	Ventricular fibrillation/vocal fremitus
V/Q scan	Ventilation/perfusion scan
VSD	Ventricular septal defect
VTE	Venous thrombo-embolic
WCC	White cell count
WBC	White blood cell
YO	Type 1 purkinje cell cytoplasmic autoantibodies (PCA-1)

Scenario 1: 'What a wheeze'

Station 1

History *10-minute station*

You are the FY1 doctor on call for the Medical Team in the Emergency Department. Miss Sarah Davis has presented to the hospital with increasing shortness of breath. She is known to have asthma and has been admitted under the Respiratory Team before.

- **You have been called to the 'majors' assessment area of the Emergency Department to take a history of both her present illness and her asthma history and present your history to the Respiratory Registrar on call.**

You will be assessed on the following areas, as well as the content and diagnostic reasoning of your history – take them into account in your presentation.

Professionalism

- Professional appearance (NHS dress code) – including general appearance, hair and jewellery
- Maintains patient and personal safety
- Polite introduction; identifies patient or interviewee correctly; confirms patient's date of birth from name band or other source
- Obtains informal consent; maintains patient's privacy
- Displays empathetic and caring attitudes and behaviours throughout.

Process

- Good organisation and structure; appropriate use of open and closed questions
- Appropriate fluency/rhythm/pace to the interview – this may change depending on environment and acute nature of the problem
- Appropriate time for the patient to respond/reply to questions
- Appropriate acknowledgement of difficult or emotional areas of the patient's history.

Communication skills

- Demonstrates caring and sympathetic attitude
- Asks open questions
- Invites patient to ask questions and answers them appropriately
- Addresses patient's ideas, concerns and expectations.

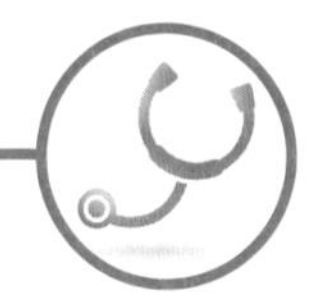

Station 2

Examination *10-minute station*

Miss Davis has an RR of 25 and O_2 sats of 95% on room air. She has had one dose of nebulised salbutamol in the Emergency Department but remains tachypnoeic. She has been transferred to the resuscitation area of the Emergency Department.

- **Please perform a focused respiratory examination of Miss Davis and present this to your Registrar.**

You will be assessed on the following areas, as well as the content and skills of your examination – take them into account in your presentation.

Professionalism

- Professional appearance; maintains infection control standards, including hand cleaning and appropriate use of gloves and aprons
- Maintains patient and personal safety
- Polite introduction; identifies patient and confirms date of birth from name band or other source
- Obtains informal consent; maintains patient privacy and dignity
- Displays empathetic and caring attitudes and behaviours throughout.

Process

- Appropriate fluency/rhythm/pace to the examination – this may change depending on environment and acute nature of the problem
- Good organisation and structure of examination; sensitive and empathetic approach
- Uses appropriate clinical techniques throughout
- Maintains privacy and dignity throughout.

Clinical communication

- Explains proposed examination/procedure; explains examination/procedure as it proceeds
- Offers information in a clear, structured and fluent manner, avoiding jargon
- Listens to patient and responds appropriately
- Demonstrates appropriate body language.

Please read the information below before presenting this case to the ST3 Medical Registrar as if you were on a busy medical take.
[NB If you have a model do not read this section]

Clinical findings

- o **Patient appears dyspnoeic at rest, and unable to complete sentences**
- o **RR 24 breaths per minute, O_2 sats 95% room air 100% on 15 O_2 l/min, BP 130/75**
- o **GCS 15**
- o **PEFR 350 (65% expected)**
- o **Peripheral capillary refill time <2 s; Pulse regular in rhythm; Carotid pulse normal in volume; JVP not elevated; Apex beat not displaced**
- o **CV examinations – heart sounds easily heard, normal**
- o **RS examination – trachea central, no chest scars, chest expansion normal and equal bilaterally, widespread expiratory wheeze throughout both lung fields, normal percussion note throughout and breath sounds audible in all areas.**

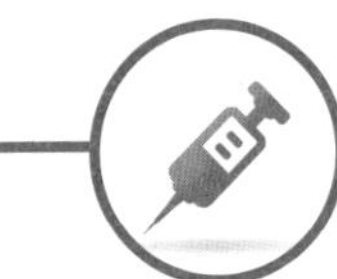

Station 3

Procedural skills *10-minute station*

Procedure

You have moved your patient to the monitored bay of the Medical Admissions Unit and while your nurse colleague is inserting an IV cannula you have been asked to administer a nebulised dose of salbutamol.

- Please demonstrate how you would set up and apply the nebuliser to the patient.

Equipment provided

- A selection of oxygen masks and nebulisers
- Oxygen supply with variable delivery
- Patient (either dummy or volunteer)
- Vials of salbutamol for nebulisation

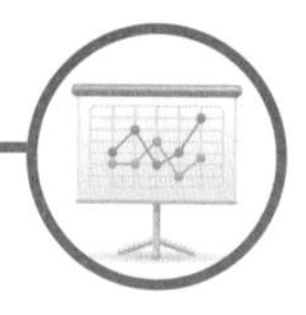

Station 4

Data interpretation *10-minute station*

As a training exercise the registrar on the team has asked you to review Miss Davies's previous lung function tests and compare them to those of some other patients on the respiratory ward.

Patient A

27-year-old woman with rheumatoid arthritis now presenting with a 6-month history of shortness of breath; FEV1: 3.0; O_2 sats on air: 92%; FVC: 3.8; transfer coefficient: grossly reduced.

Patient B

69-year-old man with 2-year history of exertional dyspnoea and an episodic cough; FEV1: 2.5; O_2 sats on air: 89%; FVC: 3.7; transfer coefficient: reduced.

Patient C

22-year-old woman with 2-month history of worsening shortness of breath and fatigue on exertion and repetitive movement; FEV1: 3.7; O_2 sats on air: 95%; FVC: 6; transfer coefficient: normal.

Patient D

23-year-old woman with 18-month history of nocturnal cough and wheeze; FEV1: 3.0; O_2 sats on air: 97%; FVC: 3.5; Transfer coefficient: normal; no increase in FEV1 with nebulised B agonist.

Which of patients A, B, C, D:

1. **Demonstrates a restrictive lung defect?**
2. **Demonstrates an obstructive lung defect?**
3. **Has type I respiratory failure?**
4. **Typically demonstrates type II respiratory failure?**
5. **Should be treated with nebulisers?**
6. **Is most likely to have a thymoma?**
7. **Is most likely to have an associated primary lung cancer?**
8. **Classically worsens their hypoxia with exertion?**
9. **May benefit from steroid therapy?**
10. **May derive benefit from other forms of immunosuppression?**

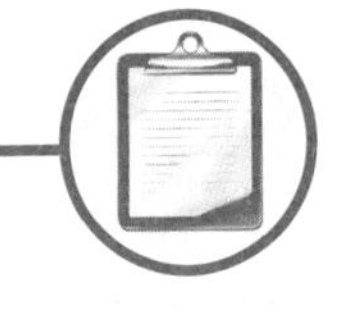

Station 5

Prescribing skills *10-minute station*

Your registrar has now asked you to prescribe appropriate medications to treat Miss Davis's asthma exacerbation.

Details

Miss Sarah Davis; DOB: 24/11/1988; No known allergies; Weight: 64 kg; Ward: MAU; Consultant: Dr Beadle

Blood results

FBC: Hb 14.4 g/dl, MCV 90 fl, WCC 13.9 $\times 10^9$/l, neutrophils 12.4 $\times 10^9$/l, platelets 122 $\times 10^9$/l

U&Es: Na+ 139 mmol/l, K+ 3.4 mmol/l, urea 4.6 mmol/l, creatinine 73 μmol/l

RBG: 5.2 mmol/l

CCa2+ 2.23 mol/l, PO4- 0.78 mmol/l, Mg 1.02 mmol/l

CXR: no pneumothorax, no focal consolidation.

ECG sinus tachycardia

Management – prescribing task

Please prescribe the following therapeutic interventions using the charts (page 368) and the BNF provided

- Oxygen
- Nebulisers
- Steroids
- Antibiotics
- Fluids

Remember: DRUG DRs Don't Forget Signing Off (page 373)

Station 6

Communication skills *10-minute station*

Miss Davis has been on inhaled therapy on the ward for 24 hours and her PEFR is now 500 l/min (best 550). Your consultant has asked you to have a discussion with her about her asthma control. Discuss any changes in her lifestyle that may help with her control.

Answers

Station 1 – History

Patient script

You are 23 years old and have been asthmatic since the age of 14. Your asthma is not well controlled and have had at least one to two admissions a year since then. The last admission was 3 months ago, when you were ventilated in intensive care. You have been previously ventilated three times. You are a current smoker of five to ten cigarettes a day and have to use inhalers three to four times a day. Your current medication is beclometasone and salbutamol inhalers. You have had six courses of steroids in the last 12 months.

You take inhalers when you are wheezy rather than every morning and night. Your normal PEFR when well is 550 l/min. You regularly wake up coughing during the night and have often missed days at work because you are very wheezy; you gave up your job in a supermarket after your last admission.

The present illness started 5 days ago with a slight head cold followed by a cough productive of green sputum and you are short of breath and wheezy, particularly at night. You feel exhausted, like before you were ventilated the last time. You have had a fever but have not noticed any blood in your sputum or chest pain.

You have no pets and do not know of anything specifically that exacerbates your asthma. You did not have hay fever or eczema as a child and you don't know any other family members who have eczema, asthma or hay fever. You live in a flat with your four siblings and your parents.

You are worried because you do not want to be admitted and would rather go home. You are very scared of being ventilated again.

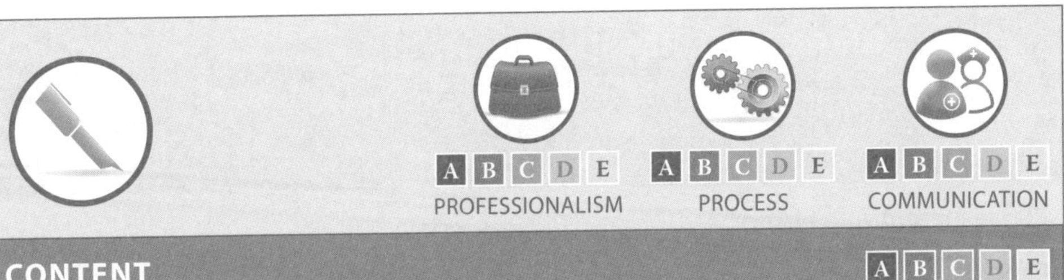

CONTENT

A B C D E

Identifies key information

- Presence of wheeze, increased shortness of breath and decreased exercise tolerance
- Presence of infective symptoms – fever, coryza, thick green sputum

Identifies key information from rest of history

History of chronic asthma

- Time of diagnosis
- Current treatment regime – inhaled steroid and PRN ß2-agonist
- Peak flow at best
- Current control – any interference with sleep, frequency of exacerbations
- Previous admissions to hospital; exacerbation requiring high dependency or intensive care – intubated 3 months ago

Includes important negatives including systemic enquiry

- Absence of chest pain and haemoptysis

Relevant factors from employment, housing, social support

- Unable to work due to poor control, lives in a small flat with a number of family members
- No environmental triggers identified

Previous medical history

- Atopy history – no eczema, no hay fever or allergic rhinitis

Social and occupational history

- Smoker, 5–10 per day
- No pets

Drug and allergic history

- Inhalers (as above), no allergies

No relevant family history

- No family history of asthma or eczema

Summarises important areas of the history back to the patient

Invites patient to ask questions and deals with them appropriately

Establishes patient's ideas, concerns and expectations

- Identifies that patient is concerned about being admitted to hospital and is worried that she may be admitted to intensive care once again

Appropriately explains to patient that she is likely to be admitted to the hospital and reassures her that treatment of her exacerbation is the priority

DIAGNOSTIC REASONING

A B C D E

Please present your history

Candidate offers a logical, well-structured account of the history

- **What is your diagnosis?**
  - Candidate offers the correct diagnosis and appropriate differentials
  - Diagnosis: this an exacerbation of asthma with a probable infective trigger, as the patient's symptoms include a cough productive of green sputum and fever.
- **How would you describe her current control of her chronic asthma?**
  - This patient obviously has very poor control of her asthma with frequent severe exacerbations. Previous admission to intensive care requiring intubation and ventilation is a key point to elicit from the history, as this will guide you to treat and monitor this patient very closely.
- **What are the key aspects to obtain in any chronic disease history?**
  - Time of diagnosis
  - Current treatment regime and contact with specialist services
  - Frequency of admissions and severity of exacerbations
  - Functional ability at best and at worst
  - Interference with activities of daily living (and sleep in the case of asthma, as nocturnal cough can be extremely disruptive)
  - Patient's understanding of her diagnosis.

GLOBAL HISTORY MARK

A B C D E

Station 2 – Examination

Patient script

If you are an actor/patient, read the patient history and physical signs fully – when the candidate comes to an abnormal site in their examination, act-out tenderness and/or volunteer the relevant physical sign.

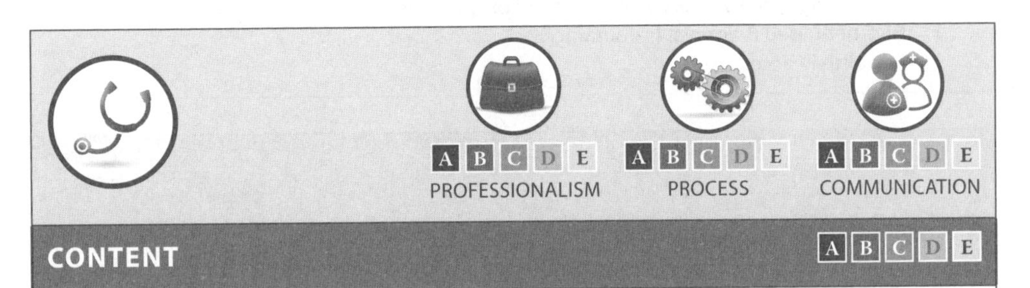

CONTENT A B C D E

Exposes and positions patient correctly and maintains comfort

- Exposes chest and ensures monitoring and oxygen are applied

Comments on wellbeing of patient

- Patient appears short of breath at rest
- Only able to complete short sentences
- Not using accessory muscle of respiration

Asks for appropriate relevant clinical observations

- Tachypneoic at 24 breaths per minute, O_2 sats 95% room air 100% on 15 l/min O_2
- BP 130/75, capillary refill <2 s, GCS 15

Focused examination

- Inspection – no scars on chest
- Palpation – chest expansion normal and equal bilaterally; trachea central
- Percussion – normal percussion note in all zones
- Auscultation – polyphonic expiratory wheeze throughout both lung fields

Completes examination by identifying relevant additional clinical signs

Completes examination by assessing PEFR: 350 (65% best)

Thanks patient, offers assistance, maintains patient's dignity and privacy until they are dressed

DIAGNOSTIC REASONING

A B C D E

Identifies correct physical signs, including important negative findings; does not identify signs that are not present.

Demonstrates a safe and sensible management plan.

- Place patient in an area where they can be monitored closely
- Apply oxygen via a reservoir mask at 15 l oxygen per minute
- Give nebulised B-agonist (salbutamol)
- Establish IV access.

GLOBAL EXAMINATION MARK

A B C D E

Station 3 – Procedural skills

NEBULISER ADMINISTRATION

Exposes and positions patient correctly and maintains comfort

- Patient sat up at >45 degrees to optimised inhaled therapy

Washes hands before giving medication

Performs the procedure correctly

- Selects correct mask and nebuliser chamber
- Selects correct dose of salbutamol (2.5 or 5 mg), checks dose, medication and date of expiry with colleague
- Removes lid from nebuliser chamber
- Pours liquid into bottom of chamber
- Reassembles chamber and attaches to oxygen mask
- Attaches to oxygen tubing
- Places facemask over patient's nose and mouth and secures
- Starts oxygen at 4–6 l/min
- Documents administration in drug chart
- Advises patient that it will take 5–7 min to complete nebuliser.

Addresses relevant post-procedure follow-up and safety issues

GLOBAL PROCEDURAL MARK

A B C D E

Station 4– Data interpretation

DATA INTERPRETATION

1 A
2 B and C
3 A
4 B and C
5 B and D
6 C
7 B
8 A
9 B, C and D
10 A and C

Patient (A) – demonstrates a restrictive lung defect with resting hypoxia and reduced transfer coefficient. In view of the history of rheumatoid arthritis, this picture would fit with fibrosing alveolitis. These patients have type I respiratory failure and classically the hypoxia worsens with exercise.

Patient (B) – the history and lung function tests suggest underlying obstructive airways disease. The reduced transfer coefficient suggests probable emphysema and excludes late-onset asthma. The data do not indicate whether there is any reversibility. This is demonstrated by repeating the FEV1 and FVC tests pre- and post-nebuliser. Demonstration of reversibility is important, as it indicates whether inhaled steroid therapy may be useful.

Patient (C) – this history is suggestive of myasthenia gravis. These patients get an obstructive lung defect, as they are unable to move their chest wall due to the neuromuscular defect. The transfer coefficient is normal, as there is no alveolar problem.

Patient (D) – this is the history and lung function test for Miss Davis. This shows a normal lung function test with symptoms suggestive of intermittent wheeze. Young patients with asthma usually have normal spirometry between exacerbations. If asthma control remains poor, then some element of chronic obstruction may develop.

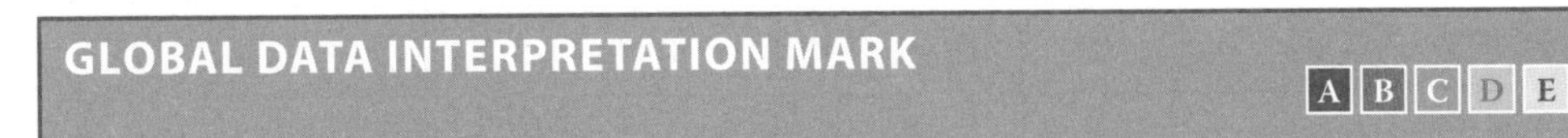

SCENARIO 1

Station 5– Prescribing skills

Check: DRUG DRs Don't Forget Signing Off (page 373)

Allergies, sensitivities and adverse drug reactions					Patient details/addressograph
No known allergies ✓		Initials MIA 224	Gender M / (F)		NHS/ Hospital No: 624011
Not possible to ascertain ☐		Date 13/01	Weight (kg)	Date	
Medicine/substance	Reaction & Severity	Initials & Date	64		Surname: DAVIS
			Height		First name: SARAH
			1.60m		
Alerts			Surface area (m²)		Date of birth: 24.01.88

IN-PATIENT MEDICATION PRESCRIPTION AND ADMINISTRATION RECORD

PasTest HOSPITAL

Consultant	Trainee Dr. Name and Bleep no.	Date of admission	Date chart reboarded	Estimated date of discharge
BEADLE	MIAH 224	13.01.12		
This chart is no. 1 of 1	Transcribing Check by Pharmacy Sign .... Date	Ward 1. MAU 2.		

Supplementary Medication charts in use: Other (please specify): 1 .... 2 ....

Epidural/PCA ☐ Syringe driver ☐ TPN ☐ Chemotherapy ☐ Insulin sliding scale ☐

Once only medications – loading doses, pre-medication, PGDs or surgical antibiotic propylaxis

Date	Time to be given	Medicine (approved name)	Dose	Route	Signature and bleep no.	Pharmacy	Time given	Given by	Checked by
13.01	STAT	PREDNISOLONE	30mg	PO	MIA 224				
13.01	STAT	SALBUTAMOL	2.5mg	NEB	MIA 224				
13.01	STAT	IPRATROPIUM	500mcg	NEB	MIA 224				
13.01	STAT	AMOXYCILLIN	500mg	PO	MIA 224				
13.01	STAT	CLARITHROMYCIN	500mg	PO	MIA 224				

As required prescriptions			Date	Time	Dose	Route	Date	Time	Dose	Route	Date	Time	Dose	Route	Date	Time	Dose	Route
Drug PARACETAMOL	Allergies Checked	Dose 1g																
Frequency	Max Dose/24 hrs 6 HR	Route PO																
Indication																		
Signature MIA 224	Pharmacy	Start 13.01																

As required prescriptions																		
			Date	Time	Dose	Route	Date	Time	Dose	Route	Date	Time	Dose	Route	Date	Time	Dose	Route
Drug SALBUTAMOL	Allergies Checked	Dose 1g																
Frequency	Max Dose/24 hrs 6 HR	Route PO																
Indication																		
Signature MIA 224	Pharmacy	Start 13.01	IF FURTHER NEEDED PLEASE CALL DOCTOR															

Thromboprophylaxis please prescribe treatment regimens in the regular medications section								
Choice of mechanical prophylaxis and leg(s) to be applied to							Enter Time	Enter details below
Graduated elastic compression stockings	Intermittend pneumatic compression device (IPC)		Leg					
			Left	Right	Both			
13.01 ☐ Start Date:	☐ End Date:	Signature and Bleep No.	☐	☐	☑			
☐ Start Date:	☐ End Date:	Signature and Bleep No.	☐	☐	☐			

Medication		Dose	Dose Change	Enter Time	Enter details below
CLEXANE		40mg			
Please ensure you have completed the VTE risk assessment form	Date	13.01.12			
	Route	SC			
	Signature	MIA 224		Instructions	Pharmacy
	Bleep no.				

Oxygen				
Target Saturation	88-92% ☐	94/98% ☑	If oxygen saturation falls below target range on prescribed oxygen, patient needs urgent clinical review. If oxygen saturation is above targent range on prescribed oxygen, ask for review.	
Other specify)			*Device: N= nasal cannula, SM = simple face mask, V = venturi, H = humidified, RM = reservoir mask, OTHER = other eg. NCPAP/NIPPV	Pharmacy
Target Saturation not applicable				

	Date Started	Date Changed	Date Changed	Enter Time	Enter details below
	13.01				
* Device	VENTURI				
% or L/min (Specify a range eg 1-12 L/min)	40%				
Signature and Bleep No.	MIA 224				

Infusion prescriptions continued										SC = subcutaneous		IVC = intravenous central IVP = intravenous peripheral		
Date & time	Route	Infusion Fluid		Medication		Duration	Rate	Prescriber's signature & bleep no.	Date given	Given by / Added by	Check by	Start time	Finish time	Pharmacy
		Name & strength	Volume	Approved name with expiry / unit number	Dose									
13/01	IV	0.9% SALINE Exp: Batch/unit no:	1 LITRE				8hr							
13/01	IV	0.9% SALINE Exp: Batch/unit no:	1 LITRE	+20mmol Kcl			8hr							

Regular prescriptions continued

Anti-infectives prescription *prescribe long term prophylaxis and anti-tuberculosis medications in regular medications section*

For 5 Days			Date 13	14	15	16	17									
Date		13/01	Medication: AMOXYCILLIN					Indication: LRTI				Signature and bleep no.: MIA 224			Pharmacy: ☐	
Route																
Times		Dose														
(06)		500mg														
09																
(12)		500mg														
18																
(22)		500mg														
24																

Regular prescriptions continued

Anti-infectives prescription *prescribe long term prophylaxis and anti-tuberculosis medications in regular medications section*

For 5 Days			Date 13	14	15	16	17									
Date		13/01	Medication: CLARITHROMYCIN					Indication: LRTI				Signature and bleep no.: MIA 224			Pharmacy: ☐	
Route		PO														
Times		Dose														
06																
(09)		500mg														
12																
18																
(22)		500mg														
24																

Regular prescriptions continued

Regular medications

		Dose			Date 13	14	15	16	17	18								
Date		13.01			Medication: PREDNISOLONE					Instructions: 5/7 ONLY				Signature and bleep no.: MIA 224			Pharmacy: ☐	
Route		PO																
Signature		MIA																
06																		
(09)		30mg			X													
12																		
18																		
22																		
24																		

Regular prescriptions continued

Regular medications

		Dose			Date 13	14	15											
Date		13.01			Medication: SALBUTAMOL					Instructions				Signature and bleep no.: MIA 224			Pharmacy: ☐	
Route		NEB																
Signature		MIA																
06		2.5mg																
10		2.5mg																
14		2.5mg																
18		2.5mg																
22		2.5mg																
02		2.5mg																

Regular prescriptions continued																			
Regular medications																			
		Dose			Date 13	14	15	16	17	18									
Date		13.01			Medication					Instructions				Signature and bleep no.			Pharmacy		
Route		NEB			IPRATROPIUM									MIA 224					
Signature		MIA																	
06																			
10		500mcg																	
14		500mcg																	
18		500mcg																	
22		500mcg																	
24																			

GLOBAL PRESCRIBING MARK

A B C D E

Station 6 – Communication skills

Patient script

You are a 23-year-old woman with asthma who was diagnosed at age 14 after having increasing wheeze, especially on exertion. You have been admitted to hospital at least six times, including an admission to the intensive care unit 3 months ago. You use both of your inhalers at least three or four times a day.

You have had to leave your university course because of frequent absences and you have become frustrated with your asthma preventing you from having a normal life. You smoke five to ten cigarettes a day and know this doesn't help your asthma, but it helps when you feel 'stressed'.

You do not know anyone with asthma and feel that no one understands how difficult it is for you. You do not visit your GP, as he just 'lectures' you about taking your inhalers. You have never had an asthma action plan and feel hopeless to prevent further exacerbations, so there is no point taking regular inhalers. You are not keen on your steroid inhalers, as you know that steroids make you fat.

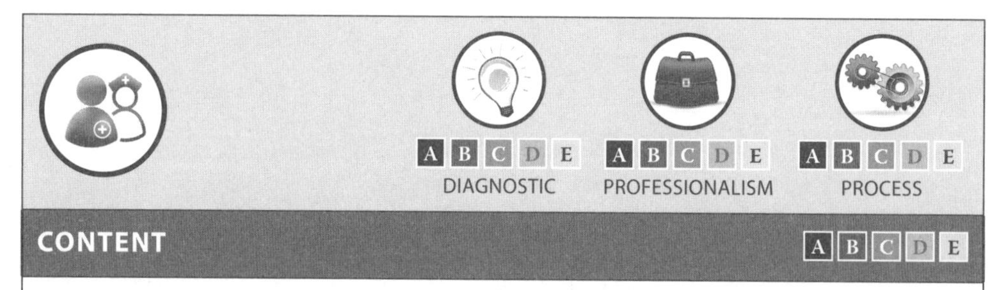

Reviews patient's current understanding of clinical situation and summarises what has happened so far

- Establishes current control of asthma
- Establishes events of this admission
- Identifies current issues regarding control
- Smoking, irregular use of inhalers, frequent admissions

Establishes patient's ideas, concerns and expectations

- Establishes patients beliefs that she is unable to control asthma
- Understanding of stepwise treatment

Explains the key important information; invites patient to ask questions and is able to deal with them appropriately

- Addresses importance of smoking cessation
- Explains escalation of stepwise therapy (and de-escalation when control is adequate)
- Explains asthma action plan and areas of support
- Deals with concern regarding inhaled steroids

Summarises important areas of the consultation back to the patient

Formally ends the consultation and ensures appropriate follow-up has been discussed

GLOBAL COMMUNICATION MARK A B C D E

Scenario 1: Reflection and consolidation

History

Miss Davis is a 23-year-old patient with chronic asthma since the age of 14. Her control is very poor, she has been ventilated in ICU three times. The last time was 3 months ago. She uses her reliever on a daily basis. She is prescribed regular inhaled steroids but does not take them regularly. She sleeps poorly and has had multiple admissions and courses of oral steroids. She is a current smoker. She has not been able to work because of her frequent exacerbations.

Her current illness started 5 days ago. She has had a cough productive of green sputum and a fever. She has been increasingly wheezy and it is not responsive to her inhaled ß2-agonist. She has no chest pain or haemoptysis. She came to hospital as she feels exhausted and is very worried that she may need ventilation once again.

Examination

Miss Davis is a young lady who, on examination, is short of breath at rest and only able to complete short sentences. She has oxygen sats of 95% in room air. She is tachypnoeic at 24 resps per minute. She is tachycardic at rest with a pulse of 102 and BP 130/75. On examination of the chest she has no evidence of pneumothorax but has widespread expiratory polyphonic wheeze.

The purpose of the examination of any patient with an acute exacerbation of asthma is to assess the severity of the exacerbation in order to ensure that appropriate treatment and escalation is provided in a timely way. Every junior doctor should be able to perform this clinical examination and stratify an exacerbation.

The assessment is based on:

- Ability to speak in full/short sentences or not at all
- RR and respiratory effort
- Oxygen saturations
- PEFR as a percentage of either best (if known) or expected
- A normal or rising pCO_2 (a sign of tiring of respiratory effort).

The exacerbation is then classified as mild, moderate, severe or life-threatening.

Investigations

The diagnosis of chronic asthma is based on history and a clinical probability of more than one of the following symptoms:

- wheeze
- breathlessness
- chest tightness
- cough

particularly if:

- symptoms worse at night and in the early morning
- symptoms occur in response to exercise, allergen exposure, cold air and after taking aspirin or beta blockers.

If the diagnosis of chronic asthma is most likely, a trial of inhaled ß2-agonist should be started.
The ability to instruct in the technique and subsequently obtain accurate PEFR in all patients presenting with wheeze and dyspnoea is a core skill for all foundation year doctors.

Management

The management of any chronic condition can be extremely challenging to both the patient and junior doctor. The key is to control symptoms with a stepwise escalation of therapy. Good control is that which enables patients with asthma to complete ADLs without interruption and to require rescue therapy only up to once per week.
Liaison with primary care and asthma specialist nurses and personalised asthma action plans facilitate patient-led therapy.

Further reading and web links
BTS/SIGN guidelines for both diagnosis, acute and chronic management of asthma:
www.brit-thoracic.org.uk/guidelines/asthma-guidelines.aspx

Scenario 2: 'Heartache'

Station 1

History *10-minute station*

You are the FY1 attached to a GP surgery. The next patient is Mr James Wright, who has made an urgent appointment to see the doctor. He has agreed to see you before seeing the GP.

- **Please take a focused history from the patient with a view to presenting the history and likely diagnosis to the GP.**

You will be assessed on the following areas, as well as the content and diagnostic reasoning of your history – take them into account in your presentation.

Professionalism

- Professional appearance (NHS dress code) – including general appearance, hair and jewellery; maintains patient and personal safety
- Polite introduction; identifies patient or interviewee correctly; confirms patient's date of birth from name band or other source
- Obtains informal consent; maintains patient's privacy
- Displays empathetic and caring attitudes and behaviours throughout.

Process

- Good organisation and structure; appropriate use of open and closed questions
- Appropriate fluency/rhythm/pace to the interview – this may change depending on environment and acute nature of the problem
- Appropriate time for the patient to respond/reply to questions
- Appropriate acknowledgement of difficult or emotional areas of the patient's history.

Communication skills

- Demonstrates caring and sympathetic attitude
- Asks open questions
- Invites patient to ask questions and answers them appropriately
- Addresses patient's ideas, concerns and expectations.

Station 2

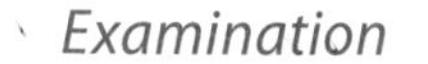

Examination *10-minute station*

After completing and presenting the history, the GP asks you to perform a focused/ appropriate examination of the patient. Mr Wright was also seen this morning by the Practice Nurse, who performed a series of clinical observations and tests on him. You may ask for these during your assessment.

- **You should present the relevant findings (given within the station) to the GP in an appropriate manner for a busy GP surgery.**

You will be assessed on the following areas, as well as the content and skills of your examination – take them into account in your presentation.

Professionalism

- Professional appearance; maintains infection control standards, including hand cleaning and appropriate use of gloves and aprons
- Maintains patient and personal safety
- Polite introduction; identifies patient and confirms date of birth from name band or other source
- Obtains informal consent; maintains patient privacy and dignity
- Displays empathetic and caring attitudes and behaviours throughout.

Process

- Appropriate fluency/rhythm/pace to the examination – this may change depending on environment and acute nature of problem
- Good organisation and structure of examination; sensitive and empathetic approach
- Uses appropriate clinical techniques throughout
- Maintains privacy and dignity throughout.

Clinical communication

- Explains proposed examination/procedure; explains examination/procedure as it proceeds
- Offers information in a clear, structured and fluent manner, avoiding jargon
- Listens to patient and responds appropriately
- Demonstrates appropriate body language.

Please read the information below before presenting this case to the GP as if you were in a busy GP surgery.
[NB If you have a model do not read this section]

Clinical findings

- o **Patient looks well**
- o **Feet to face: peri-orbital xanthelasma; no other obvious stigmata of CV disease**
- o **HR 88 bpm, BP 164/98 mmHg, RR 14 bpm, O_2 sats 97% on air, temperature 36.5 °C CBG 6.8 mmol/l**
- o **Height 1.80 m, weight 98 kg, BMI $98/(1.8)^2 = 30.3$ kg/m^2; urinalysis – WCC nil, protein negative, blood negative, nitrites negative, glucose +**
- o **General examination – fingers of right hand heavily tar stained; no anaemia, no tendon xanthoma**
- o **RS and CV examinations – no abnormal chest signs, no features of arrhythmia, cardiac valvular dysfunction, or features of heart failure.**

Station 3

Data interpretation *10-minute station*

The GP prescribes Mr Wright aspirin 75 mg od, bisoprolol 5 mg od and glyceryl trinitrate (GTN) spray 2 puffs PRN. However, Mr Wright fails to collect his prescription and 10 days later is admitted to the local hospital with a diagnosis of acute coronary syndrome (ACS).

- **The on-call cardiology ST4 presents you with a number of statements concerning the admission ECG and chest radiograph of Mr Wright. Please indicate whether the statements are TRUE (T) or FALSE (F).**

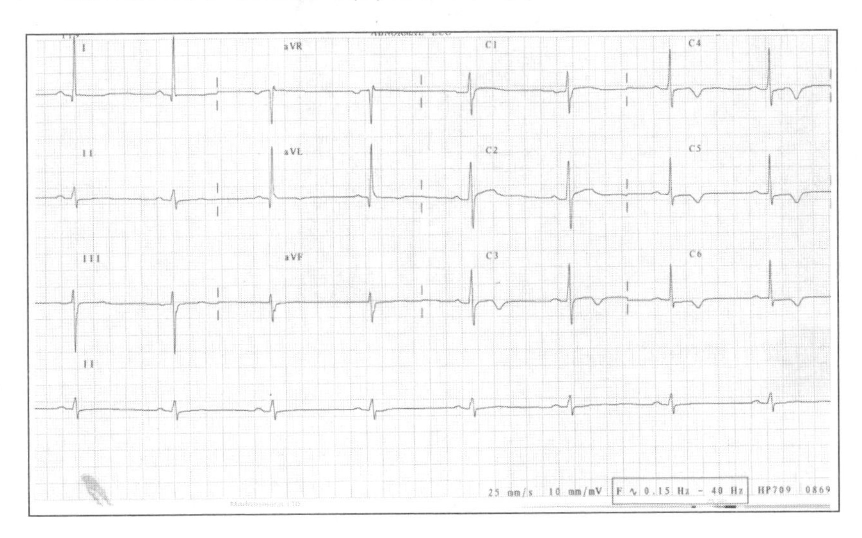

Figure 2.1 Mr Wright's ECG

1. The rhythm is consistent with sinus bradycardia.
2. The P wave indicates that there is right atrial hypertrophy.
3. The PR interval indicates that there is first-degree heart block.
4. The axis is deviated to the right.
5. There is evidence of a left bundle branch block pattern.
6. There is evidence of an old inferior MI.
7. There is evidence of acute septolateral ischaemia.
8. There is abnormal R wave progression.
9. There are changes consistent with the voltage criteria of left ventricular hypertrophy.
10. If the patient's 12-hour troponin was 0.96 iu/l, this would indicate that he had suffered an acute non-STEMI.

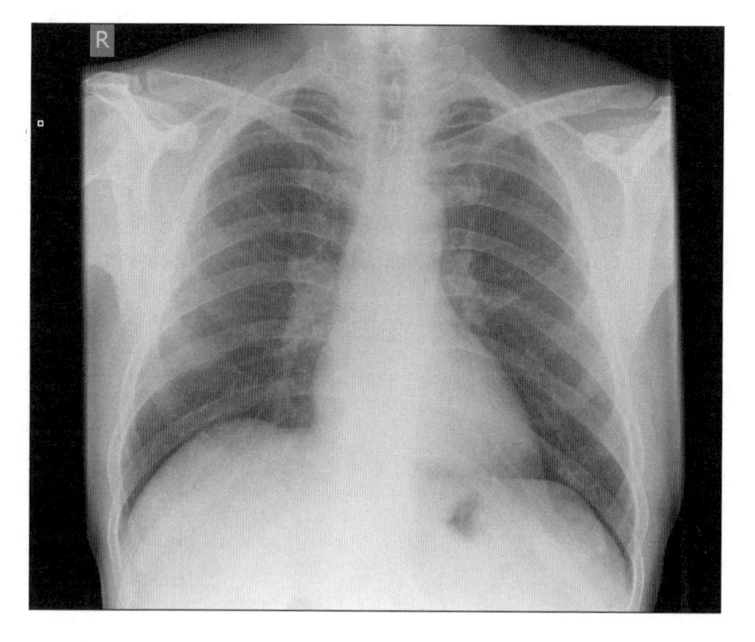

Figure 2.2 Mr Wright's chest radiograph

1 There is evidence of left atrial hypertrophy.

2 The cardiothoracic ratio is increased.

3 There is calcification of the aortic valve.

4 There is evidence of a right pleural effusion.

5 The left hilum is abnormal.

6 The thoracic aorta is 'unfolded'.

7 There is fluid in the horizontal fissure.

8 There are multiple Kerley B lines.

9 There is evidence of asbestos exposure.

10 This chest radiograph is consistent with biventricular failure.

Station 4

Prescribing skills *10-minute station*

- Mr Wright is admitted to the CCU awaiting his 12-hour troponin. Using the charts and the BNF provided please write up Mr Wright's regular medications and the hospital ACS protocol.

Details

Mr James Wright; DOB: 14/04/1964; Ward: CCU; Consultant: Dr Agrawal; Hospital No.: 6172099; Weight: 98 kg; U&Es: normal; RBG: 6.7 mmol/; Total cholesterol: 8.9 mmol/l

Regular medications

Aspirin 75 mg od; Bisoprolol 5 mg od; GTN spray 2 puffs PRN

ACS protocol

IV access
Cardiac monitor
Oxygen via nasal cannulae or mask (maintain sats at 96–98%)

To be given after ECG confirmation of diagnosis:

Aspirin 300 mg stat (in this case already given); followed by aspirin 75 mg od (lifelong)
Clopidogrel 300 mg (in this case already given); followed by clopidogrel 75 mg od (1 year)
Fondaparinux 2.5 mg sc – stat; followed by fondaparinux 2.5 mg od for 48 hours
Lansoprazole 30 mg od

Lipids: total cholesterol >6.0 mmol/l; atorvastatin 20 mg od
Blood glucose: start insulin sliding scale if RBG >11 mmol/l

If ongoing or severe pain:
Diamorphine 2.5–5 mg IV with metoclopramide 10 mg IV – stat
Consider addition of enoxaparin, bivalirudin or glycoprotein inhibitor
Discuss with cardiologist regarding transfer for PCI

To write up on PRN side
Diamorphine 2.5–5 mg IV (only)
Metoclopramide 10 mg IV (only)
GTN spray 2 puffs sl
Paracetamol 1 g max (po) qds

Remember: DRUG DRs **D**on't **F**orget **S**igning **O**ff (page 373)

Station 5

Communication skills *10-minute station*

- You are the FY1 on the cardiology firm under which Mr Wright has been admitted. The Nursing Sister on the CCU is concerned that Mr Wright shows little or no understanding of his medications and condition. She asks you to explain these issues to him. Investigations have confirmed a troponin <0.05 iu/l, total cholesterol 8.9 mmol/l, RBG 6.7 mmol/l and BMI 31.6. Please explain the diagnosis, possible further management and the medications that have been prescribed.

Answers

Station 1 – History

Patient script

You are Mr James Wright, 47 years old, DOB 14 April 1964. You have been previously fit and well but 'never see a doctor and don't really look after yourself'. Over the past 3–4 months you have been suffering with increasingly frequent and severe episodes of chest pain. Initially you thought the pains were 'muscle strains' but they have got slowly worse. Initially the pains lasted less than 20–30 seconds at a time and came on once or twice a week. They would take your breath away sometimes but were never prolonged and were always when you were exerting yourself, eg lifting heavy boxes in the factory. More recently the pains have been lasting for up to 2–3 minutes and come on when you are walking in the park with your dog. They have never come on at rest and have never been prolonged. You get pains nearly every day – hence the urgent appointment that your wife made for you today.

You have never had any nausea, vomiting, sweats, clamminess, loss of consciousness or dizziness, but the pains often make you feel 'unwell' and you have to sit on a park bench or a low wall for a few minutes until they go away.

Cardiovascular risk factors: your grandfather and father both died in their 60s of 'heart problems', and your older brother had a 'heart by-pass' operation last year aged 49 years. You smoke 40–50 cigarettes a day and have done so for many years. You often drink 15–20 pints at the weekend but little during the week. You had a blood pressure check several years ago at a local supermarket health promotion day; you were told it was 150 over something but never got it checked again. You do not know about your cholesterol and have never had symptoms suggestive of a stroke, peripheral vascular disease or ischaemic heart disease (IHD).

Medications: you take 'handfuls' of indigestion tablets, including Zantac®, and occasional paracetamol but no other regular medications; you have no known allergies.

SHx: you are married with three children, aged 7, 11 and 14 years. You are the foreman in a large textile factory and are responsible for the day-to-day running of the entire shop floor. This is very stressful. You bought a large house at the end of 2008, but have subsequently had to take a pay cut and have been left with mounting debts.

Ideas and concerns: you think you may have heart problems, as these are the same symptoms as your father and brother described in the past. You hope you have not had a heart attack over the last few weeks.

Expectations: you are hoping the doctor can confirm or refute your worries and if it is a heart problem 'start you on the right medicines'. You suppose you'll have to lose some weight and stop smoking as well.

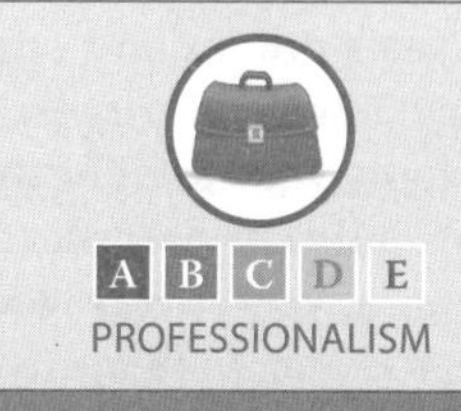

A B C D E PROFESSIONALISM

A B C D E PROCESS

A B C D E COMMUNICATION

CONTENT

A B C D E

Identifies key information

- Pain – chronological progression, onset, frequency, duration, character, radiation, relieving and exacerbating factors
- Associated features – shortness of breath, nausea and vomiting, dizziness, presyncope and syncope, feeling unwell, washed out, palpitations

Identifies important negatives, including systemic enquiry

- No radiation to the back (thoracic aortic aneurysm)
- No features of heart failure – peripheral oedema, orthopnoea, PND, shortness of breath, wheeze, dry cough, frothy white sputum
- No features suggestive of gastrointestinal or hepatobiliary disease
- Excludes other systemic symptoms

Identifies key information from rest of the history

- Cardiovascular risk – FHx, known IHD, stroke or PVD, diabetes mellitus, hypertension, smoking, alcohol, others
- Relevant facts about employment, housing, social support, life stressors

Completing the patient history

- Drug and allergic history: Zantac and indigestion tablets, occasional paracetamol
- Allergies: NKDA
- Previous medical history: nil known
- Social and occupational history: as above

Summarises important areas of the history back to the patient

Invites patient to ask questions and is able to deal with them appropriately

Establishes patient's ideas, concerns and expectations

DIAGNOSTIC REASONING

A B C D E

Please present your history

- Candidate offers a logical, well-structured account of the history

What is your diagnosis?

- Candidate offers the correct diagnosis and appropriate differentials
- Diagnosis: unstable angina/IHD – the patient has not suffered a prolonged or severe episode in recent days, excluding a diagnosis of ACS or MI
- Differentials: although the usual differentials may be offered, they are unlikely in this very clear-cut history, eg basal pneumonia, upper abdominal causes (gallstones, peptic ulcer disease)

If you were the GP what immediate therapeutic management would you initiate?

- Include aspirin, GTN spray, anti-anginal, eg β blocker

What lifestyle changes would you recommend?

- Weight loss, exercise, smoking cessation, reduced alcohol intake, address life stressors (job, money worries)

What other interventions might you consider?

- Referral for further investigation, lipids assessment

Demonstrates safe, sensible and appropriate management plan

Demonstrates clear and logical diagnostic reasoning

GLOBAL HISTORY MARK

A B C D E

Station 2– Examination

Patient script

If you are an actor/patient, read the patient history and physical signs fully – when the candidate comes to an abnormal site in their examination, act out tenderness and/or volunteer the relevant physical sign.

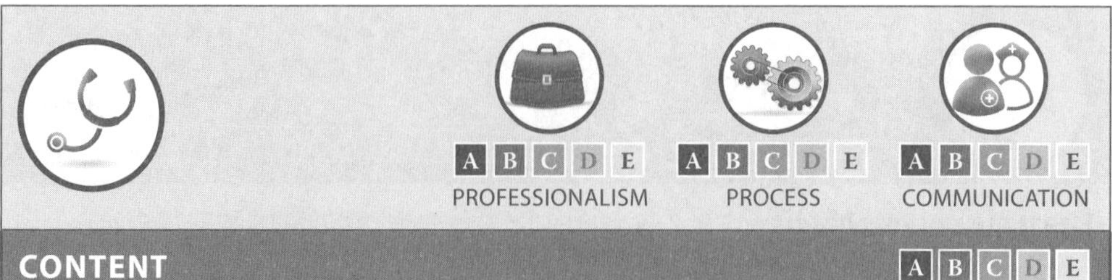

CONTENT

A B C D E

Exposes and positions patient correctly and maintains comfort

Comments on wellbeing of patient, ie well or unwell

'Feet to face'

- Observes, and comments on patient and surroundings from foot of bed – evidence of previous cardiac surgery, eg sternotomy, JVP, anaemia, colour/perfusion.

Asks for appropriate/relevant clinical observations

- BP 164/98 mmHg, RR 14 bpm, O_2 sats 97% on air, temperature 36.5 °C, CBG 6.8 mmol/l,
- Urinalysis: WCC nil, protein negative, blood negative, nitrites negative, glucose +
- Height 1.80 m, weight 98 kg, BMI $98/(1.8)^2 = 30.3$ kg/m^2.

General/systemic examination

- Hands and upper limbs: tar staining, perfusion of hands, anaemia, stigmata of hyperlipidaemia; comments on general signs, eg clubbing, leukonychai
- Face and neck: including signs of anaemia, peri-orbital xanthelasma, central cyanosis.

Focused examination

- **Inspection:**
- Sternotomy scar, JVP – makes appropriate assessment including correct positioning of patient, correct technique; comments correctly on JVP.
- **Palpation:**
- Carotid pulse – comments on character and presence of bruits
- Apex beat – position and character
- Assesses and comments on heaves and thrills
- **Auscultation:** listens in correct areas, assesses for radiation, manoeuvres patient correctly, appropriate use of stethoscope – bell and diaphragm.

Completes examination by identifying relevant additional clinical signs and formally completing assessment

- Signs of left and right heart failure, including bibasal crackles, pleural effusions, peripheral oedema; hepatomegaly/ascites
- Signs of PVD and generalised atherosclerosis, including AAA, peripheral pulses and abdominal bruits.

Thanks patient, offers assistance, maintains patient's dignity and privacy until they are dressed

DIAGNOSTIC REASONING

A B C D E

Correctly identifies the relevant physical signs, including important negative findings

Demonstrates safe, sensible and appropriate management plan, including

- Anti-platelet treatment
- Anti-anginals
- Lipid-lowering agents, primarily statins
- Anti-hypertensives: given his age, race and new-onset IHD, ACEI or β blockade should be considered
- Nicotine replacement therapy.

Demonstrates clear and logical diagnostic reasoning

GLOBAL EXAMINATION MARK

A B C D E

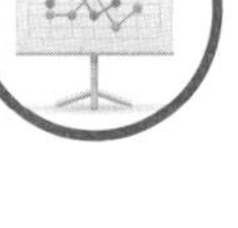

Station 3 – Data interpretation

1. **TRUE – the rate is 300/6 = 50 bpm**
2. **FALSE – the P wave is slightly notched but is less than 3 mm broad; this is more suggestive of left atrial compared with right atrial enlargement; if broader this would be consistent with P mitrale**
3. **TRUE – the PR interval is 5 mm; borderline first-degree heart block**
4. **FALSE – there is marked left axis deviation (LAD); lead I is positive, lead II is isoelectric, lead III is negative (ie leads I and III are pointing away from one another = 'leaving' one another = LAD)**
5. **FALSE – the QRS complex has a normal width (<3 mm) and does not demonstrate any features suggestive of LBBB**
6. **FALSE – there are no features suggestive of an old MI, eg Q waves**
7. **TRUE – there are inverted Q waves from V2 to V6, extending up to a VL**
8. **TRUE – the R wave should be small in amplitude in V1 and increase in size across the chest leads to V4 or V5, then drop away slightly to V6; there are relatively tall R waves from V2 to V5, with equal amplitude**
9. **FALSE – there are no voltage criteria suggestive of the LVH**
10. **TRUE – patients presenting with features of ACS are divided first by their ECG findings STEMI vs non-STEMI or unstable angina; non-STEMI and unstable angina are subsequently subdivided by the 12-hour troponin level; a positive result (in context) is suggestive of a non-STEMI; cardiac (tachyarrhythmias) and non-cardiac pathologies (chronic renal impairment or PE) may also increase the troponin level**

Figure 2.2 is a normal CXT

When assessing a CXR, as with all images, it is important to have a structured approach, considering each aspect in turn, and to know the normal appearance. Always start by checking that the **patient details** are correct for your patient. Is it **PA** (posteroroanterior – X-ray plate against the chest) or **AP** – in the latter the heart appears magnified, and technically, one should not comment on the cardiac size. Is there any **rotation** – in a well-centred film the clavicles are horizontal, directly opposing one another, clearly seen along their entire length, and equally placed on either side of the vertebral column, which should be perpendicular to them. If the film is under-**penetrated** (the focus of the X-rays is in front of the plate), the heart and lung markings appear very dense and the vertebrae are not seen. In over-penetrated views (X rays focussed behind the plate), lung markings and vertebrae become very prominent (occasionally, used to give lesions in the lung more definition).

The **left heart border** is made up (from superior to inferior) of the aortic knuckle, the left pulmonary artery, the left atrial appendage and the left ventricle. It is intimately related to the lingual lobe, a part of the upper lobe, of the left lung - with consolidation of the lingual lobe, the left heart border becomes hazy and difficult to define. The **right heart border** is made up of the superior vena cava and the right atrium. It is intimately related to the right middle lobe and consolidation within this lobe causes loss of definition of this border. The **heart size** on a PA film should be less than half of the thoracic cavity at its widest point, ie this cardiothoracic ratio (CTR) should be < 0.50.

The upper lobe of the **left lung** (incorporating the lingual lobe) lies anteriorly and the lower lobe posteriorly. The **right lung** has upper, middle and lower lobes; the horizontal fissure becomes visible on X-ray when fluid filled. The lungs are both divided radiologically into the **upper zone** (incorporates the apices and extends from the apex to the 2nd anterior rib), **midzone** (extends from the 2nd to 4th anterior ribs) and **lower zone** (extends from the 4th to the 6th anterior ribs).

Both **costodiaphragmatic angles** must be included on a CXR: if not, it should be repeated before commenting on the lungs. The right **hemidiaphragm** should lie 1–2 cm higher than the left. Blunting or loss of an angle implies an effusion. The left hemidiaphragm usually has an underlying gastric bubble: do not confuse this with a pneumoperitoneum caused by perforation of a viscus.

Two features must be present to diagnose **hyperexpansion** of the lung fields: (a) there should be no more than **six anterior ribs** seen on a PA film (unless a deep inspiration has been taken). The ribs, in a hyperextended view, often look 'flattened' or very horizontal, as do the hemidiaphragms, (b) the precise way of establishing hyperexpansion is to draw a line between the costodiaphragmatic angle and the cardiodiaphragmatic angle. In the normal CXR, a **perpendicular** drawn from the mid-point of the hemidiaphragm to the original line should be **1.0 cm or more**: if less, the hemidiaphragms are 'flattened' and the lung fields hyperexpanded.

Comment on whether the **ribs** and other **bones** look normal or osteopenic, and whether there is evidence of arthritis, fractures or other abnormality. The rib spacing is greatly reduced with underlying lung collapse and is termed 'crowding'. Check the **soft tissues** for the breast, and other shadows, air (surgical emphysema) and calcification.

GLOBAL DATA INTERPRETATION MARK

A B C D E

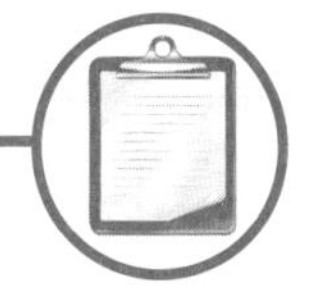

Station 4 – Prescribing skills

Check: DRUG DRs Don't Forget Signing Off (page 373)

Allergies, sensitivities and adverse drug reactions			Patient details/addressograph
No known allergies ✓		Initials AF 007	NHS/ Hospital No: 6172099
Not possible to ascertain ☐		Date 21.11.11	
Medicine/substance	Reaction & Severity	Initials & Date	Surname: WRIGHT
			First name: JAMES
Alerts			Date of birth: 14.04.64

Gender (M) / F	
Weight (kg)	Date
98	
Height	
1.80m	
Surface area (m²)	

IN-PATIENT MEDICATION PRESCRIPTION AND ADMINISTRATION RECORD

PasTest HOSPITAL

Consultant	Trainee Dr. Name and Bleep no.	Date of admission	Date chart reboarded	Estimated date of discharge
AGRAWAL	FEATHER 007	21.11.11		
This chart is no. .... of	Transcribing Check by Pharmacy Sign .... Date	Ward 1. HDU 2.		

Supplementary Medication charts in use: Other (please specify): 1 .... 2 ....

Epidural/PCA ☐ Syringe driver ☐ TPN ☐ Chemotherapy ☐ Insulin sliding scale ☐

Once only medications – loading doses, pre-medication, PGDs or surgical antibiotic propylaxis

Date	Time to be given	Medicine (approved name)	Dose	Route	Signature and bleep no.	Pharmacy	Time given	Given by	Checked by
21.11	18.00	FONDAPARINUX	2.5mg	SC	AF 007				

Regular prescriptions continued

Regular medications

	Dose			Date													
				21	22	23	24	25	26	27							
Date	21.11			Medication					Instructions				Signature and bleep no.			Pharmacy	
Route	SC			FONDAPRINUX									AF 007			☐	
Signature	AF																
06																	
(09)	2.5mg																
12																	
18																	
22																	
24																	

Regular prescriptions continued

Regular medications

	Dose			Date													
				22	23	24											
Date	21.11			Medication					Instructions				Signature and bleep no.			Pharmacy	
Route	PO			LANSOPRAZOLE									AF 007			☐	
Signature	AF																
06																	
(09)	30mg																
12																	
18																	
22																	
24																	

Regular prescriptions continued

Regular medications

	Dose			Date													
				22	23	24											
Date	21.11			Medication					Instructions				Signature and bleep no.			Pharmacy	
Route	PO			ASPIRIN									AF 007			☐	
Signature	AF																
06																	
(09)	75mg																
12																	
18																	
22																	
24																	

Regular prescriptions continued

Regular medications

	Dose			Date													
				22	23	24											
Date	21.11			Medication					Instructions				Signature and bleep no.			Pharmacy	
Route	PO			CLOPIDOGREL									AF 007			☐	
Signature	AF																
06																	
(09)	75mg																
12																	
18																	
22																	
24																	

Regular prescriptions continued																		
Regular medications																		
		Dose			Date													
					22	23	24											
Date		21.11			Medication					Instructions				Signature and bleep no.			Pharmacy	
Route		PO			BISOPROLOL									AF 007			☐	
Signature		AF																
06																		
(09)		5mg																
12																		
18																		
22																		
24																		

Regular prescriptions continued																		
Regular medications																		
		Dose			Date													
					22	23	24											
Date		21.11			Medication					Instructions				Signature and bleep no.			Pharmacy	
Route		PO			ATORVASTATIN									AF 007			☐	
Signature		AF																
06																		
(09)		20mg																
12																		
18																		
22																		
24																		

Regular prescriptions							
Oral anticoagulation follow the anticoagulation guidelines available on the intranet							
Indication	Target INR	Baseline INR (if applicable)	Duration of therapy	Date of anticoagulation follow-up appointment (clinic or other)*	Anticoagulant record book given or updated. Sign and date	Date patient counselled and sign	
			Date therapy started				

* A follow-up appointment must be booked with the anti-coagulant clinic or enhanced provider of primary care services. If not, the TTA will not be dispensed

Initiating warfarin	Perform baseline coagulation screen, LFTs, U&Es and FBC	Prescribe initiation dose as per guidelines	CHECK INR ON DAY 3	FOLLOW DOSING ALGORITHM IN GUIDELINE
Continuing warfarin	Maintenance therapy	FOLLOW MAINTENANCE DOSING ALGORITHM IN GUIDELINE		

Do not use the initiation protocol for patients already on warfarin. More frequent INR monitoring may be required for patients on interacting drug(s)

Medication				Date														
1				INR														
Route	Frequency OD	Time 18.00	Start	Dose														
			Stop	Dr sign														
Signature		Bleep no.	Pharmacy	Given														

Initiating warfarin – Reduced dosing regimen in red. Refer to anticoagulation policy																		
Day	One	Two	Three							Four and above								
INR	<1.4	No test	<2.0	2.0-2.1	2.2-2.5	2.6-2.9	3.0-3.3	3.4-4.0	>4.0	<1.4	1.4-1.5	1.6-1.7	1.8-1.9	2.0-2.3	2.4-3.0	3.1-4.0	4.1-4.5	>4.5
Dose mg	10 5	10 5	10	5	4	3	2	1	0	9	8	7	6	5	4	3	Miss 1 day	Miss 2 day

Thromboprophylaxis please prescribe treatment regimens in the regular medications section

Choice of mechanical prophylaxis and leg(s) to be applied to						Enter Time	Enter details below
Graduated elastic compression stockings	Intermittend pneumatic compression device (IPC)		Leg				
			Left	Right	Both		
21/11 ☑ Start Date:	☐ End Date:	Signature and Bleep No.	☐	☐	☑		
Start Date:	End Date:	Signature and Bleep No.	☐	☐	☐		

Medication		Dose	Dose Change	Enter Time	Enter details below
Please ensure you have completed the VTE risk assessment form	Date				
	Route				
	Signature			Instructions: ON ACS PROTOCOL	Pharmacy ☐
	Bleep no.				

Oxygen

Target Saturation	88-92% ☐	94/98% ☑	If oxygen saturation falls below target range on prescribed oxygen, patient needs urgent clinical review. If oxygen saturation is above targent range on prescribed oxygen, ask for review.
Other specify)			*Device: N= nasal cannula, SM = simple face mask, V = venturi, H = humidified, RM = reservoir mask, OTHER = other eg. NCPAP/NIPPV — Pharmacy ☐
Target Saturation not applicable ☐			

	Date Changed	Date Changed	Enter Time	Enter details below
	21/11			
Device	NASAL CANNULAE			
% or L/min (specify a range eg 1-21 L/min)	1-2L/MIN			
Signature and Bleep no.	AF			

As required medications

Medication				Date
MORPHINE				
Indication				Time
Dose: 25-5Mg	Route: IV	Maximum frequency / dose: as reqd.	Start date: 21/11	Dose
			Stop date	Route
Signature: AF			Bleep no.: 007	Given
Additional instructions: IV ONLY				Pharmacy ☐

As required medications

Medication	METOCLOPRAMIDE
Indication	
Dose	10 mg
Route	IV
Maximum frequency / dose	8 hour
Start date	21/11
Stop date	
Signature	AF
Bleep no.	007
Additional instructions:	
Pharmacy	☐

Date / Time / Dose / Route / Given

As required medications

Medication	PARACETAMOL
Indication	
Dose	1g
Route	PO
Maximum frequency / dose	6 hour
Start date	21/11
Stop date	
Signature	AF
Bleep no.	007
Additional instructions:	
Pharmacy	☐

Date / Time / Dose / Route / Given

As required medications

Medication	GTN SPRAY
Indication	
Dose	1-2 PUFF
Route	S/L
Maximum frequency / dose	
Start date	21/11
Stop date	
Signature	AF
Bleep no.	007
Additional instructions:	
Pharmacy	☐

Date / Time / Dose / Route / Given

GLOBAL PRESCRIBING MARK

A B C D E

Station 5 – Communication skills

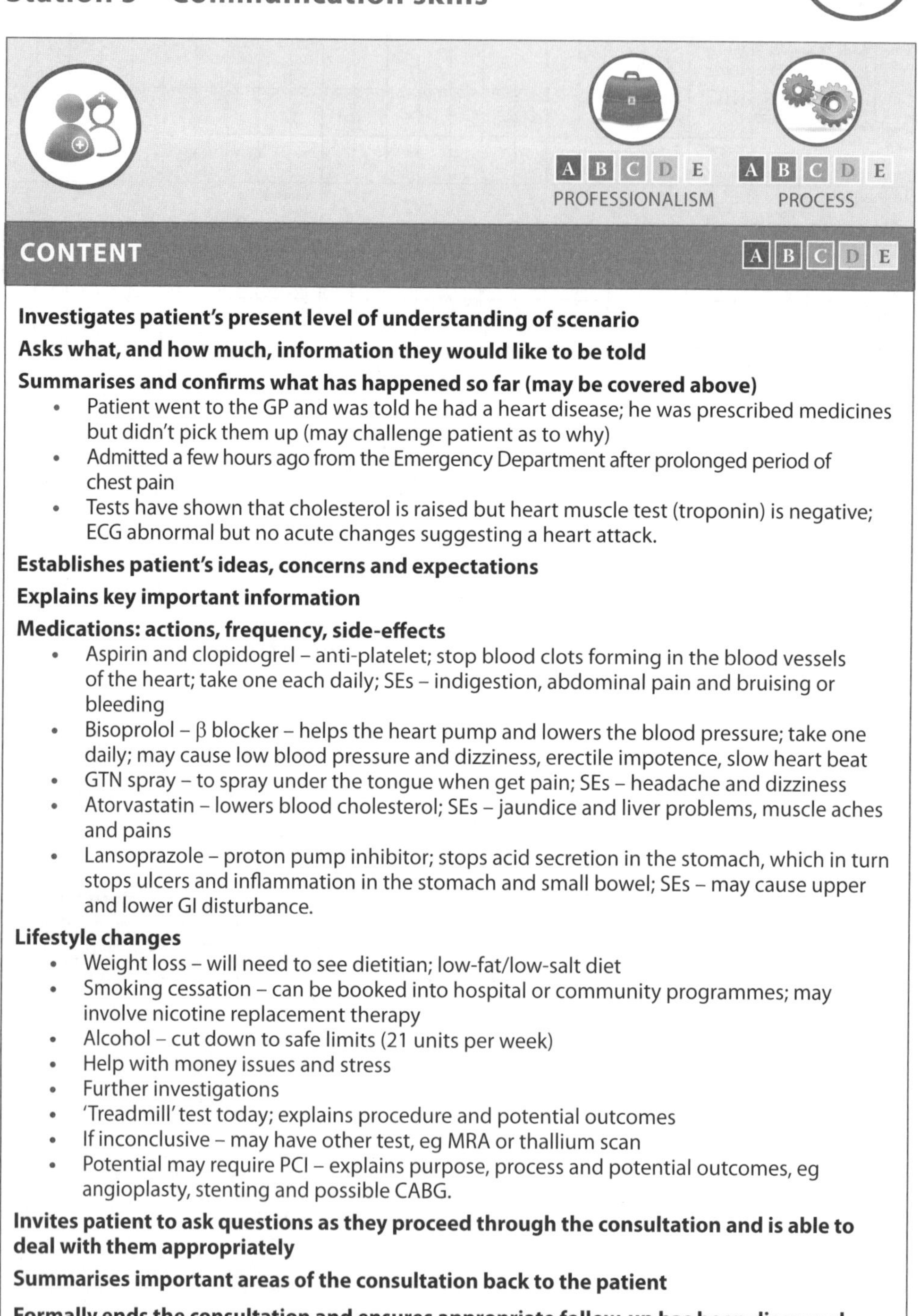

A B C D E
PROFESSIONALISM

A B C D E
PROCESS

CONTENT A B C D E

Investigates patient's present level of understanding of scenario

Asks what, and how much, information they would like to be told

Summarises and confirms what has happened so far (may be covered above)

- Patient went to the GP and was told he had a heart disease; he was prescribed medicines but didn't pick them up (may challenge patient as to why)
- Admitted a few hours ago from the Emergency Department after prolonged period of chest pain
- Tests have shown that cholesterol is raised but heart muscle test (troponin) is negative; ECG abnormal but no acute changes suggesting a heart attack.

Establishes patient's ideas, concerns and expectations

Explains key important information

Medications: actions, frequency, side-effects

- Aspirin and clopidogrel – anti-platelet; stop blood clots forming in the blood vessels of the heart; take one each daily; SEs – indigestion, abdominal pain and bruising or bleeding
- Bisoprolol – β blocker – helps the heart pump and lowers the blood pressure; take one daily; may cause low blood pressure and dizziness, erectile impotence, slow heart beat
- GTN spray – to spray under the tongue when get pain; SEs – headache and dizziness
- Atorvastatin – lowers blood cholesterol; SEs – jaundice and liver problems, muscle aches and pains
- Lansoprazole – proton pump inhibitor; stops acid secretion in the stomach, which in turn stops ulcers and inflammation in the stomach and small bowel; SEs – may cause upper and lower GI disturbance.

Lifestyle changes

- Weight loss – will need to see dietitian; low-fat/low-salt diet
- Smoking cessation – can be booked into hospital or community programmes; may involve nicotine replacement therapy
- Alcohol – cut down to safe limits (21 units per week)
- Help with money issues and stress
- Further investigations
- 'Treadmill' test today; explains procedure and potential outcomes
- If inconclusive – may have other test, eg MRA or thallium scan
- Potential may require PCI – explains purpose, process and potential outcomes, eg angioplasty, stenting and possible CABG.

Invites patient to ask questions as they proceed through the consultation and is able to deal with them appropriately

Summarises important areas of the consultation back to the patient

Formally ends the consultation and ensures appropriate follow-up has been discussed

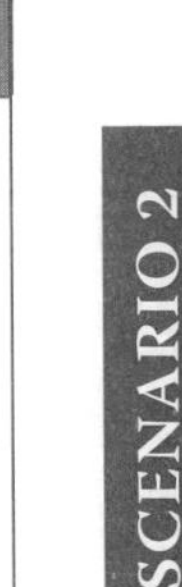

DIAGNOSTIC REASONING

A B C D E

- **What questions might you ask a patient before asking them to do an exercise tolerance test?**
  - Do they understand and want the test?
  - Do they understand the possible implications of a positive test?
  - Are they able to walk and run?
  - What is their normal exercise tolerance?
  - Do they have any contraindications to the test, eg severe aortic valve disease, recent MI.
- **What are the contraindications to a patient having an MRA scan?**
  - Absolute: metallic implants/prostheses of any kind, unable to lie flat because of severe respiratory or cardiac disease
  - Relative: claustrophobia.

Demonstrates safe, sensible and appropriate management plan

Demonstrates clear and logical diagnostic reasoning

GLOBAL COMMUNICATION MARK

A B C D E

Scenario 2: Reflection and consolidation

History

Mr Wright is a 46-year-old man who presents today with features suggestive of unstable angina. Of note he is a life-long smoker, has untreated hypertension and has a very strong family history of IHD and premature death. He now presents with a 3- to 4-month history of angina-like chest pain. Initially the pains lasted 20–30 seconds and came on once or twice week. They were always associated with exertion such as lifting heavy objects at work, but the pains were never at rest or prolonged and there were no associated features of note. More recently the pains have become more frequent – now once a day – and last for a few minutes. They often come on when he is walking his dog in the park but are always relieved with sitting and resting. No other significant cardiovascular (eg suggestive of heart failure), respiratory or systemic symptoms.

The patient's cardiovascular risk factors include:

- His brother has just had CABG surgery aged 49 years and his father and grandfather died in their 60s of IHD.
- He is a known heavy smoker – 40–50 cigarettes per day for many years.
- He has hypertension – his blood pressure was measured at 150/something at a local health promotion day, 2 years ago, but he never sought treatment.
- He has a very stressful job, and has significant financial worries at the present time.

Other risk factors are negative or unknown.

Examination

On examination of this middle-aged gentleman, who presented with unstable chest pain, he looked well. The general examination was remarkable only for heavily-tar-stained fingers of the right hand and peri-orbital xanthelasma. There were no other stigmata of generalised systemic or cardiovascular disease. His pulse was 88 regular and his BP was 164/98 mmHg. His RR, and his O_2 sats and CBG was 6.8 mmol/l were normal.
His height is 1.80 m, weight 98 kg and BMI $98/(1.8)^2 = 30.3$ kg/m^2.
His urinalysis was remarkable only for 1+ of glycosuria.
Cardiovascular and respiratory examinations were essentially otherwise normal with no features of heart failure or valvular dysfunction.

Data interpretation

In a patient presenting with ACS, the following routine investigations should be checked:

- Bloods: FBC, U&Es, RBG, cholesterol, 12-hour troponin
- Chest X-ray: need to ensure there are no features of heart failure, calcified valves or cardiomegaly, or respiratory disease, eg features of COPD (chronic smoker)
- ECG: checking for signs of hypertensive and/or IHD, eg arrhythmia, heart block, left axis deviation, ST segment and T wave changes, left bundle branch block; voltage criteria of LVH.

Management

Before prescribing the medications of an ACS protocol, important factors to consider include:

- Patient's haemodynamic status: BP, HR
- Renal function and urine output
- Bleeding risk (consider CRUSADE score)
- Risk of further ischaemia and complications (GRACE or similar score) – consider acute transfer for PCI.

Acute ACS protocol, including fondaparinux or low molecular weight heparin, aspirin and clopidogrel, anti-anginals (β blockers, nitrates)
Secondary prophylaxis: statins, anti-platelets, anti-hypertensives
Further investigations according to GRACE or similar score – may need inpatient MRA, ETT, PCI.

Further reading and web links
www.sign.ac.uk/pdf/sign93.pdf
www.nice.org.uk/nicemedia/live/12949/47924/47924.pdf

Scenario 3: 'Tummy pain'

Station 1

History *10-minute station*

You are the surgical FY1 doctor on call for general surgery. Your Registrar has asked you to assess Ms Laura Barnard, a 19-year-old female patient who has arrived on the admissions ward having been referred by her GP with abdominal pain.

- **Take a full history with a view to diagnosing the cause of her pain. You will be asked to present your history at the end of the station.**

You will be assessed on the following areas, as well as the content and diagnostic reasoning of your history – take them into account in your presentation.

Professionalism

- Professional appearance (NHS dress code) – including general appearance, hair and jewellery
- Maintains patient and personal safety
- Polite introduction; identifies patient or interviewee correctly; confirms patient's date of birth from name band or other source
- Obtains informal consent; maintains patient's privacy
- Displays empathetic and caring attitudes and behaviours throughout.

Process

- Good organisation and structure; appropriate use of open and closed questions
- Appropriate fluency/rhythm/pace to the interview – this may change depending on environment and acute nature of the problem
- Appropriate time for the patient to respond/reply to questions
- Appropriate acknowledgement of difficult or emotional areas of the patient's history.

Communication skills

- Demonstrates caring and sympathetic attitude
- Asks open questions
- Invites patient to ask questions and answers them appropriately
- Addresses patient's ideas, concerns and expectations.

Station 2

Examination *10-minute station*

After presenting your history to the Registrar, you both agree that Ms Barnard may have appendicitis.

- **Please perform an appropriate, focused examination of this patient, including any specific clinical tests to help confirm the diagnosis. A full set of observations have been taken which you may ask for.**
- **After you have completed your examination you should turn the page for a summary of the examination findings, which you should read. You will then be asked to present the relevant findings.**

You will be assessed on the following areas, as well as the content and skills of your examination – take them into account in your presentation.

Professionalism

- Professional appearance; maintains infection control standards, including hand cleaning and appropriate use of gloves and aprons
- Maintains patient and personal safety
- Polite introduction; identifies patient and confirms date of birth from name band or other source
- Obtains informal consent; maintains patient privacy and dignity
- Displays empathetic and caring attitudes and behaviours throughout.

Process

- Appropriate fluency/rhythm/pace to the examination – this may change depending on environment and acute nature of problem
- Good organisation and structure of examination; sensitive and empathetic approach
- Uses appropriate clinical techniques throughout
- Maintains privacy and dignity throughout.

Clinical communication

- Explains proposed examination/procedure; explains examination/procedure as it proceeds
- Offers information in a clear, structured and fluent manner, avoiding jargon
- Listens to patient and responds appropriately
- Demonstrates appropriate body language.

Please read the information below before presenting the examination findings. ***[NB If you have a model do not read this section]***

Clinical findings

- o **Patient looks uncomfortable**
- o **Feet to face – no specific findings**
- o **Observations – HR 111 bpm, BP 108/56 mmHg, RR 17 bpm, O_2 sats 99% on air, temperature 37.3, CBG 6.6 mmol/l**
- o **Height 1.64 m, weight 68 kg, BMI $68/(1.44)^2 = 25.3$ kg/m$^{2;}$ urinalysis – WCC nil, protein 1+, blood negative, nitrites negative, leucocytes negative, βHCG negative**
- o **General examination – no specific examination findings except for tachycardia**
- o **Abdominal examination – tenderness in right lower quadrant, maximally tender overlying McBurney's point, percussion and rebound tenderness, bowel sounds present and normal, Rovsing's positive, hernial orifices normal, DRG – no tenderness, soft stool in rectum.**

Station 3

Data interpretation *5-minute station*

Ms Barnard has a CT scan of the abdomen shown below.

- **Please label the structures on 3.1a and b.**

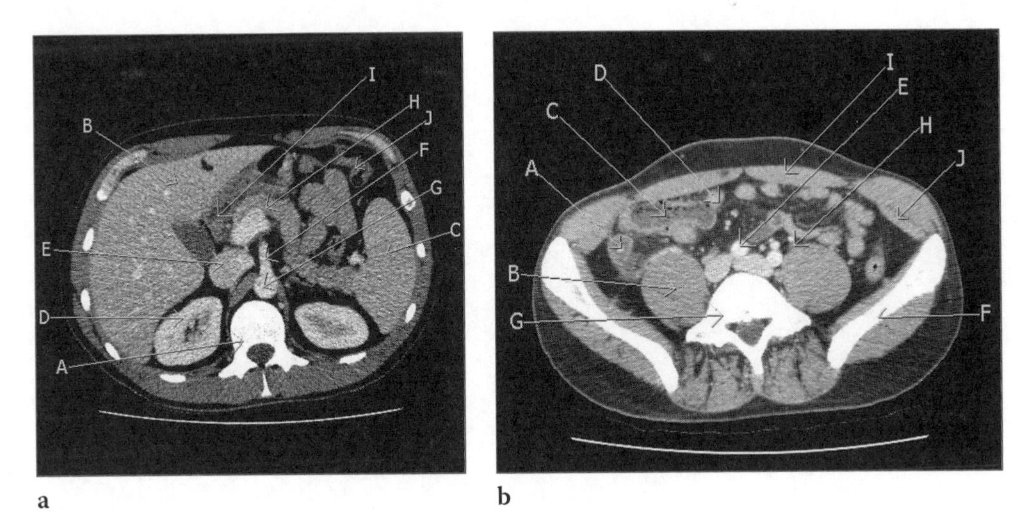

a b

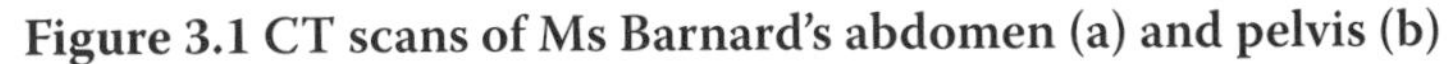

Figure 3.1 CT scans of Ms Barnard's abdomen (a) and pelvis (b)

Station 4

Prescribing skills *10-minute station*

Ms Barnard has been booked for a laparoscopic appendicectomy on the emergency operating list the following morning. Of note she is not on any regular medications, but she requires analgesia and antibiotics.

- **Using the charts below and a copy of the BNF, prescribe the appropriate medications for this patient.**

Remember: DRUG DRs Don't Forget Signing Off (page 373)

Station 5

Procedural skills *10-minute station*

Procedure

The Staff Nurse comes to tell you that Ms Barnard is still reporting some pain in spite of the oral analgesia that was given to her about an hour ago. Your Registrar suggests that she be given morphine 5 mg and cyclizine 50 mg as intramuscular injections. He suggests that you administer the drug and will supervise you performing the procedure.

- **Using the equipment provided, administer the injections. Follow the instructions as the station proceeds.**

Equipment:

- **Glass ampoules:**
  - **Morphine 10 mg in 1 ml**
  - **Cyclizine 50 mg in 1 ml**
- **Gloves**
- **Syringes (2 ml, 5 ml, 10 ml)**
- **Needles (orange, blue, green, white)**
- **Sharps bin**
- **Alcohol swab**
- **Cotton wool swab.**

Station 6

Clinical communication skills *10-minute station*

As part of your foundation training workplace-based assessments, your Registrar has suggested you may wish to use consent of Ms Barnard as a case-based discussion (CbD).

Part 1:

- **What are the risks associated with all operations under general anaesthesia?**
- **What are the risks and complications specific to a laparoscopic appendicectomy?**

Part 2:

Now that you have talked through and identified the issues above, your Registrar will use preoperative consent as a case-based discussion.

Answers

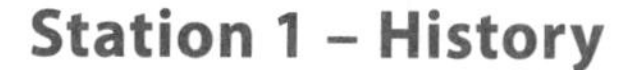

Station 1 – History

Patient script

You are Ms Laura Barnard (DOB 6 December 1992), a 19-year-old geography student. You have always been fit and well and have no previous medical or surgical problems.

Two days ago you began to develop central abdominal pain, which has now settled to the right lower abdomen. The pain is severe (7/10) and sharp in nature. It is a constant pain and nothing seems to ease it, although you are slightly more comfortable when lying still. You have not wanted to eat anything in the last 24 hours, and have vomited twice since last night. You opened your bowels normally yesterday.

You have never had anything like this before.

You have not had any urinary symptoms, such as increased frequency, pain or blood when passing urine. Your last menstrual period was 2 weeks ago and you have had no abnormal vaginal discharge and you are not currently sexually active (last sexual partner 12 months ago).

You smoke 5–10/day, and drink quite heavily at the weekend (20–30 units on some weekends – mainly vodka). You live in halls of residence at university.

You take no regular medications, and are not aware of any allergies.

You are otherwise well.

You are not aware of any family history.

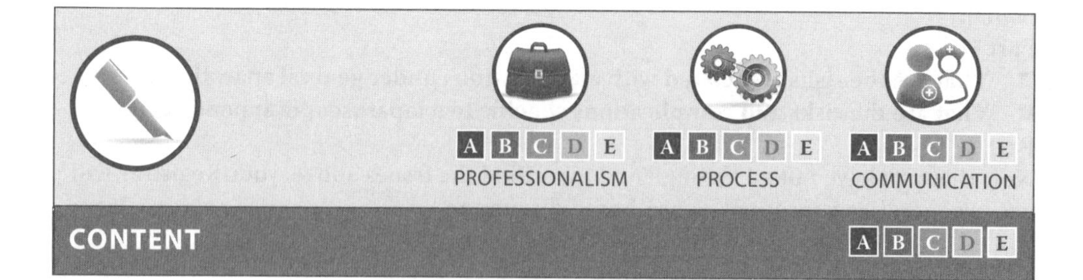

Identifies key information
- Pain – sharp, constant, severe, worsening over 2 days, migration from central to RIF, no relieving and exacerbating factors
- Associated features – nausea and vomiting, pyrexia
- Poor appetite

Identifies important negatives, including systemic enquiry
- Normal bowel movement
- No urinary symptoms
- LMP two weeks ago, no PV discharge, not sexually active.
- No previous episodes

Identifies key information from rest of the history
- No previous surgical or medical history
- Relevant factors from employment, housing, social support

Completing the patient history
- Previous medical history: nil
- Social and occupational history: smokes <10/day, moderate alcohol intake
- Drug and allergic history: nil
- Family history

Summarises important areas of the history back to the patient

Invites patient to ask questions and is able to deal with them appropriately

Establishes patient's ideas, concerns and expectations

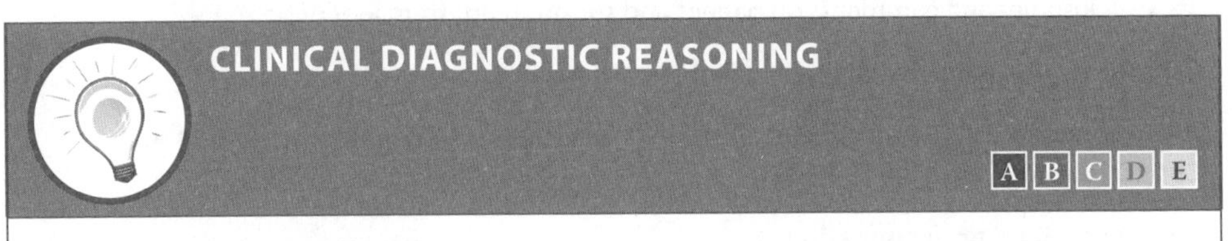

- **Please present your history**
  - Candidate offers a logical, well-structured account of the history
- **What is your diagnosis?**
  - Candidate offers the correct diagnosis and appropriate differentials
  - Diagnosis: acute appendicitis
  - Differentials: urinary tract infection, inflammatory bowel disease, biliary colic/cholecystitis, gynaecological causes (pelvic inflammatory disease, ovarian torsion)

Demonstrates safe, sensible and appropriate management plan

Demonstrates clear and logical diagnostic reasoning

GLOBAL HISTORY MARK

A B C D E

Station 2 – Examination

Patient script

If you are an actor/patient, read the patient history and physical signs fully – when the candidate comes to an abnormal site in their examination, act-out tenderness and/or volunteer the relevant physical sign.

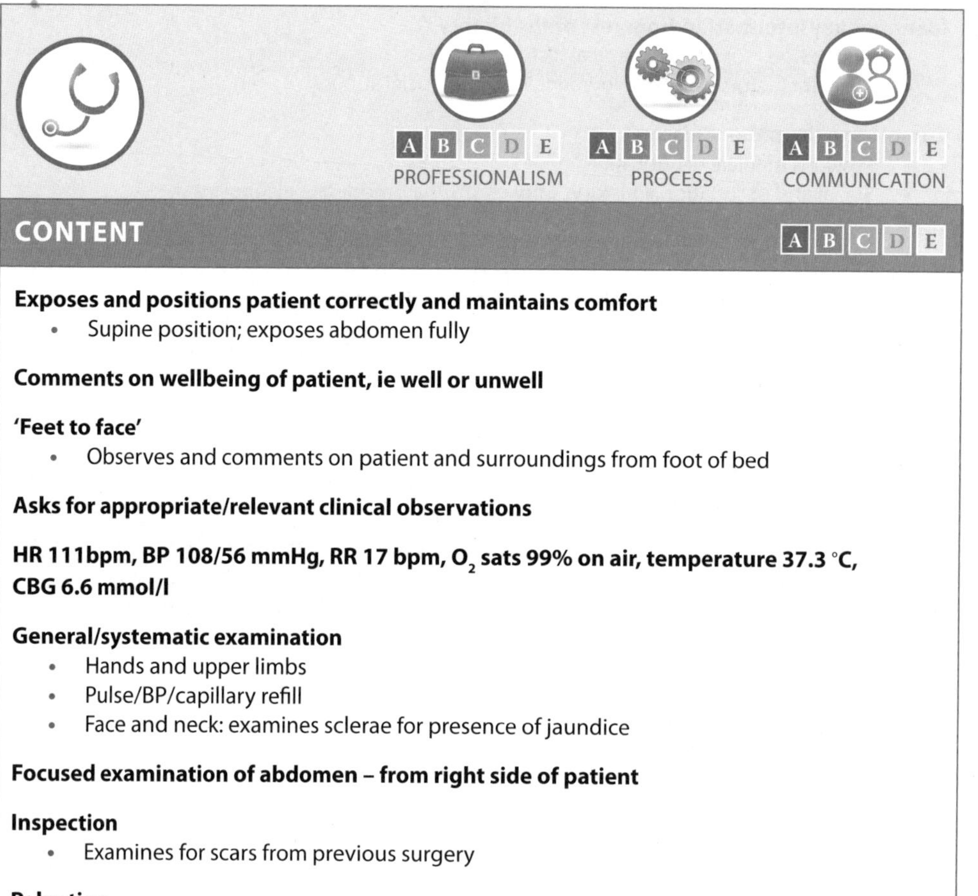

CONTENT A B C D E

Exposes and positions patient correctly and maintains comfort

- Supine position; exposes abdomen fully

Comments on wellbeing of patient, ie well or unwell

'Feet to face'

- Observes and comments on patient and surroundings from foot of bed

Asks for appropriate/relevant clinical observations

HR 111bpm, BP 108/56 mmHg, RR 17 bpm, O_2 sats 99% on air, temperature 37.3 °C, CBG 6.6 mmol/l

General/systematic examination

- Hands and upper limbs
- Pulse/BP/capillary refill
- Face and neck: examines sclerae for presence of jaundice

Focused examination of abdomen – from right side of patient

Inspection

- Examines for scars from previous surgery

Palpation

- Identifies area of maximal tenderness – starts away from this site
- Superficial and deep palpation in systematic manner
- Comments on areas of guarding or rigidity, and attempts to elicit rebound tenderness in right iliac fossa
- Attempts to elicit Rovsing's sign (RIF pain on LIF palpation)
- Attempts to elicit psoas and obturator sign:

- The **psoas sign** is performed by passively extending the right hip with the patient lying on their side, or flexing the hip when lying supine. Pain on these movements may be caused by irritation of the iliopsoas muscles by an acutely inflamed appendix (especially if orientated retrocaecally) or by a psoas abscess
- The **obturator sign** is performed by passively flexing and internally rotating the right hip (with knee flexed) and may cause pain due to an acutely inflamed appendix irritating the obturator internus muscle.

Percussion

- Elicits percussion tenderness over McBurney's point

Auscultation

- Presence and quality of bowel sounds

Completes examination by identifying relevant additional clinical signs and formally completing assessment

- Digital rectal examination
- External genitalia and hernial orifices

Asks for appropriate relevant clinical observations and bedside tests

- Pyrexia, tachycardia, hypotension
- Urinalysis to investigate for urinary or renal tract disease, pregnancy test

Thanks patient, offers assistance, maintains patient's dignity and privacy until they are dressed

SCENARIO 3

CLINICAL DIAGNOSTIC REASONING

A B C D E

Correctly identifies the relevant physical signs, including important negative findings:

- Tachycardia
- Tenderness in right iliac fossa, maximally at McBurneys point
- Percussion tenderness
- Rebound tenderness
- Bowel sounds present
- Rovsings positive

■ **What is your management plan?**

- Investigations – WCC, CRP, U&Es, urinalysis including βHCG
- Analgesia and anti-emetic; IV fluid and antibiotics
- Maintain nil by mouth
- Senior review; consent for appendicectomy

GLOBAL EXAMINATION MARK

A B C D E

Station 3–Data interpretation

a. **Abdominal CT**
   - A. Vertebral body
   - B. Liver
   - C. Spleen
   - D. Right kidney
   - E. Inferior vena cava
   - F. Superior mesenteric artery
   - G. Abdominal aorta
   - H. Pancreas
   - I. Duodenum
   - J. Transverse colon

b. **Pelvic CT**
   - A. Enlarged appendix, with central high attenuation appendicolith
   - B. Psoas muscle
   - C. Caecum
   - D. Terminal ileum
   - E. Right common iliac artery
   - F. Ilium
   - G. Body of fifth lumbar vertebra
   - H. Left ureter
   - I. Rectus abdominis muscle
   - J. Transverus abdominis muscle

GLOBAL DATA INTERPRETATION MARK

A B C D E

Station 4 – Prescribing skills

Check: DRUG DRs Don't Forget Signing Off (page 373)

Allergies, sensitivities and adverse drug reactions			Patient details/addressograph
No known allergies ✓	Initials AF	Gender M / (F)	NHS/ Hospital No: 631149
Not possible to ascertain ☐	Date 13/01	Weight (kg): 67 / Date	Surname: BARNARD
Medicine/substance	Reaction & Severity	Initials & Date	First name: LAURA
		Height: 1.62m	
Alerts		Surface area (m²)	Date of birth: 06.12.92

IN-PATIENT MEDICATION PRESCRIPTION AND ADMINISTRATION RECORD

PasTest HOSPITAL

Consultant	Trainee Dr. Name and Bleep no.	Date of admission	Date chart reboarded	Estimated date of discharge
FRANKS	Feather 214	13.01.12		
This chart is no. .... of	Transcribing Check by Pharmacy Sign .... Date	Ward CUMBERLAND 1. .... 2.		

Supplementary Medication charts in use: Other (please specify): 1 .... 2 ....

Epidural/PCA ☐ Syringe driver ☐ TPN ☐ Chemotherapy ☐ Insulin sliding scale ☐

Once only medications – loading doses, pre-medication, PGDs or surgical antibiotic propylaxis

Date	Time to be given	Medicine (approved name)	Dose	Route	Signature and bleep no.	Pharmacy	Time given	Given by	Checked by
13.01	STAT	CO-AMOXICLAV	1.2g	IV	AF 214				
	TO								
	INDUCTION								

Thromboprophylaxis please prescribe treatment regimens in the regular medications section

Choice of mechanical prophylaxis and leg(s) to be applied to			Leg: Left	Leg: Right	Leg: Both	Enter Time	Enter details below
Graduated elastic compression stockings	Intermittend pneumatic compression device (IPC)						
✓ 13.01 Start Date:	☐ End Date:	Signature and Bleep No.	☐	☐	✓		
☐ Start Date:	☐ End Date:	Signature and Bleep No.	☐	☐	☐		

Medication		Dose	Dose Change	Enter Time	Enter details below
CLEXANE		40mg			
Please ensure you have completed the VTE risk assessment form	Date	13.01.12			
	Route	SC			
	Signature	AF 214		Instructions	Pharmacy ☐
	Bleep no.				

SCENARIO 3

Infusion prescriptions continued										SC = subcutaneous		IVC = intravenous central IVP = intravenous peripheral		
Date & time	Route	Infusion Fluid: Name & strength	Infusion Fluid: Volume	Medication: Approved name with expiry / unit number	Medication: Dose	Duration	Rate	Prescriber's signature & bleep no.	Date given	Given by / Added by	Check by	Start time	Finish time	Pharmacy
13/01	IV	0.9% SALINE Exp: Batch/unit no:	1 LITRE				8°	DRW 214						
13/01	IV	0.9% SALINE Exp: Batch/unit no:	1 LITRE	+20mmol KCl			8°	DRW 214						

Regular prescriptions continued

Anti-infectives prescription *prescribe long term prophylaxis and anti-tuberculosis medications in regular medications section*

For 1 Day

Date: 13, 14, 15

Date	13/01	Medication	Indication	Signature and bleep no.	Pharmacy
Route	IV	CO-AMOXICLAV	APPENDICITIS	AF 214	☐

Times	Dose	13	14	15
06				
(09)	1.2g		☐	——
(12)	1.2g		☒	——
18				
(22)	1.2g	☐	☒	——
24				

2 doses of post-op-only

As required prescriptions

			Date	Time	Dose	Route	Date	Time	Dose	Route	Date	Time	Dose	Route	Date	Time	Dose	Route
Drug: PARACETAMOL	Allergies Checked	Dose: 1g																
Frequency: MAX 6 HOURLY	Max Dose/24 hrs: 4g	Route: PO																
Indication																		
Signature: AF 214	Pharmacy	Start: 13.01																

As required prescriptions

			Date	Time	Dose	Route	Date	Time	Dose	Route	Date	Time	Dose	Route	Date	Time	Dose	Route
Drug: CODEINE PHOSPHATE	Allergies Checked	Dose: 30mg																
Frequency: 6 HOURLY	Max Dose/24 hrs: 60mg	Route: PO																
Indication																		
Signature: AF 214	Pharmacy	Start: 13.01																

As required prescriptions

			Date	Time	Dose	Route	Date	Time	Dose	Route	Date	Time	Dose	Route	Date	Time	Dose	Route
Drug: MORPHINE	Allergies Checked	Dose: 2.5mg																
Frequency	Max Dose/24 hrs	Route: S/C IM/IV																
Indication																		
Signature: AF 214	Pharmacy	Start: 13.01																

As required prescriptions			Date	Time	Dose	Route	Date	Time	Dose	Route	Date	Time	Dose	Route	Date	Time	Dose	Route
Drug METOCLOPRAMIDE	Allergies Checked	Dose 10MG																
Frequency 8 HOURLY	Max Dose/24 hrs	Route S/C IM/IV																
Indication																		
Signature AF 214	Pharmacy	Start 13.01																

As required prescriptions			Date	Time	Dose	Route	Date	Time	Dose	Route	Date	Time	Dose	Route	Date	Time	Dose	Route
Drug CYCLIZINE	Allergies Checked	Dose 50MG																
Frequency	Max Dose/24 hrs	Route S/C IM/IV																
Indication																		
Signature AF 214	Pharmacy	Start 13.01																

SCENARIO 3

GLOBAL PRESCRIBING MARK A B C D E

Station 5–Procedural skills

Intramuscular injection

A B C D E PROFESSIONALISM

A B C D E PROCESS

CONTENT A B C D E

Identifies and sets out correct equipment; maintains aseptic technique throughout

Preparation

- Checks ampoules for correct drug, dose and expiry date
- Wearing gloves, safely breaks glass ampoule
- Draws up drug into 1 ml syringe using correct drawing-up needle
- Places orange or blue intramuscular needle on syringe

Exposes and positions patient correctly and maintains comfort

- Appropriate choice of site for IM injection, including gluteal region, deltoid region, vastus lateralis region

Process

- Washes hands and applies gloves
- Cleans area with alcohol swab and allows to dry for 1 minute
- Identifies injection site
- Inserts needle at 90° to skin; inserts to hilt and pulls back plunger to confirm no aspiration of blood
- Delivers injection of appropriate dose (0.5 ml morphine/1 ml cyclizine) and removes syringe
- May apply cotton wool swab if any bleeding

Disposes of all sharps and other items correctly

GLOBAL PROCEDURE MARK

A B C D E

Station 6–Clinical communication skills

Part 1: Risks of general anaesthesia

Appendicectomy is performed under general anaesthesia as the abdominal musculature and peritoneum must be pharmacologically relaxed in order to facilitate the surgery. The operation can be performed 'open' or via a laparoscopic technique.

General anaesthesia is often associated with postoperative nausea, and patients will often require anti-emetics to be prescribed. Intubation with an endotracheal tube can lead to a sore throat. Prolonged periods of mechanical ventilation (not normally encountered in short surgery such as appendicectomy) is associated with increased risk of postoperative chest infection due to atelectasis, as well as venous thromboembolic events such as deep vein thrombosis and pulmonary embolism.

Complications of laparoscopic appendicectomy?

For a specific operation, the risks and complications can be considered as:

Immediate: Blood loss (+/– transfusion); nerve injury; bowel injury or perforation with need for bowel resection.

Early: wound infection; abscess formation; paralytic ileus.

Late: inguinal hernia; adhesions.

Part 2:

Patient script

You have been told that you have appendicitis, and are aware that surgery is required. You are concerned about the recovery period, how long you will be in hospital, when you can return to university and what happens if they find a normal appendix.

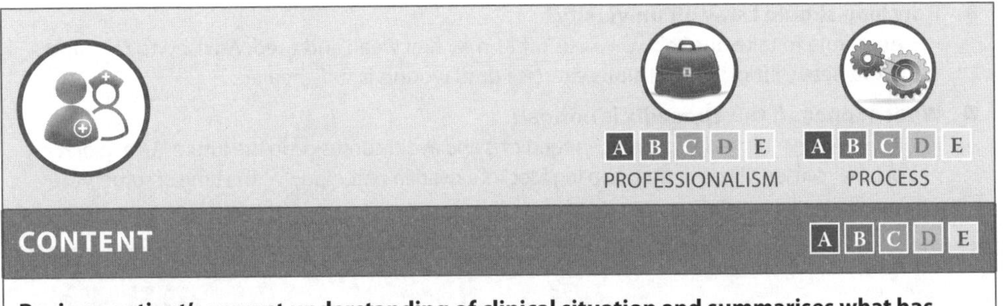

CONTENT A B C D E

Reviews patient's current understanding of clinical situation and summarises what has happened so far

- Establishes diagnosis of appendicitis and need for surgery

Establishes patient's ideas, concerns and expectations

- Explains that appendicitis is common, and surgery is safe and 'routine'
- Explains that surgery can be 'open' or laparoscopic
- Explains operation takes approx 30 minutes to 1 hour but can be variable

Explains the key important information; invites patient to ask questions and is able to deal with them appropriately

- Explains reasons for operation – to treat appendicitis by removal of appendix
- Talks about risks and complications of general anaesthesia.
- Discusses common complications of appendicectomy

Summarises important areas of the consultation back to the patient

Formally ends the consultation and ensures appropriate follow-up has been discussed

CLINICAL DIAGNOSTIC REASONING

A B C D E

- **How long will I need to stay in hospital?**
  - Explains may be able to go home the following day. Will be reviewed by the surgical team to ensure the pain is well controlled, the wound appears healthy and enquire about bowel movements.
- **How long should I stay off university?**
  - Advisable to take one to two weeks off as may feel weak and tired. Advised to rest, and avoid heavy lifting or strenuous exercise until wound is fully healed.
- **What happens if the appendix is normal?**
  - It will still be removed to prevent appendicitis and avoid confusion in the future. An exploration of other causes will be undertaken (eg Meckel's, ovarian pathology) at the time of surgery

GLOBAL COMMUNICATION MARK

A B C D E

Scenario 3: Reflection and consolidation

History

Appendicitis is one of the most common acute surgical problems and affects people of all ages. Patients will often present with a classical history characterised by central or non-specific abdominal pain that settles to the right iliac fossa and is associated with anorexia, nausea and vomiting and low-grade fever. Other non-specific features such as diarrhoea are not uncommon.

Examination

Appendicitis is a clinical diagnosis, and an experienced surgeon will make the diagnosis with confidence based on the history and examination findings. Localised peritonism in the right iliac fossa is often found, with guarding and rebound tenderness. Additional tests such as Rovsings, psoas and obturator may reinforce the initial findings.

Investigations

An inflammatory response may be noted from laboratory tests (raised WCC with 'left shift' (neutrophilia) and CRP), but the absence of raised inflammatory markers does not exclude the diagnosis. Imaging investigations (CT or USS) are generally reserved for patients in whom there is diagnostic uncertainty, and may delay surgery. Diagnostic laparoscopy is increasingly performed in patients with equivocal diagnosis, especially in women with a gynaecological differential diagnosis.

Treatment

Appendicectomy is the treatment for appendicitis, and surgery should not be delayed, owing to the increased risk of perforation of the appendix and consequent clinical deterioration. Antibiotics are generally prescribed while patients are awaiting surgery and continued for several days postoperatively depending on the presence of perforation and the degree of intraperitoneal contamination.

Scenario 4: 'Party girl'

Station 1

History *10-minute station*

You are the FY1 working in the neurology clinic of your local district hospital. You have been asked to see the next patient, Ms Joanna Kelly, who has been referred by her GP for '?seizures'.

- **Please take a diagnostic history from the patient with a view to presenting the history and likely diagnosis to the consultant neurologist.**

You will be assessed on the following areas, as well as the content and diagnostic reasoning of your history – take them into account in your presentation.

Professionalism

- Professional appearance (NHS dress code) – including general appearance, hair and jewellery
- Maintains patient and personal safety
- Polite introduction; identifies patient or interviewee correctly; confirms patient's date of birth from name band or other source
- Obtains informal consent; maintains patient's privacy
- Displays empathetic and caring attitudes and behaviours throughout.

Process

- Good organisation and structure; appropriate use of open and closed questions
- Appropriate fluency/rhythm/pace to the interview – this may change depending on environment and acute nature of problem
- Appropriate time for the patient to respond/reply to questions
- Appropriate acknowledgement of difficult or emotional areas of the patient's history.

Communication skills

- Demonstrates caring and sympathetic attitude
- Asks open questions
- Invites patient to ask questions and answers them appropriately
- Addresses patient's ideas, concerns and expectations.

Station 2

Examination *10-minute station*

After completing and presenting the history, the Consultant asks you to perform a formal, complete neurological examination of Ms Kelly's cranial nerves and cerebellar system.

- **You should present the relevant findings (given within the station) to the Consultant in an appropriate manner for a busy outpatient clinic.**

To complete this station you will need an appropriate neurological testing kit.

You will be assessed on the following areas, as well as the content and skills of your examination – take them into account in your presentation.

Professionalism

- Professional appearance; maintains infection control standards, including hand cleaning and appropriate use of gloves and aprons
- Maintains patient and personal safety
- Polite introduction; identifies patient and confirms date of birth from name band or other source
- Obtains informal consent; maintains patient privacy and dignity
- Displays empathetic and caring attitudes and behaviours throughout.

Process

- Appropriate fluency/rhythm/pace to the examination – this may change depending on environment and acute nature of problem
- Good organisation and structure of examination; sensitive and empathetic approach
- Uses appropriate clinical techniques throughout
- Maintains privacy and dignity throughout.

Clinical communication

- Explains proposed examination/procedure: explains examination/procedure as it proceeds
- Offers information in a clear, structured and fluent manner, avoiding jargon
- Listens to patient and responds appropriately
- Demonstrates appropriate body language.

Please read the information below before presenting this case to the Consultant as if you were in a busy outpatient clinic.
[NB If you have a model do not read this section]

Clinical findings

- o Patient looks well
- o Feet to face – peri-orbital xanthelasma, no other obvious stigmata of CV disease
- o Observations – HR 88 bpm, BP 164/98 mmHg, RR 14 bpm, O_2 sats 97% on air, temperature 36.5 °C, CBG 6.8 mmol/l
- o Height 1.80 m, weight 98 kg, BMI $98/(1.8)^2 = 30.3$ kg/m^2; urinalysis – WCC nil, protein negative, blood negative, nitrites negative, glucose +
- o General examination – fingers of right hand heavily tar stained, no anaemia, no tendon xanthoma
- o CV examination – no features of arrhythmia, cardiac valvular dysfunction, or features of heart failure.

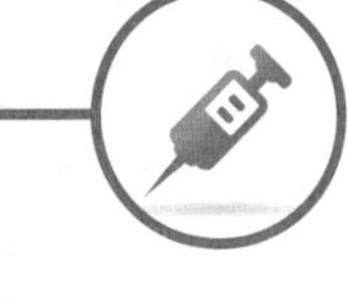

Station 3

Procedural skills *10-minute station*

Procedure

Several weeks later Ms Kelly is brought into the Emergency Department having had two tonic-clonic seizures while at a night club. You are the FY1 on call for general medicine and have been asked to clerk the patient. However, as you enter the 'resus' room she starts to have another seizure. Unfortunately all the nursing and medical staff are dealing with several patients who have been brought in from a major road traffic accident.

- **Using the equipment provided, secure her airway, oxygenation and position her safely while she is having the seizure. Follow the instructions as the station proceeds.**

Equipment provided

- ResusAnni or similar manikin
- Variety of oxygen-delivery systems, including Hudson mask, nebuliser mask, venturi (28%) mask, non-rebreath mask, nasal prongs
- Oxygen tubing and oxygen cylinder or oxygen point on the wall
- Guedel's airway and nasal airway (variety of sizes)
- Intubation set – endotracheal tube various sizes, oxygen bag/system to attach to ET tube.

SCENARIO 4

Station 4

Prescribing skills *10-minute station*

YOU MAY USE A CALCULATOR IN THIS STATION

Despite several doses of diazepam, Ms Kelly continues to have some seizure activity. You are asked to write up a phenytoin infusion. The nurse notes that at her outpatient clinic appointment Ms Kelly was 62 kg. She has normal renal function, is on no other medications and has no known drug allergies.

- **Using the charts below and a copy of the BNF, calculate and write out a loading and maintenance dose of phenytoin (note: the infusion rate needs to be set in millilitres per hour; the loading does is to be placed in 50 ml 0.9% saline and the maintenance dose in 250 ml 0.9% saline) and an appropriate fluid regime for 24 hours.**

Details

Ms Joanna Kelly; Hospital number P010267; DOB: 05/10/1988; No known drug allergies; Weight: 62 kg; Ward: ITU; Consultant: Dr Khan

Remember: DRUG DRs Don't Forget Signing Off (page 373)

Station 5

Clinical communication skills *10-minute station*

Ms Kelly is recovering on the general ward having spent 2 days in the ICU. You are asked by your Registrar to talk to Ms Kelly to gauge her understanding of her condition and to explain to her the future management of the condition.

- **Explore with Ms Kelly her present understanding of her condition and her lifestyle, and explain to her the future management of the condition, addressing any of her concerns.**

Answers

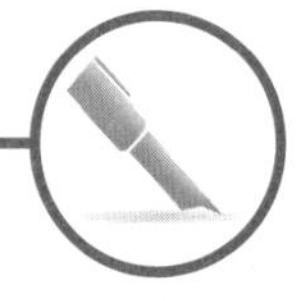

Station 1 – History

Patient script

You are Ms Joanna Kelly, 23 years old, DOB 5 October 1988. You have been previously fit and well with no health problems of note. Over the past 2–3 months you have had several funny episodes during sleep that have really worried you and left you feeling very distressed.

The first episode was just after a 'big night out' with friends on your birthday. You remember coming home and getting into bed after taking off your make-up. You woke up about 9 hours later feeling 'terrible'. You had a severe headache, felt 'battered and bruised' and ached all over. Your flatmate thought you had brought a boyfriend home as you were 'bashing against the wall' for several minutes. You thought you just had a hangover and didn't think much about that episode. But looking back, you now realise you may have bitten your tongue (as it was sore and cut on one side) and had wet the bed.

Since then you have had three similar episodes, all occurring at night. You wake up feeling terrible, with a headache and feeling like all your muscles are aching and burning. You wet the bed during two of these episodes.

However, 3 days ago you had a 'funny turn' in the toilet at work that really frightened you. You were sitting on the toilet, 'going for a wee' when you suddenly felt 'strange' as if 'I wasn't there'. The next thing you remember is work colleagues trying to drag you out of the cubicle. According to them, you groaned and then collapsed onto the floor. They couldn't get you to open the door and had to break the lock. They told you that you were lying on the floor shaking and frothing at the mouth, and that you had gone dark purple in the face. The shaking stopped on its own after about 2 minutes and you woke up after another minute or two. You felt very tired and sleepy but insisted they just put you in a taxi home. At home you lay on the sofa for about 3 or 4 hours and felt back to normal once your flatmate returned at about 7:30 pm.

In between these episodes you have been very well and have had no headache, blurred vision, dizziness, speech or communication problems. Your arms and legs limbs feel normal and you have been otherwise systemically well.

Risk factors

You were born by caesarean section and were a well baby and child. As far as you know you never had a seizure as a child. You have never had suffered any major head injuries or been involved in any recent car accidents or trauma.

Medication – no regular medications other than the oral contraceptive pill; no known drug allergies.

Smoking – 10–20 cigarettes per day (5 years or so); marijuana at weekends – commonly one or two joints.

Alcohol – you drink quite heavily and enjoy partying most nights. You drink white wine and gin and tonics and it is not unusual for you to drink two bottles of wine in an evening and several double gin and tonics.

Drugs – at the weekends (and on some weekdays) you regularly use cocaine. You may snort two to three lines in an evening. You also use ecstasy and marijuana but don't inject or smoke heroin or other drugs.

Occupation – you work as a clerk in a large city law firm and although you don't earn that much, the lawyers and other city workers you socialise with buy you lots of the alcohol and drugs you take.

Your life is quite chaotic and you often have memory lapses after going out. You have woken up several times in bed with men you've met at parties. You were infected with chlamydia by one and have recently been on a course of antibiotics to treat this.

You are single, having split up with a long-term partner several months ago. You live with a college friend.

Ideas and concerns – you have looked up your symptoms on the internet and are worried you may have a brain tumour.

Expectations – you hope you can have a brain scan and that you will be OK. When asked you realise that you may have had seizures or fits, but think is the result of the tumour.

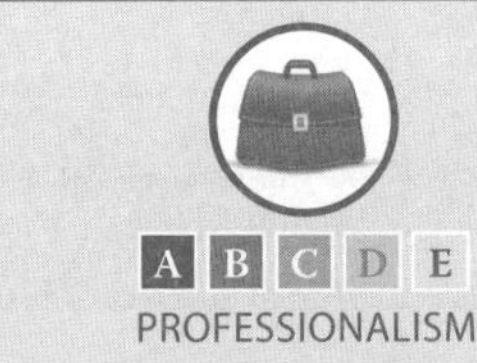

A B C D E PROFESSIONALISM

A B C D E PROCESS

A B C D E COMMUNICATION

CONTENT

A B C D E

Identifies key information

- Onset, duration/progression and frequency of episodes
- Warning symptoms/aura prior to episodes
- During the episode
- Post-episode symptoms

Identifies key information from rest of the history, including risk factors for seizures

- Childhood seizures and birth injury
- Recent head trauma/brain injury
- Medications – on OCP only
- Alcohol excess
- Smoking – cigarettes
- Illicit drug use – cocaine and marijuana

Includes important negatives, including systemic enquiry

- Excludes features of raised intracranial pressure
- Excludes other neurological deficit – higher functions (speech, language, swallowing, vision, hearing, memory), limbs – motor and sensory deficit

Completing the patient history

- Drug and allergic history: OCP
- Allergies: NKDA
- Previous medical history: nil of note
- Occupational history: as above
- Chaotic lifestyle

Summarises important areas of the history back to the patient

Invites patient to ask questions and is able to deal with them appropriately

Establishes patient's ideas, concerns and expectations

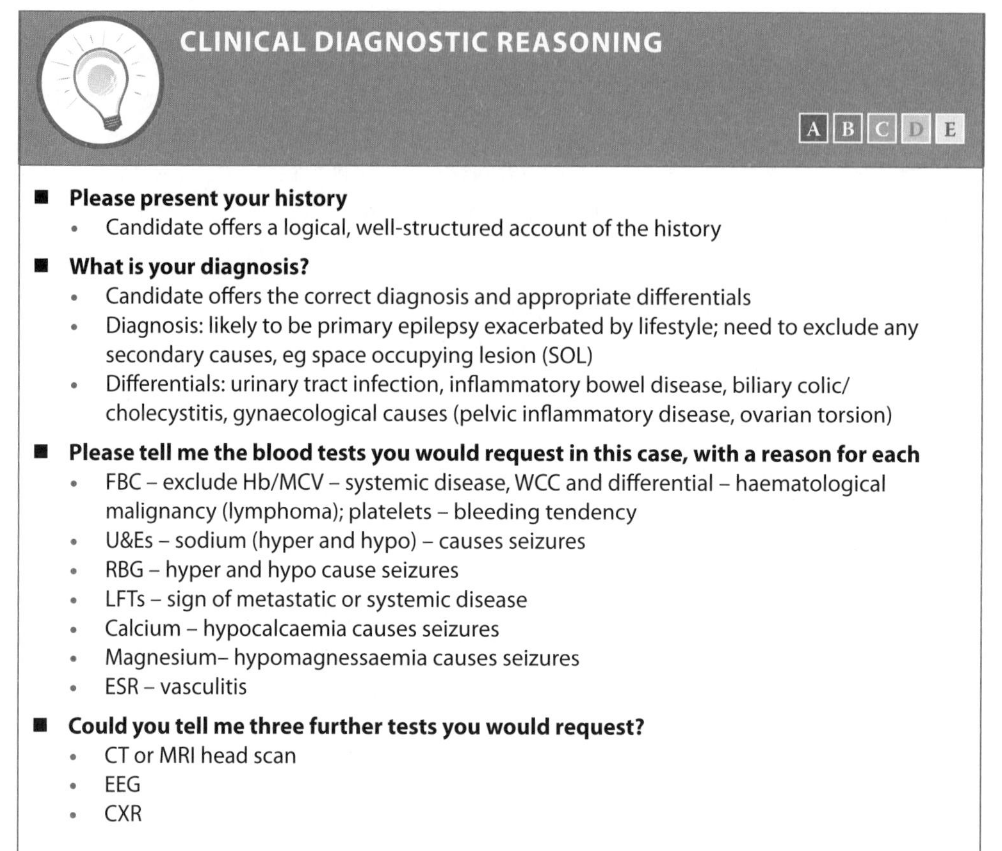

CLINICAL DIAGNOSTIC REASONING

A B C D E

- **Please present your history**
  - Candidate offers a logical, well-structured account of the history
- **What is your diagnosis?**
  - Candidate offers the correct diagnosis and appropriate differentials
  - Diagnosis: likely to be primary epilepsy exacerbated by lifestyle; need to exclude any secondary causes, eg space occupying lesion (SOL)
  - Differentials: urinary tract infection, inflammatory bowel disease, biliary colic/cholecystitis, gynaecological causes (pelvic inflammatory disease, ovarian torsion)
- **Please tell me the blood tests you would request in this case, with a reason for each**
  - FBC – exclude Hb/MCV – systemic disease, WCC and differential – haematological malignancy (lymphoma); platelets – bleeding tendency
  - U&Es – sodium (hyper and hypo) – causes seizures
  - RBG – hyper and hypo cause seizures
  - LFTs – sign of metastatic or systemic disease
  - Calcium – hypocalcaemia causes seizures
  - Magnesium– hypomagnessaemia causes seizures
  - ESR – vasculitis
- **Could you tell me three further tests you would request?**
  - CT or MRI head scan
  - EEG
  - CXR

Demonstrates safe, sensible and appropriate management plan

Demonstrates clear and logical diagnostic reasoning

GLOBAL HISTORY MARK

A B C D E

Station 2 – Examination

Patient script

If you are an actor/patient, read the patient history and physical signs fully – when the candidate comes to an abnormal site in their examination, act-out tenderness and/or volunteer the relevant physical sign.

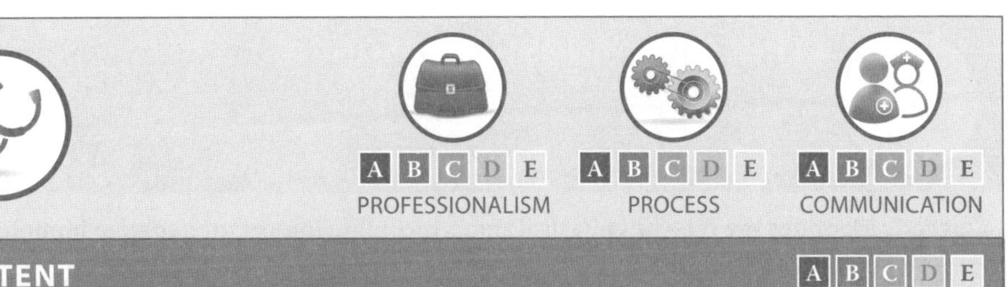

CONTENT

A B C D E

Exposes and positions patient correctly and maintains comfort

- Comments on wellbeing of patient, ie well or unwell
- 'Feet to face' – observes, and comments on patient and surroundings from foot of bed – no signs of neurological deficit (hemiparesis), facial asymmetry, speech abnormalities; mobility aids – wheelchair, walking stick

Asks for appropriate relevant clinical observations

- HR, BP, CBG and GCS or AVPU

Examination of cranial nerves

- I – olfactory – demonstrates how to assess sense of smell (appropriate technique)
- EYES – II, III, IV and VI (optic, oculomotor, trochlear, abducens)
- Looks and comments on both eyes – appearance, absence of obvious palsies
- Visual acuity – using Snellen chart; visual fields; EOM of both eyes
- Pupillary responses – PERL (direct and consensual) and accommodation
- Ophthalmoscopy (both eyes) – specifically comments on presence/absence of papilloedema
- V (trigeminal) – motor examination – assesses muscles of mastication; sensory – assesses LT in the three divisions of the face; explains how to do corneal reflex
- VII – (facial) motor – asks patient to smile, blow out cheeks, shut eyes tightly, look up at the ceiling (observing symmetry of forehead)
- IX/X – (glossopharyngeal and vagus) – observes palate elevation, listens to patient's speech and assesses swallow
- XI – accessory – motor assessment of trapezius and sternocleidomastoid
- XII – hypoglossal – observes tongue within mouth; asks patient to stick tongue out

Assessment of the cerebellar system

- Observation – looks and comments on patient sitting straight with no obvious truncal ataxia
- Assesses
- Hands – dysdiadokokinesia; Intention tremor and past pointing
- Upper limbs – mentions need to assess hypotonia and hyporeflexia (examiner asks them to move on)
- Face – nystagmus (tests in both directions), speech
- Gait – asks patient to stand up and walk; guides patient, watching they don't fall.

Thanks patient, offers assistance, maintains patient's dignity and privacy until they are dressed

CLINICAL DIAGNOSTIC REASONING

A B C D E

Correctly identifies the relevant physical signs, including important negative findings

Correctly identifies the abnormalities of speech and gait associated with cerebellar disease:

- Speech – slow, slurred and staccato
- Gait (classically) – wide based, and ataxic (sensory ataxia is high stepping, slapping gait)

Correctly describes the management steps in this case – the same as any other long-term condition:

- Education, Education, Education – educate patient, family and friends, work colleagues
- Assess and treat risks or exacerbating factors – lifestyle changes are very important in this case
- Multidisciplinary team members – a specialist nurse and perhaps a support group where the patient could talk to similar women of her own age may be useful
- Medications – the simple rule in epilepsy – 'the fewest anti-epileptics at the lowest effective doses' – depending on the patient – medications to consider would include sodium valproate, carbamazepine, lamotrigine and topiramate (see References for details).

Demonstrates safe, sensible and appropriate management plan

Demonstrates clear and logical diagnostic reasoning

GLOBAL EXAMINATION MARK

A B C D E

Station 3 – Procedural skills

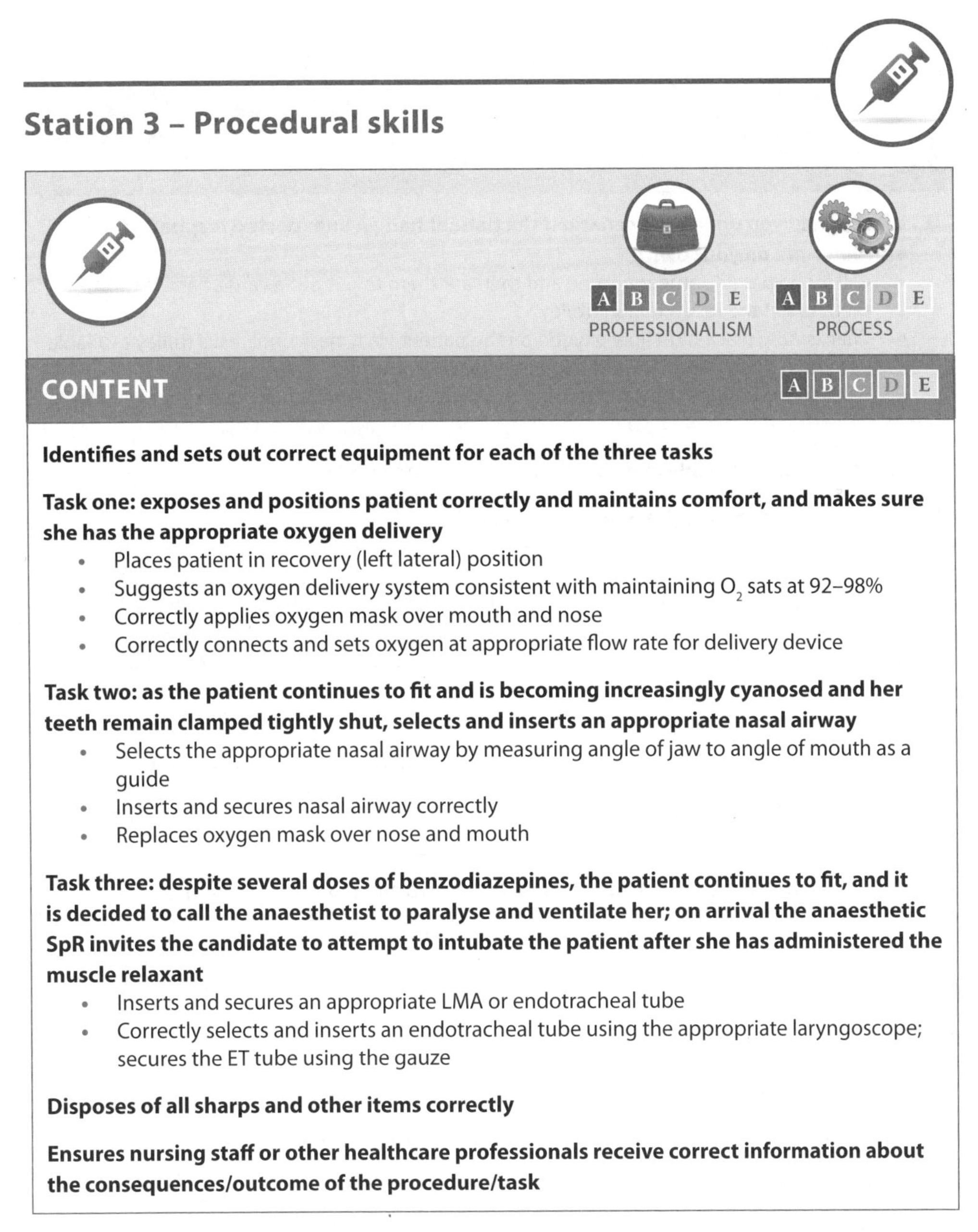

A B C D E PROFESSIONALISM

A B C D E PROCESS

CONTENT A B C D E

Identifies and sets out correct equipment for each of the three tasks

Task one: exposes and positions patient correctly and maintains comfort, and makes sure she has the appropriate oxygen delivery

- Places patient in recovery (left lateral) position
- Suggests an oxygen delivery system consistent with maintaining O_2 sats at 92–98%
- Correctly applies oxygen mask over mouth and nose
- Correctly connects and sets oxygen at appropriate flow rate for delivery device

Task two: as the patient continues to fit and is becoming increasingly cyanosed and her teeth remain clamped tightly shut, selects and inserts an appropriate nasal airway

- Selects the appropriate nasal airway by measuring angle of jaw to angle of mouth as a guide
- Inserts and secures nasal airway correctly
- Replaces oxygen mask over nose and mouth

Task three: despite several doses of benzodiazepines, the patient continues to fit, and it is decided to call the anaesthetist to paralyse and ventilate her; on arrival the anaesthetic SpR invites the candidate to attempt to intubate the patient after she has administered the muscle relaxant

- Inserts and secures an appropriate LMA or endotracheal tube
- Correctly selects and inserts an endotracheal tube using the appropriate laryngoscope; secures the ET tube using the gauze

Disposes of all sharps and other items correctly

Ensures nursing staff or other healthcare professionals receive correct information about the consequences/outcome of the procedure/task

CLINICAL DIAGNOSTIC REASONING

A B C D E

- **What would you do in this scenario if the patient had an unexpected respiratory arrest and you were on your own?**
  - Call for help until someone came and then ask them to put out a cardiac arrest call; get them to get the resuscitation trolley
  - Checks ABC; place high flow oxygen on the patient via a mask until resus trolley available
  - Assemble a bag and mask with high flow oxygen attached
  - Proceed to ventilate the patient using the bag and mask until anaesthetist or similar help arrived.

Demonstrates safe, sensible and appropriate management plan

Demonstrates clear and logical diagnostic reasoning

GLOBAL PROCEDURE MARK

A B C D E

Station 4 – Prescribing skills

Check: DRUG DRs Don't Forget Signing Off (page 373)

CALCULATION

Phenytoin infusion

Loading dose = 15 mg/kg = 62 × 15 = 930 mg

Make up 930 mg to 50 ml with 0.9 % saline = (930/50) = 18.6 mg/ml

By the BNF, the maximum rate is 50 mg/min and by calculation there are 18.6 mg/ml

Thus, infusion rate should be set at 50/18.6 = 2.7 ml/min × 60 = 162 ml/h

Maintenance dose = 5 mg/kg = 62 × 5 = 310 mg made up to 250 ml with 0.9% saline = (310/250) = 1.24 mg/ml

The maintenance dose should run over the next 24 hours – 250 ml running over 24 hours – thus infusion rate should be set at 250/24 = 10.4 ml/h

Allergies, sensitivities and adverse drug reactions						Patient details/addressograph
No known allergies ✓		Initials AF	Gender M / (F)			NHS/ Hospital No: P010267
Not possible to ascertain ☐		Date 21.11.11	Weight (kg)	Date		
Medicine/substance	Reaction & Severity	Initials & Date	62			Surname: KELLY
			Height			First name: JOANNA
			1.65m			
Alerts			Surface area (m²)			Date of birth: 5.10.88

As required medications						
Medication DIAZEPAM				Date		
Indication				Time		
Dose 2-10 mg	Route IV	Maximum frequency / dose as reqd.	Start date 21/11	Dose		
			Stop date	Route		
Signature AF			Bleep no. 089	Given		
Additional instructions:					Pharmacy ☐	

As required medications						
Medication PARACETAMOL				Date		
Indication				Time		
Dose 1g	Route PO/PR	Maximum frequency / dose	Start date 21/11	Dose		
			Stop date	Route		
Signature AF			Bleep no. 089	Given		
Additional instructions:					Pharmacy ☐	

21/11 Infusion prescriptions continued										SC = subcutaneous		IVC = intravenous central IVP = intravenous peripheral		
Date & time	Route	Infusion Fluid		Medication		Duration	Rate	Prescriber's signature & bleep no.	Date given	Given by / Added by	Check by	Start time	Finish time	Pharmacy
		Name & strength	Volume	Approved name with expiry / unit number	Dose									
21/11	IVP	LOADING INFUSION: PHENYTOIN 930mg made up to 50ml with 0.9% saline - to run 162ml/hr. RF 089												
21/11	IVP	MAINTENANCE INFUSION: PHENYTOIN 310mg made up to 250ml with 0.9% saline - to run 10.4ml/hr. RF 089												
21/11	IVP	0.9% SALINE Exp: Batch/unit no:	1 LITRE	+20mmol KCl		8 hour		AF 089						
21/11	IVP	0.9% SALINE Exp: Batch/unit no:	1 LITRE			8 hour		AF 089						
21/11	IVP	0.9% SALINE Exp: Batch/unit no:	1 LITRE	+20mmol KCl		8 hour		AF 089						

SCENARIO 4

GLOBAL PRESCRIBING MARK

A B C D E

Station 5 – Clinical communication skills

Patient script

You are recovering on the ward after being transferred this morning from the intensive care unit. You are feeling very frightened and realise that you must stop your present way of life and take your medications. The consultant in the intensive therapy unit was quite 'brutal' this morning and told you 'to change your ways or you might die the next time'.

Ideas: you know your 'partying' has contributed to your seizures and you are willing to stop drinking so heavily and stop taking illicit drugs if it will help. Concerns: you are frightened that you will be left with epilepsy for life and that you won't be able to drive or do other 'normal' things again.

Expectations: you are willing to accept the advice given and realise you will need to take the medications offered regularly.

You are happy to accept advice but should challenge any medical jargon or concepts you don't feel have been fully explained.

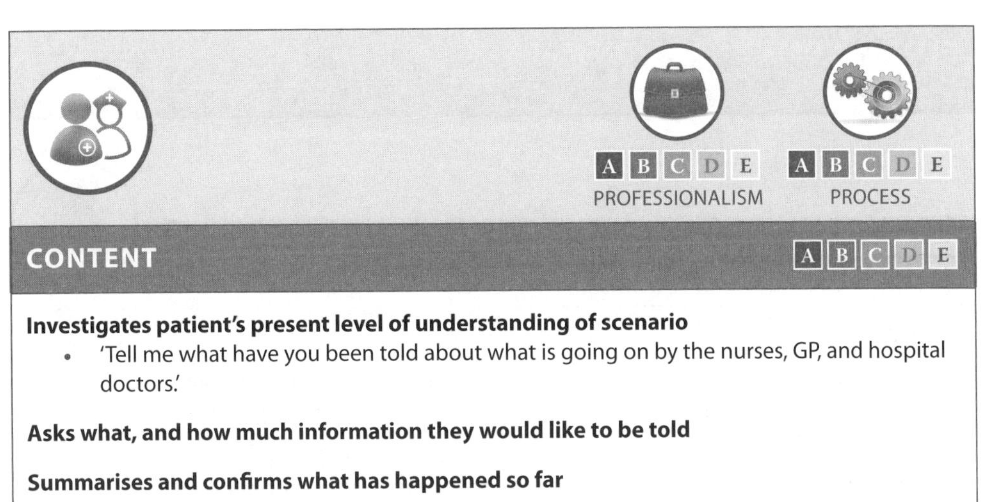

Investigates patient's present level of understanding of scenario

- 'Tell me what have you been told about what is going on by the nurses, GP, and hospital doctors.'

Asks what, and how much information they would like to be told

Summarises and confirms what has happened so far

Establishes patient's ideas, concerns and expectations

Explains the key, important information

Lifestyle changes

- Reduce alcohol intake to safe levels
- Stop illicit drug taking

Drug adherence – confirms what drugs she is taking and her previous adherence

Explores barriers to adherence

Invites patient to ask questions as they proceed through the consultation and is able to deal with them appropriately

Summarises important areas of the consultation back to the patient

Formally ends the consultation and ensures appropriate follow-up has been discussed

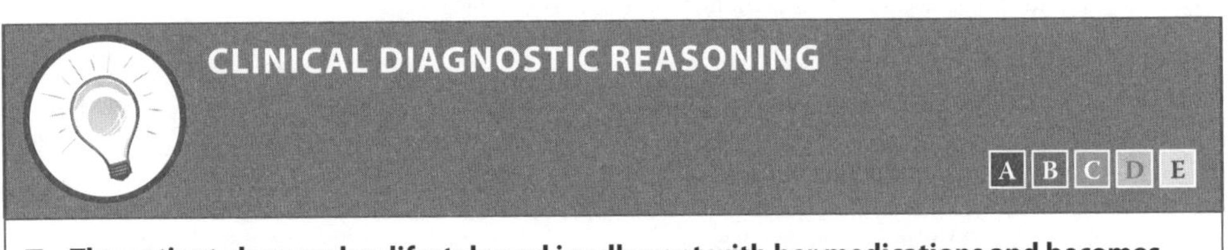

- **The patient changes her lifestyle and is adherent with her medications and becomes 'fit-free' – how long before she can drive a car again?**
  - One year fit-free from date of last seizure or three years of nocturnal seizures; laws are different for commercial vehicles
- **Please tell me three antibiotics that may interact with phenytoin and other anti-epileptic medications?**
  - Clarithromycin, Metronidazole, Isoniazide, Ciprofloxacin, Trimethoprin, Sulfonomides, Rifamycins

GLOBAL COMMUNICATION MARK

A B C D E

Scenario 4: Reflection and consolidation

History

Ms Joanna Kelly is a 23-year-old woman who was previously fit and well with no significant medical history. She now presents with a 2- to 3-month history of several worrying episodes during sleep. The first episode was after her birthday celebration with friends. She remembers coming home and getting into bed after taking off her make-up but then woke about 9 hours later feeling 'terrible'. She had a severe headache, felt 'battered and bruised' and ached all over. Her flatmate thought she had brought a boyfriend home as she was 'bashing against the wall' for several minutes. She thinks she may have bitten her tongue and had wet the bed. Since then she has had three similar episodes, all occurring at night. She wakes feeling terrible, with a headache and feeling like her muscles are aching and burning. She wet the bed on two of these episodes. Three days ago she had a 'funny turn' in the toilet at work during the daytime. She was passing urine when she suddenly felt 'strange' as if 'she wasn't there'. The next thing she remembers is work colleagues trying to drag her out of the cubicle. According to them, she groaned and then collapsed onto the floor. They report she was lying on the floor shaking and frothing at the mouth, and that she had gone dark purple in the face. The shaking stopped on its own after about 2 minutes and she woke up after another minute or two. She insisted they just put you in a taxi home but once at home she just lay on the sofa for about 3 or 4 hours, feeling back to normal on return of her flatmate at about 1930 hours.
In between these episodes the patient has been very well and she has had no headache, blurred vision, dizziness, speech or communication problems. Her arms and legs limbs feel normal and she has been otherwise systemically well.
Risk factors:

- Born by caesarean section
- Well baby and child
- No known childhood seizures
- No major head injuries, car accidents or trauma.

Medications:

- No regular medications other than the oral contraceptive pill
- No known drug allergies.

Lifestyle factors:

- Smoking – 10–20 cigarettes per day (5 years or so); marijuana at weekends – commonly one or two joints
- Alcohol – heavy intake – up to 20–30 units at parties in an evening
- Illicit drug taking – at the weekends (and on some weekdays) regularly uses cocaine – two to three lines; also ecstasy and marijuana use.

Examination

On examination of this right-handed young woman in the outpatient clinic she was tired and slightly 'haggard', but her vital observations including heart rate, blood pressure, temperature and blood glucose were all within normal limits. Examination of her cranial nerves including speech and swallowing were all normal, as was assessment of her cerebellar function.

Data Interpretation

The definitive investigations in this case are primarily used to exclude secondary causes of seizures including blood tests – FBC, U&Es, glucose, calcium and magnesium, LFTs and ESR; radiology including CXR and CT head scan; EEG is unlikely to be useful unless seizure activity is captured. Other tests may include an ECG if a cardiac cause was suspected from the history and examination.

Management

This patient requires lifestyle advice and counselling about her drug and alcohol behaviours.
She needs reassurance that statistically she will become fit-free and lead a totally normal life within the next 5 years, if she changes her lifestyle and is adherent to her medications.
She should be cared for by an expert team, and they will review her on a regular basis until she is fit-free and happy with her management.

Further reading and web links
www.epilepsy.org.uk/info/driving/agencies-license-categories#standards

Scenario 5: 'Diarrhoea and vomiting'

Station 1:

History *10-minute station*

You are the FY1 on-call with the acute medical team. The next patient is Mr John Dennison who has been brought into the Emergency department by ambulance with diarrhoea and vomiting. He is very confused and you have been asked to take a history from the patient's son, Mr Gerry Dennison.

- **Please take a focussed history with a view to presenting the history and likely diagnosis to the Medical Registrar.**

You will be assessed on the following areas, as well as the content of your history and communication stations – take them into account in your presentation.

Professionalism

- Professional appearance (NHS dress code) – including general appearance, hair and jewellery; maintains patient and personal safety
- Polite introduction; identifies patient or interviewee correctly; confirms patient's date of birth from name band or other source
- Obtains informal consent; maintains patient's privacy
- Displays empathetic and caring attitudes and behaviours throughout.

Process

- Organisation and structure; appropriate use of open and closed questions
- Appropriate fluency/rhythm/pace to the interview – this may change depending on environment and acute nature of the problem
- Allows appropriate time for patient to respond/reply to questions
- Appropriately acknowledges difficult or emotional areas of the patient's history.

Communication skills

- Demonstrates caring and sympathetic attitude
- Asks open questions
- Invites patient to ask questions and answers them appropriately
- Addresses patient's ideas, concerns and expectations.

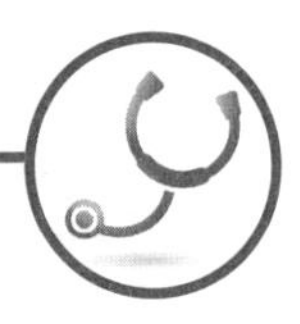

Station 2

Examination *10-minute station*

The CMT2 examines the patient whilst you are taking the history from the son. He then asks you to perform a focussed examination of the patient. Given the history he asks you to include the following elements:

Signs of uraemia

Signs of chronic renal disease and/or renal replacement therapy

Fluid status

Assessment of the abdomen.

Mr Dennison is in the resus area and is attached to a cardiac monitor. The nurse has recorded Mr Dennison's observations on the chart. You may ask for these during your assessment.

- **Once you have completed your assessment you should present the relevant findings (given within the station) to the CMT2 in an appropriate manner for a busy medical on-call.**

You will be assessed on the following areas, as well as the content and skills of your examination – take them into account in your presentation.

Professionalism

- Professional appearance (NHS dress code) – including general appearance, hair and jewellery; maintains patient and personal safety
- Polite introduction; identifies patient or interviewee correctly; confirms patient's date of birth from name band or other source
- Obtains informal consent; maintains patient's privacy
- Displays empathetic and caring attitudes and behaviours throughout.

Process

- Appropriate fluency/rhythm/pace to the examination – this may change depending on environment and acute nature of problem
- Good organisation and structure of examination; sensitive and empathetic approach
- Appropriate clinical techniques used throughout
- Maintains privacy and dignity throughout.

Clinical Communication

- Explains proposed examination/procedure: explains examination/procedure as it proceeds
- Offers information in a clear, structured and fluent manner, avoiding jargon
- Listens to patient and responds appropriately
- Demonstrates appropriate body language.

Please read the information below before presenting this case to the CMT2 as if you were on a busy medical take.
[NB If you have a model do not read this section]

Clinical findings

- Grossly unwell looking elderly patient; extremely dehydrated as evidence by – poor skin turgor, dry, cracked tongue, JVP is not seen
- No recorded urine output at the present time; no features of nephrotic syndrome or renal replacement therapy; no oedema or ascites
- He is very confused and agitated AMTS = 2/10; has twitching of the limbs and asterixis – features of uraemia; is being monitored and is wearing nasal oxygen
- Vital observations include HR 132bpm, BP = 85/58 mmHg, RR 24bpm, O_2 sats 84% on air, Temperature 39.5°C, CBG 6.4 mmol/l; Urine output – none recorded at the present time
- Abdominal examination – soft, distended, no ascites, no organomegaly, no palpable kidneys or bladder, no signs of renal replacement therapy; BS – active sounds; DRE – liquid yellow stool; large smooth benign feeling prostate
- CV examinations – heart sounds easily heard, no third heart sound, no rubs.
- RS examination– no signs of pulmonary oedema, no effusions. Reduced BS at the bases, nil focal

Station 3

Data Interpretation *10-minute station*

Part 1: The patient's intial investigation results are shown below.

- **Please list the abnormalities and the inferred/confirmed diagnoses. 5-minutes**

FBC: Hb 10.4g/dl, MCV 91fl, WCC 27.8 × 10^9/l, Neutrophils 23.3 × 10^9/l, Platelets 24 × 10^9/l
U&Es: Na^+ 165 mmol/l, K^+ 2.9 mmol/l, Urea 45.9 mmol/l, Creatinine 555 µmol/l
RBG: 5.9 mmol/l
Coagulation: INR 1.9, APTT 64 secs
LFTs: ALB 26 g/l, TBil 6.5iu/l, ALT 32iu/l, AST 23iu/l, Alk Phos 212iu/l
CCa^{2+} 2.23 mol/l, PO_4^{2-} 0.78 mmol/l

ABGs (on 2 l/minute) pH 7.08, PaO_2 8.9 kPa, Sats 89%, $PaCO_2$ 6.9 kPa, Bicarb 9.9 mmol/l, BXS -14.9 mmol/l

Part 2: EMQ - Theme: Gastroenteritis - causative organisms 5-minutes

A *Bacillus cereus*
B *Campylobacter jejuni*
C *Clostridium difficile*
D *Crytosporidium*
E *Entamoeba histolytica*
F *Escheria coli*
G *Giardia Lamblia*
H *Salmonella enteritidis*
I *Shigella*
J *Yersinia*

■ **The following patients have all presented with gastroenteritis. Please choose the most likely cause from the above list. The items may be used once, more than once or not at all.**

1 A 64-year-old man is seen by his GP at home, 3–4 hours after re-heating the previously refrigerated remains of a Chinese takeaway meal. He has had profuse vomiting but no abdominal pain or diarrhoea. The GP gives him an intramuscular injection of an anti-emetic and reassures him that it should all resolve over night, which it does.

2 A 79-year-old man is admitted to hospital from a nursing home with profuse, offensive green-coloured diarrhoea. Of note he has recently been treated for a series of urinary tract infections in the community with trimethoprim, nalidixic acid and augmentin. He improves after ten days with oral metronidazole.

3 An 85-year-old man presents in the Emergency Department with a 48-hour history of a high fever, vomiting, crampy abdominal pains and profuse watery diarrhoea. Of note he was celebrating his birthday two evenings ago and had some pork chops that 'smelt and tasted rather peculiar'. Blood cultures grow a gram negative, motile rod-shaped bacteria. His symptoms improve with intravenous fluids and ciprofloxacin.

4 A 39-year-old man and his wife are seen by their GP with profuse watery diarrhoea containing blood and mucous, a week after returning from Cambodia and Vietnam. They admit to eating 'street food' wherever they went but tried to ensure it was well cooked and clean. Stool samples reveal trophozoites and cysts. They improve with metronidazole and paramomycin.

5 A 91-year-old man is admitted to the Emergency department from a nursing home with profuse vomiting and diarrhoea. Of note several of the residents have been similarly unwell after a Sunday lunch of roast lamb. He is severely unwell and dehydrated, BP 80/60 mm Hg and pulse 123 bpm. He is anuric and U&Es reveal Na 156 mmol/l, K^+ 2.2 mmol/l, Urea 34.9 mmol/l, Creatinine 1024 μmol/l. Blood cultures grow a gram negative rod shaped bacterium. Despite intravenous fluids and antibiotics he dies 12-hours later.

Station 4

Prescribing Skills *10-minute station*

■ **Using the BNF and the drug chart provided (page 368), write up his regular medications (where appropriate) and the prescribed antibiotics and fluids for this patient.**

Mr John Dennison; Number 2009767; DOB 14.11.33; Ward: Acacia; Consultant: Dr Dawes; Weight approx 60 kg; Drug Allergies: Nil Known

U&Es: Na^+ 165 mmol/l, K^+ 2.9 mmol/l, Urea 45.9 mmol/l, Creatinine 555 μmol/l eGFR = 22 ml/min/1.73m^2

Stat side
Ciprofloxacin 500 mg IV
Metoclopramide 10 mg IV

Regular side
Ciprofloxacin 500 mg twice a day for 7 days
Tiotropium 18 μg once a day
Budesonide / Fometerol inhaler 2 puffs twice a day
Tamulosin 400 μg once a day
Bendroflumethaizide 2.5 mg once a day
Ramipril 5 mg once a day
Amlodipine 10 mg once a day

PRN side
Paracetamol 1 g max four times per day (6 hourly)
Metoclopramide 10 mg max three times per day (8 hourly)

Fluids – it has been left to you to prescribe the fluids – type, volume and rate

Remember: DRUG DRs Don't Forget Signing Off (page 373)

Station 5 – Clinical Communication Skills

- You have been asked by the ST5 to discuss the CPR status of the patient as if the ST5 were the patient's son. 10-minute station

On the ward Mr Dennison remains very confused on the ward with profuse watery diarrhoea.

His most recent vital signs:

BP 90/50 mmHg – he has had 4 litres in 8 hours; HR 120bpm; O_2 sats – 91% on 2 l/min; RR 29 bpm; CBG 5.7 mmol/l; UO – last 5 hours 14 ml, 23 ml, 14 ml, 15 ml, 7 ml

Repeat ABGs: pH 7.13, Pa O_2 11.1 kPa, Pa CO_2 5.9 kPa, Bicarb 11.9 mmol/l, BX – 12.6 mmol/l

Station 6 –Confirming Death and Writing the Death Certificate

Despite further fluid resuscitation and IV antibiotics, Mr Dennison continues to deteriorate. He becomes increasingly 'chesty' and starts to cough up thick yellow sputum. 36-hours later he dies.

The cause of the diarrhoea had been identified as a strain of *E. coli.*

Part 1: Confirmation of Death 5-minutes

- You are taken to see Mr Dennison's body by the ward nursing sister who asks you to demonstrate to her how you would confirm the patient is dead
- Using the Resus Annie or a similar manikin demonstrate how to confirm a patient's death. You should talk to the examiner as you proceed. Record your findings in the space provided below as if this was the medical notes.

Equipment necessary

- Resus Annie or similar manikin
- Pen torch
- Stethoscope

PATIENT DETAILS

Mr John Dennison; Number 2009767; DOB 14.11.33; Ward: Acacia; Consultant: Dr Dawes

Part 2. Writing the death certificate 5-minutes

After discussion with the coroner's clerk, it is agreed a death certificate can be issued with the causes of death recorded as

1a – Bronchopneumonia
1b – Acute renal failure
1c – *E. coli* diarrhoea
2 – Hypertension and benign prostatic hypertrophy

- Please write the death certificate for this patient using the certificate shown overleaf. You should use the patient's details and information given in part 1.

COUNTERFOIL

For use of Medical Practitioner who should complete in all cases

Name of deceased ....

Date of death..........................

Age ....

Place of death ....

Last seen alive by me ....

Postmortem/ Coroner* 1 2 3 4

Whether seen after death a b c

Cause of death*
I a) ....
b) ....
c) ....

II ....

Employment?

Further information offered ....

Signature ....

Date ....

*Ring appropriate digit(s) and letter

Births and Deaths registration act 1953
(form prescribed by the registration of births and deaths regulations 1987)

MEDICAL CERTIFICATE OF CAUSE OF DEATH

For use only by a Registered Medical Practitioner WHO HAS BEEN IN ATTENDANCE during the deceased's last illness and to be delivered by him forthwith to the Register of Births and Deaths

Registrar to enter No. of Death entry ....

PasTest HOSPITAL

Name of deceased ....

Date of death as stated to me .... Age as stated to me..........................

Place of death ....

Last seen alive by me..........................

1 The certified cause of death takes account of information obtained from post-mortem.
2 Information from post mortem may be available later.
3 Post-mortem not being held.
4 I have reported this death to the Coroner for further action. (see overleaf)

Please ring appropriate digits and letter

a Seen after death by me
b Seen after death by another medical practitioner but not by me
c Not seen after death by a medical practitioner

CAUSE OF DEATH

The condition thought to be the 'underlying cause of death' should appear in the lowest completed line of part 1.

1 (a) Disease or condition directly leading to death* ....

(b) Other disease or condition, if any, leading to (a) ....

(b) Other disease or condition, if any, leading to (b) ....

II Other significant conditions contributing to the death but not related to the disease or condition causing it.
....

These particulars not to be entered in death register
Approximate interval between onset and death
....

The death might have been due to or contributed to by the employment followed at some time by the deceased. Please tick where applicable ☐

*This does not mean the mode of dying, such has heart failure, asphyxia, asthenia, etc, it means the disease, injury, or complication which caused death.

I hearby certify that I was in medical attendance during the above named deceased's last illness, and that the particulars and cause of death above written are true to the best of my knowledge and belief.

Signature ....

Residence ....

Qualifications as registered by General Medical Council ....

Date ....

For deaths in hospital: Please give the name of the consultant responsible for the above named as a patient ....

(Form prescribed by the Registration of Births and Deaths Regulations 1987)

NOTICE TO INFORMANT

I hereby give notice that I have this day signed a medical certificate of cause of death of
....

Signature ....

Date ....

This notice is to be delivered by the informant to the registrar of births and deaths for the sub-district in which the death occurred.

The certifying medical practitioner must give this notice to the person who is qualified and liable to act as informant for the registration of death (see list overleaf). Where the informant intends giving information for the registration outside of the area where the death occurred, this notice may be handed to the informant's agent.

DUTIES OF INFORMANT

Failure to deliver this notice to the registrar renders the informant liable to prosecution. The death cannot be registered until the medical certificate has reached the registrar. When the death is registered the informant must be prepared to give to the registrar the following particulars relating to the deceased:

1. The date and time of death.
2. The full name and surname (and the maiden surname if the deceased was a woman who had married).
3. The date and place of birth.
4. The occupation (and if applicable the name and occupation of the deceased's spouse or civil partner).
5. The usual address.
6. Whether the deceased was in receipt of a pension or allowance from public funds.
7. If the deceased was married or in a civil partnership, the date of birth of the surviving spouse or civil partner.

THE DECEASED'S MEDICAL CARD SHOULD BE DELIVERED TO THE REGISTRAR

SCENARIO 5

Answers

Station 1 – History

Patient's son's script

You are Mr Gerry Dennison, the eldest son of the patient, Mr John Dennison, age 78 years, DOB 14.11.33. Your father was a relatively well, older man until about 5-years ago. He is a retired car factory worker and lives on the third floor of a council block with your mum, who is well. They manage just about and don't have any carers, other than me and my wife. I've got two younger brothers who live abroad, one in Australia and one in Texas, USA.

In the past five years things have started to catch up with him. He was a 'work hard – play hard' type of man who was a heavy drinker in his younger years (often drinking > 40 pints per week) and a lifelong smoker, smoking 30–40 cigarettes per day until about 2–3 years ago. His normal exercise tolerance is about 200 yards to the pub, which 'he takes very slowly'.

Over the last 5-years he has had problems with high blood pressure, emphysema and prostate problems. 'They are unable to operate on his prostate because of his chest and his blood pressure'. He takes multiple tablets and inhalers but isn't as good as he should be at taking them all. Over the last two winters he has had several admissions for chest problems, one requiring a 'breathing mask' 'you know the really tight one over the face' (NIV). If asked you tell the doctor that he has never been in the intensive care unit or needed 'a tube down the throat' to breathe.

He was brought into the ED this afternoon by ambulance after becoming increasingly unwell over the past week. Over the past 5–6 days he has been 'laid low' with a 'tummy bug'. He told me that he thinks it was due to a kebab he had on the way home from the pub last weekend. During this period he has had horrible, smelly diarrhoea, at least 10–15 times per day. It is loose, yellowish fluid like motions, that he is unable to hold and he's messed the bed several times over the last few days. He had vomiting for about the first 24–48 hours but this seems to have settled now. I didn't see, nor did anyone mention to me that there was any blood in the vomit.

He's not been able to keep any food or drink down for the entire week and is becoming worse and worse. I'm not sure if he's had abdominal pain but he hasn't mentioned it. No other contacts suffering with diarrhoea, no foreign travel.

Over the last 2 days or so I can't remember him going to 'pass water' – he may have been incontinent but I didn't notice; I've not noticed him being jaundiced/yellow.

Today he's been very confused, biting people, shouting and being very aggressive. 'He's looked a right mess this morning, like he was on his way out' and that's when I decided to ring for an ambulance. The thing that frightened me was the confusion and that he began to 'twitch'.

Medications – [only if asked – you have a list]

Tiotropium 18 mcg od **No known drug allergies**

Budesonide/fometerol inhaler

Tamulosin

Bendroflumethiazide 2.5 mg od

Ramipril 5 mg od

Amlodipine 10 mg o.d.

PMH

'Emphysema', high blood pressure, prostate problems;

No history of stroke, heart problems, diabetes mellitus, kidney disease;

Surgical history – appendicectomy (when a child), nil else.

Ideas and concerns – You know he's very ill; you are really worried about your dad, he's been getting increasingly unwell for the past few years and you think this time he may have just tipped a bit too far.

Expectations – you just hope it isn't too late and that you (the doctors) can get him better.

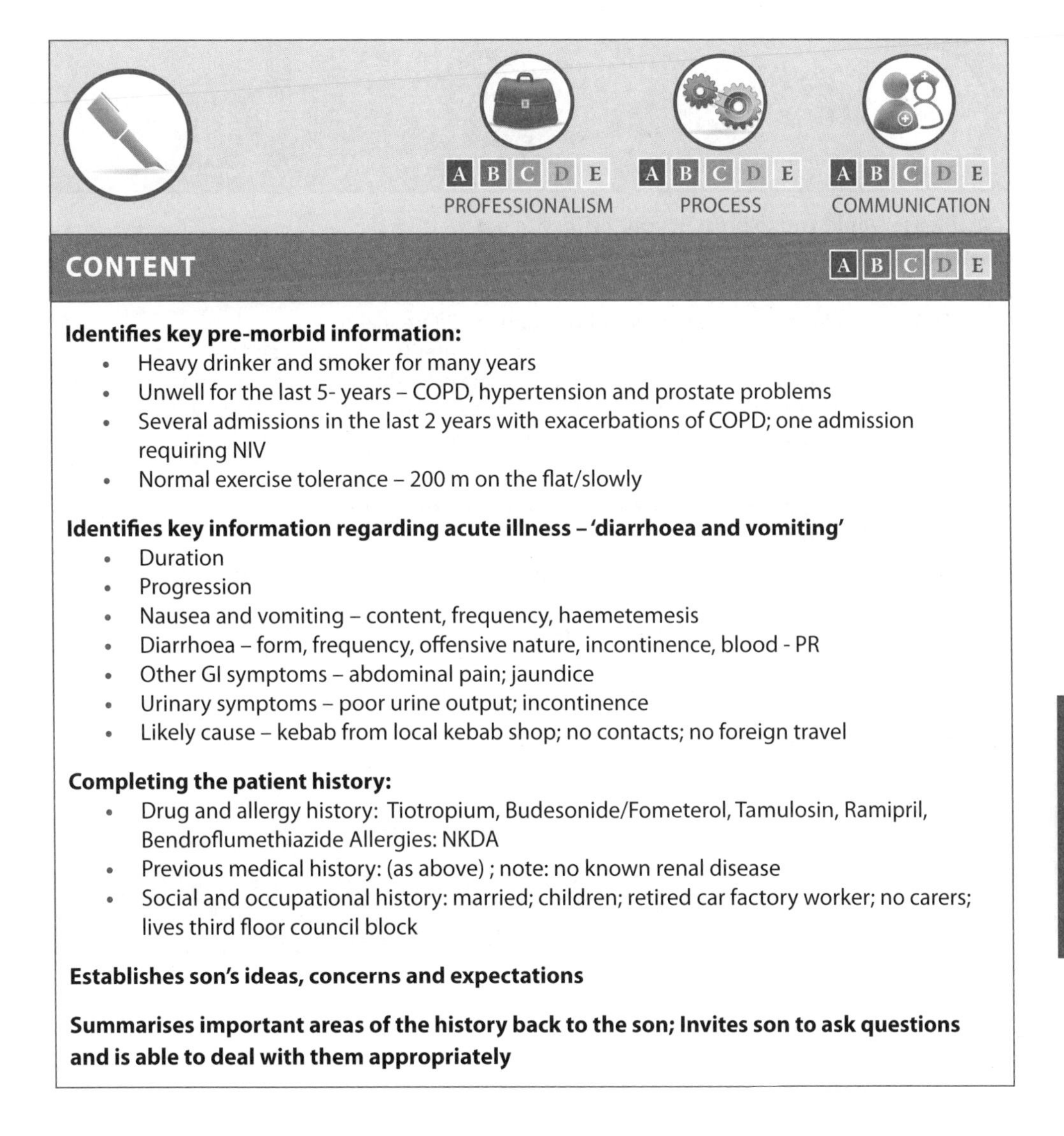

A B C D E
PROFESSIONALISM

A B C D E
PROCESS

A B C D E
COMMUNICATION

CONTENT A B C D E

Identifies key pre-morbid information:

- Heavy drinker and smoker for many years
- Unwell for the last 5- years – COPD, hypertension and prostate problems
- Several admissions in the last 2 years with exacerbations of COPD; one admission requiring NIV
- Normal exercise tolerance – 200 m on the flat/slowly

Identifies key information regarding acute illness – 'diarrhoea and vomiting'

- Duration
- Progression
- Nausea and vomiting – content, frequency, haemetemesis
- Diarrhoea – form, frequency, offensive nature, incontinence, blood - PR
- Other GI symptoms – abdominal pain; jaundice
- Urinary symptoms – poor urine output; incontinence
- Likely cause – kebab from local kebab shop; no contacts; no foreign travel

Completing the patient history:

- Drug and allergy history: Tiotropium, Budesonide/Fometerol, Tamulosin, Ramipril, Bendroflumethiazide Allergies: NKDA
- Previous medical history: (as above) ; note: no known renal disease
- Social and occupational history: married; children; retired car factory worker; no carers; lives third floor council block

Establishes son's ideas, concerns and expectations

Summarises important areas of the history back to the son; Invites son to ask questions and is able to deal with them appropriately

CLINICAL DIAGNOSTIC REASONING

A B C D E

- **Please would you to present your history to me.**

Candidate offers a logical, well-structured account of the history

- **Would you to offer me the likely diagnosis and differentials**

Candidate offers the correct diagnosis and appropriate differentials:
Diagnosis: the patient has presented with acute gastroenteritis (diarrhoea and vomiting), after eating a kebab from a local kebab shop. He has become incontinent of faeces and possibly urine, although worryingly he has had little or no urinary output in the last few days; nothing to eat or drink in the last week; candidate expresses concern around likely acute renal impairment or kidney injury (AKI)

- **Can you tell me three likely microbiological causes of this presentation**

E. coli, Campylobacter, Salmonellosis,

- **Examiner asks: Could you tell me three further tests you would request.**
    - Bloods – FBC, U&Es, RBG, LFTs and amylase
    - Microbiology – Blood and stool cultures
    - Radiology – Plain AXR and erect CXR
    - ABGs and ECG

The candidate demonstrates

- Safe, sensible and appropriate management plan
- Focussed, knowledgeable diagnostic process

GLOBAL HISTORY MARK

A B C D E

Station 2 – Examination

Patient script

If you are an actor/patient, read the patient history and physical signs fully – when the candidate comes to an abnormal site in their examination, act-out tenderness and/or volunteer the relevant physical sign.

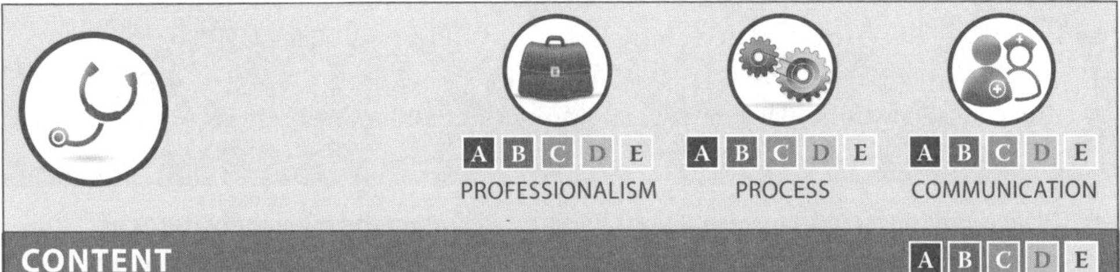

CONTENT A B C D E

Exposes and positions patient correctly and maintains comfort:
Comments on wellbeing of patient ie well or unwell
'Feet to face' – Observes, and comments on patient and surroundings from foot of bed – Colour/perfusion, hydration, position (curled up/lying flat/sitting up). Infusions; monitor
Comments patient does not have features of uraemia from end of bed including – uraemic frost, pigmentation, hiccups.
Asks for **appropriate / relevant clinical observations** – only give results if asked for individually HR 132bpm, BP = 85/58 mmHg, RR 24bpm, O2 sats 84% on air, Temperature 39.5°C ; Urine output – nil recorded at the present time; urinalysis – nil available, CBG 6.4 mmol/l

General/Systemic examination:

- **Hands and upper limbs:** including: tar staining, perfusion of hands, comments on general signs eg clubbing
- Chronic renal disease – anaemia; leukonychia
- Uraemia – asterixis
- Upper limb/hands oedema (?nephrotic)
- **Face and Neck:** including – signs of dehydration, anaemia, central cyanosis, JVP (fluid status); face swelling (nephrotic)

Focussed examination of the abdomen:

- Inspection: scars, distention,
- Palpation and percussion: comments on and excludes signs of peritonism,
- Organomegaly – specifically comments on kidneys and bladder; presence/absence ascites
- Excludes renal transplant/CAPD lines
- Auscultation: bowel sounds

Candidate asks to perform DRE – Examiner asks 'for what reason' – answers – to assess faeces, prostate: size and consistency
Completes examination by identifying relevant additional clinical signs and formally completing assessment
- CV – Specifically comments on JVP, Pericardial rub (uraemia)
- RS – Pulmonary oedema; effusions
- Peripheral oedema

Thanks patient; offers assistance; maintains patient's dignity and privacy until they are dressed/ comfortable.

CLINICAL DIAGNOSTIC REASONING

A B C D E

- **Please would you like to present your findings, including the relevant features concerning his fluid status, signs of uraemia, renal replacement therapy, abdominal assessment**

Candidate – identifies correct physical signs including important negative findings.
- Confirms patient is very unwell
- Uraemia – asterixis, confusion, muscle twitching
- Fluid status – grossly dehydrated – JVP not seen, dry mouth, poor skin turgor, no urine output since admission
- No features of renal replacement therapy, nephrotic syndrome
- Abdomen – no signs of peritonism; bowel sounds 'colitic' / active

Presentation is succinct, clear, well paced and well organised

- **Given the clinical findings could you list three acute interventions you would arrange for this gentleman in the Emergency Department**

Demonstrates safe, sensible and appropriate management plan; recognises:
(a) Hypotension/tachycardia/Pyrexia ie septic/hypovolaemic shock –
- Intravenous access (consider CVL)
- Insertion of urinary catheter
- Strict fluid balance – input/output charts
- Antipyretics/cooling

(b) Infective diarrhoea
- Isolation in high dependency area/barrier nursing

(c) The patient is very ill - Senior review asap; CPR status; possible ITU review

The candidate demonstrates
- Safe, sensible and appropriate management plan
- Focussed, knowledgeable diagnostic process

GLOBAL EXAMINATION MARK

A B C D E

Station 3 – Data Interpretation

Part 1: Answers

Abnormalities	Suggestive of (inferred / confirmed diagnosis
1. Hb 10.4 g/dl, MCV 91fl = Normocytic anaema	Suggestive of anaemia of chronic disease Chronic renal impairment
2. WCC 27.8 x 10^9/l, Neutrophils 23.3 x 10^9/l – Neutrophilic leucocytosis	Suggestive/confirms likely bacterial gastro-enteritis
3. Platelets 24 x 10^9/l – thrombocytopaenia	In this context suggestive of possible DIC
4. INR 1.9, APTT 64 secs – marked coagulopathy	Given the platelet count, this is highly suggestive of DIC
5. Na^+ 165 mmol/l – hypernatraemia	Consistent with gross dehydration
6. K^+ 2.9 mmol/l – hypokalaemia	Consistent with profuse vomiting and diarrhoea
7. Urea 45.9 mmol/l, creatinine 555 µmol/l – grossly elevated urea and creatinine show marked renal impairment	The urea: creatinine ratio is approximately (11:7) suggestive of pre-renal impairment – this confirms marked dehydration.
8. ALB 26 g/l – Hypoalbuminaemia	Due to acute severe illness or may be chronic disease eg renal
9. Low pH and Bicarbonate, with negative base excess	Severe metabolic acidosis
10. PaO_2 8.9 kPa, Sats 89%, $PaCO_2$ 6.9 kPa, - hypoxia and hypercapnia	Type II respiratory failure consistent with probable underlying COPD

Part 2: Answers

(1) A (2) C (3) H (4) E (5) F

GLOBAL DATA INTERPRETATION MARK A B C D E

SCENARIO 5

STATION 4 – Prescribing skills

Check: DRUG DRs Don't Forget Signing Off (page 373)

Allergies, sensitivities and adverse drug reactions					Patient details/addressograph
No known allergies ✓		Initials AF	Gender (M)/ F		NHS/ Hospital No: 2009767
Not possible to ascertain ☐		Date 21.11.11	Weight (kg)	Date	
Medicine/substance	Reaction & Severity	Initials & Date	60		Surname: DENNISON
			Height		First name: JOHN
Alerts			Surface area (m²)		Date of birth: 14.11.33

IN-PATIENT MEDICATION PRESCRIPTION AND ADMINISTRATION RECORD — PasTest HOSPITAL

Consultant	Trainee Dr. Name and Bleep no.	Date of admission	Date chart reboarded	Estimated date of discharge
DAWES	FEATHER 601	21.11.11		
This chart is no. .... of	Transcribing Check by Pharmacy Sign .... Date	Ward 1. ACACIA 2.		

Supplementary Medication charts in use: Other (please specify): 1 .... 2 ....

Epidural/PCA ☐ Syringe driver ☐ TPN ☐ Chemotherapy ☐ Insulin sliding scale ☐

Once only medications – loading doses, pre-medication, PGDs or surgical antibiotic propylaxis

Date	Time to be given	Medicine (approved name)	Dose	Route	Signature and bleep no.	Pharmacy	Time given	Given by	Checked by
21.11	16.00	CIPROFLOXACIN	500mg	IV	AF 601				
21.11	16.00	METOCLOPRAMIDE	10mg	IV	AF 601				
21.11	16.00	HYDROCORTISONE	200mg	IV	AF 601				

SCENARIO 5

Regular prescriptions continued

Regular medications

Date	21.11.11	Medication	Instructions	Signature and bleep no.	Pharmacy
Route	LNH	TIOTROPIUM	NOT WITH NEBULISER	AF 601	☐
Signature	AF				

Time	Dose	21	22	23	24	25	26	27							
06															
(09)	18 MICROGRAMS	X	X	X	X	X									
12															
18															
22															
24															

Date	21.11.11	Medication	Instructions	Signature and bleep no.	Pharmacy
Route	LNH	BUDESONIDE 100/ FORMOTEROL 6	NOT WITH NEBULISER	AF 601	☐
Signature	AF				

Time	Dose	21	22	23	24	25	26	27							
06															
(09)	2 PUFFS	X	X	X	X	X									
12															
(18)	2 PUFFS	X	X	X	X	X									
22															
24															

Date	21.11.11	Medication	Instructions	Signature and bleep no.	Pharmacy
Route	PO	TAMSULOSIN	NOT WHILST ↓BP POOR RENAL FUNCTION	AF 601	☐
Signature	AF				

Time	Dose	21	22	23	24	25	26	27							
06															
(09)	400 MICROGRAMS	X	X	X	X	X									
12															
18															
22															
24															

Date	21.11.11	Medication	Instructions	Signature and bleep no.	Pharmacy
Route	PO	BENDROFLUMETHIAZIDE	NOT WHILST HYPOTENSIVE POOR RENAL FUNCTION	AF 601	☐
Signature	AF				

Time	Dose	21	22	23	24	25	26	27							
06															
(09)	2.5 mg	X	X	X	X	X									
12															
18															
22															
24															

Date	21.11.11	Medication	Instructions	Signature and bleep no.	Pharmacy
Route	PO	RAMIPRIL	NOT WHILST ↓BP/ POOR RENAL FUNCTION	AF 601	☐
Signature	AF				

Time	Dose	21	22	23	24	25	26	27							
06															
(09)	5 mg	X	X	X	X	X									
12															
18															
22															
24															

SCENARIO 5

Regular prescriptions continued

Regular medications

	Dose			Date 21	22	23	24	25	26	27							

Date	21.11.11	Medication	Instructions	Signature and bleep no.	Pharmacy
Route	PO	AMLODIPINE	NOT WHILST HYPOTENSIVE	AF 601	☐
Signature	AF				

Time	Dose
06	
(09)	10mg
12	
18	
22	
24	

Date	21.11.11	Medication	Instructions	Signature and bleep no.	Pharmacy
Route	NEB	SALBUTAMOL		AF 601	☐
Signature	AF				

Time	Dose
06	2.5mg
10	2.5mg
14	2.5mg
18	2.5mg
22	2.5mg
24	2.5mg

Date	21.11.11	Medication	Instructions	Signature and bleep no.	Pharmacy
Route	NEB	IPATROPIUM		AF 601	☐
Signature	AF				

Time	Dose
06	X
10	500 MICROGRAMS
14	500 MICROGRAMS
18	500 MICROGRAMS
22	500 MICROGRAMS
24	X

Date	21.11.11	Medication	Instructions	Signature and bleep no.	Pharmacy
Route	IV	HYDROCORTISONE		AF 601	☐
Signature	AF				

Time	Dose
(06)	200MG
(12)	200MG
(18)	200MG
22	
(24)	200MG

Regular prescriptions continued

Regular medications

Date	21/11	Medication	Instructions	Signature and bleep no.	Pharmacy
Route	IV	CIPROFLOXACIN	SEVERE SEPSIS	AF 601	☐
Times	Dose				

Date			21	22	23	24	25	26	27
06									
09		500mg							
12									
18									
22		500mg							
24									

SCENARIO 5

Regular prescriptions						
Oral anticoagulation follow the anticoagulation guidelines available on the intranet						
Indication	Target INR	Baseline INR (if applicable)	Duration of therapy Date therapy started	Date of anticoagulation follow-up appointment (clinic or other)*	Anticoagulant record book given or updated. Sign and date	Date patient counselled and sign

* A follow-up appointment must be booked with the anti-coagulant clinic or enhanced provider of primary care services. If not, the TTA will not be dispensed

Initiating warfarin	Perform baseline coagulation screen, LFTs, U&Es and FBC	Prescribe initiation dose as per guidelines	CHECK INR ON DAY 3	FOLLOW DOSING ALGORITHM IN GUIDELINE
Continuing warfarin	Maintenance therapy	FOLLOW MAINTENANCE DOSING ALGORITHM IN GUIDELINE		

Do not use the initiation protocol for patients already on warfarin. More frequent INR monitoring may be required for patients on interacting drug(s)

Medication				Date														
1				INR														
Route	Frequency OD	Time 18.00	Start	Dose														
			Stop	Dr sign														
Signature		Bleep no.	Pharmacy	Given														

Initiating warfarin – Reduced dosing regimen in red. Refer to anticoagulation policy

Day	One	Two	Three							Four and above								
INR	<1.4	No test	<2.0	2.0-2.1	2.2-2.5	2.6-2.9	3.0-3.3	3.4-4.0	>4.0	<1.4	1.4-1.5	1.6-1.7	1.8-1.9	2.0-2.3	2.4-3.0	3.1-4.0	4.1-4.5	>4.5
Dose mg	10 5	10 5	10	5	4	3	2	1	0	9	8	7	6	5	4	3	Miss 1 day	Miss 2 day

Thromboprophylaxis please prescribe treatment regimens in the regular medications section

Choice of mechanical prophylaxis and leg(s) to be applied to						Enter Time	Enter details below
Graduated elastic compression stockings (circled)	Intermittend pneumatic compression device (IPC)		Leg				
			Left	Right	Both (circled)		
21/11 ☐ Start Date:	☐ End Date:	Signature and Bleep No.	☐	☐	☐		
☐ Start Date:	☐ End Date:	Signature and Bleep No.	☐	☐	☐		

Medication		Dose	Dose Change	Enter Time	Enter details below
Please ensure you have completed the VTE risk assessment form	Date				
	Route				
	Signature			Instructions NOT FOR HEPARIN - D.I.C	Pharmacy ☐
	Bleep no.				

Oxygen				
Target Saturation	88-92% ☑	94/98% ☐	If oxygen saturation falls below target range on prescribed oxygen, patient needs urgent clinical review. If oxygen saturation is above targent range on prescribed oxygen, ask for review.	
Other specify)			*Device: N= nasal cannula, SM = simple face mask, V = venturi, H = humidified, RM = reservoir mask, OTHER = other eg. NCPAP/NIPPV	Pharmacy ☐
Target Saturation not applicable ☐				

	Date Started	Date Changed	Enter Time	Enter details below
Device	VENTURI			
% or L/min (specify a range eg 1-21 L/min)	28%			
Signature and Bleep no.	AF 601			

SCENARIO 5

21/11 Infusion prescriptions continued										SC = subcutaneous		IVC = intravenous central IVP = intravenous peripheral		
Date & time	Route	Infusion Fluid		Medication		Duration	Rate	Prescriber's signature & bleep no.	Date given	Given by / Added by	Check by	Start time	Finish time	Pharmacy
		Name & strength	Volume	Approved name with expiry / unit number	Dose									
21/11	IVP	0.9% SALINE Exp: Batch/unit no:	1 LITRE	+20mmol HCl		30 minutes		AF 601						
21/11	IVP	0.9% SALINE Exp: Batch/unit no:	1 LITRE	+40mmol HCl		1 hour		AF 601						
21/11	IVP	0.9% SALINE Exp: Batch/unit no:	1 LITRE	+40mmol HCl		2 hour		AF 601						
21/11	IVP	0.9% SALINE Exp: Batch/unit no:	1 LITRE	+40mmol HCl		2 hour		AF 601						
21/11	IVP	0.9% SALINE Exp: Batch/unit no:	1 LITRE	+20mmol HCl		4 hour		AF 601						
21/11	IVP	0.9% SALINE Exp: Batch/unit no:	1 LITRE	+20mmol HCl		4 hour		AF 601						
21/11	IVP	0.9% SALINE Exp: Batch/unit no:	1 LITRE	+20mmol HCl		6 hour		AF 601						
21/11	IVP	0.9% SALINE Exp: Batch/unit no:	1 LITRE	+20mmol HCl		8 hour		AF 601						
		TO MAINTAIN - BP > 100 SYSTOLIC; HR < 100 BPM; U.O > 0.5 ml/kg/HR >30ML/HR												

SCENARIO 5

As required medications					
Medication: METOCLOPRAMIDE					Date
Indication					Time
Dose: 10 mg	Route: IM/ IV	Maximum frequency / dose: 8 hour	Start date: 21/11		Dose
			Stop date		Route
Signature: AF			Bleep no.: 601		Given
Additional instructions:				Pharmacy	

As required medications					
Medication: PARACETAMOL					Date
Indication					Time
Dose: 1g	Route: PO	Maximum frequency / dose: 6 hour	Start date: 21/11		Dose
			Stop date		Route
Signature: AF			Bleep no.: 601		Given
Additional instructions:				Pharmacy	

As required medications					
Medication: SALBUTAMOL					Date
Indication					Time
Dose: 2.5 mg	Route: Neb	Maximum frequency / dose	Start date: 21/11		Dose
			Stop date		Route
Signature: AF			Bleep no.: 601		Given
Additional instructions:				Pharmacy	

GLOBAL PRESCRIBING MARK

A B C D E

SCENARIO 5

Station 5 – Clinical Communication Skills

Patient's son's script

You should ask the candidate to role play this scenario as if you are the patient's son. You may need to remind the doctor that you have met already this evening as it was he/she who took the initial details of your father's illness from you.

Ideas and concerns – You realise that your father is gravely ill and that he may die. This was discussed earlier with the more senior doctor. You are concerned that he is just going to be left to die and that the doctors and nurses have already given up on him.

Expectations – you hope that everyone will do everything they can to save your dad

If asked directly, you will provide the following information:

- **Your father has always been a very private man and has never discussed 'if he got seriously ill what he would like done'**
- **He has never mentioned anything about an advanced directive (this term will need to be explained to you before you can comment)**
- **He has never discussed resuscitation.**

If explained appropriately you are happy to accept the doctors recommendations but are very concerned that

(a) He will not suffer

(b) Everyone will do everything they can to help him

If asked you agree that he should not be placed on a ventilator machine or receive 'resuscitation'.

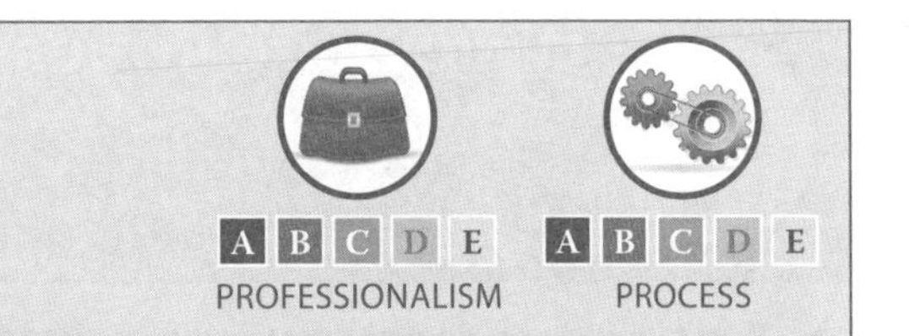

CONTENT

A B C D E

Investigates son's present level of understanding of scenario

Tell me what have you been told about what is going on by the nurses, GP, and hospital doctors?

Asks what, and how much information they would like to be told
Confirms the topics they are going to discuss –

- Future management
- What would be appropriate if Mr Dennison senior deteriorates and becomes increasingly unwell
- Resuscitation status.

Summarises and confirms what has happened so far including patient's present clinical status

- Mr Dennsion is seriously unwell
- Remains in a serious condition despite all the treatment including fluids and antibiotics.
- Now in multi-organ failure (as evidenced by data above); discusses and acknowledges this carries a very poor prognosis.

Ascertains whether Mr Dennison has ever discussed

- What he would want to happen if this situation (he was seriously ill) ever arose
- Intensive care/assisted ventilation (machines to help him breath)
- Resuscitation
- Has he made an advanced directive – this needs to be explained appropriately and satisfactorily
- Discusses management – continue with oxygen, fluids and antibiotics
- May escalate to include non-invasive ventilation but not beyond.
- Confirms ITU and other more sophisticated / invasive therapies will probably not change the prognosis
- Confirms that the team think that CPR will be futile
- Negotiates and confirms outcomes around management, escalation and CPR.

Establishes son's ideas, concerns and expectations
Invites son to ask questions as they proceed through the consultation; able to deal with them appropriately

Summarises important areas of the consultation back to the son and waits for confirmation and acknowledgement of correct summary

Formally ends the consultation.

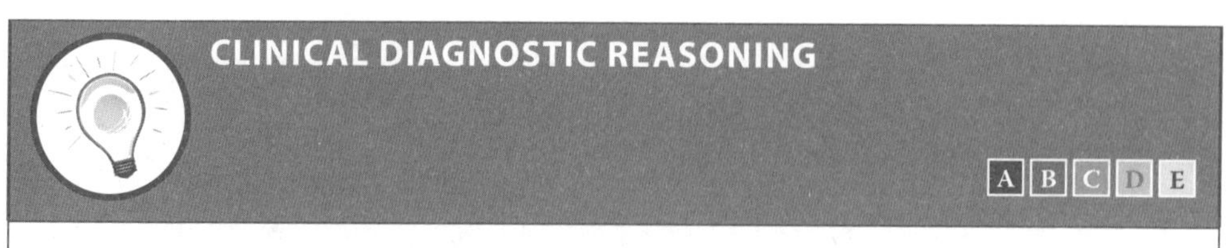

- **What would you do once you had completed the discussion with the son?**
  - Record my conversation and outcomes in the medical notes. It is good practice to ask the person you have had the conversation with to read and sign the record as true.
  - Ask a senior (Registrar or above) to sign a copy of the DNAR form with appropriate interventions highlighted.
  - Ensure nursing staff are aware of decsions and management plan.

The candidate demonstrates

- Safe, sensible and appropriate management plan
- Focussed, knowledgeable diagnostic process

GLOBAL COMMUNICATION MARK

A B C D E

Station 6 – Confirming Death and Writing the Death Certificate

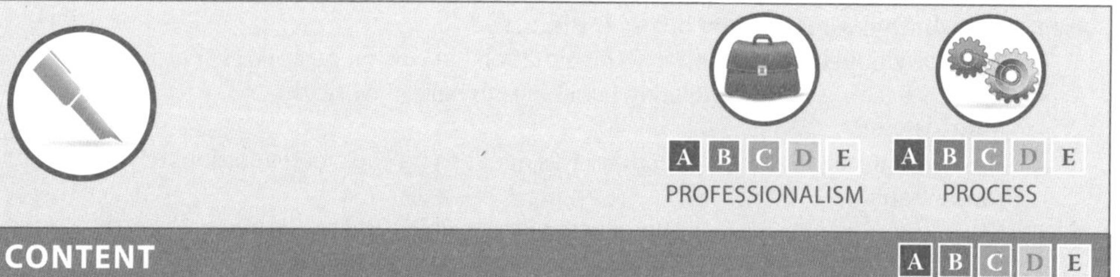

CONTENT

A B C D E

- Identifies correct equipment for the task
- Candidate states – If relatives or carers were present would introduce him/herself and ask them to just step outside whilst they certify the patient
- Identifies patient by medical notes versus wrist band
- Performs sternal rub and shouts out patient's name
- May acknowledge patient is cold to the touch and shows signs of muscle rigidity (rigor mortis)
- Palpates carotid pulse for 30 seconds–1 minute
- Opens eyelids and shines pentorch light into both pupils looking for any response
- Auscultates the chest for 1 minute listening first for breath sounds bilaterally and then heart sounds
- If candidate mentions other manoeuvres eg performing ophthalmoscopy looking for 'railroading of vessels', **examiner stops them**
- Closes patient's eyelids again and covers patient with sheet or shroud
- Does all in a fluent and professional manner

COUNTERFOIL

For use of Medical Practitioner who should complete in all cases

Name of deceased JOHN DENNISON

Date of death 22/11/11

Age 78

Place of death ACACIA WARD ST JUDES

Last seen alive by me 22/11/11

Postmortem/ Coroner* 1 2 (3) 4

Whether seen after death (a) b c

Cause of death*
I a) BRONCHOPNEUMONIA
b) ACUTE KIDNEY INJURY
c) E. COLI DIARRHOEA

II BPH, HYPERTENSION

Employment?

Further information offered

Signature ADAM FEATHER

Date 22/11/11

*Ring appropriate digit(s) and letter

Births and Deaths registration act 1953
(form prescribed by the registration of births and deaths regulations 1987)

MEDICAL CERTIFICATE OF CAUSE OF DEATH

For use only by a Registered Medical Practitioner WHO HAS BEEN IN ATTENDANCE during the deceased's last illness and to be delivered by him forthwith to the Register of Births and Deaths

Registrar to enter No. of Death entry ....

Name of deceased JOHN DENNISON

Date of death as stated to me 22 NOVEMBER 2011 Age as stated to me 78

Place of death ACACIA WARD, ST JUDES UNIVERSITY HOSPITAL NHS TRUST

Last seen alive by me 22 NOVEMBER 2011

PasTest HOSPITAL

1 The certified cause of death takes account of information obtained from post-mortem.
2 Information from post mortem may be available later.
(3) Post-mortem not being held.
4 I have reported this death to the Coroner for further action. (see overleaf)

Please ring appropriate digits and letter

(a) Seen after death by me
b Seen after death by another medical practitioner but not by me
c Not seen after death by a medical practitioner

CAUSE OF DEATH

The condition thought to be the 'underlying cause of death' should appear in the lowest completed line of part 1.

1 (a) Disease or condition directly leading to death* BRONCHOPNEUMONIA

(b) Other disease or condition, if any, leading to (a) ACUTE KIDNEY INJURY

(b) Other disease or condition, if any, leading to (b) E. COLI DIARRHOEA

II Other significant conditions contributing to the death but not related to the disease or condition causing it.
HYPERTENSION; BENIGN PROSTATIC HYPERTROPHY

These particulars not to be entered in death register
Approximate interval between onset and death

The death might have been due to or contributed to by the employment followed at some time by the deceased. Please tick where applicable ☐

*This does not mean the mode of dying, such has heart failure, asphyxia, asthenia, etc, it means the disease, injury, or complication which caused death.

I hearby certify that I was in medical attendance during the above named deceased's last illness, and that the particulars and cause of death above written are true to the best of my knowledge and belief.

Signature ADAM FEATHER

Residence ST JUDES HOSPITAL

Qualifications as registered by General Medical Council ....

Date 22/11/11

For deaths in hospital: Please give the name of the consultant responsible for the above named as a patient DR DAWES

(Form prescribed by the Registration of Births and Deaths Regulations 1987)

NOTICE TO INFORMANT

I hereby give notice that I have this day signed a medical certificate of cause of death of JOHN DENNISON

Signature ADAM FEATHER

Date 22/11/11

This notice is to be delivered by the informant to the registrar of births and deaths for the sub-district in which the death occurred.

The certifying medical practitioner must give this notice to the person who is qualified and liable to act as informant for the registration of death (see list overleaf). Where the informant intends giving information for the registration outside of the area where the death occurred, this notice may be handed to the informant's agent.

DUTIES OF INFORMANT

Failure to deliver this notice to the registrar renders the informant liable to prosecution. The death cannot be registered until the medical certificate has reached the registrar. When the death is registered the informant must be prepared to give to the registrar the following particulars relating to the deceased:

1. The date and time of death.
2. The full name and surname (and the maiden surname if the deceased was a woman who had married).
3. The date and place of birth.
4. The occupation (and if applicable the name and occupation of the deceased's spouse or civil partner).
5. The usual address.
6. Whether the deceased was in receipt of a pension or allowance from public funds.
7. If the deceased was married or in a civil partnership, the date of birth of the surviving spouse or civil partner.

THE DECEASED'S MEDICAL CARD SHOULD BE DELIVERED TO THE REGISTRAR

SCENARIO 5

Part 2: Writing the Death Certificate 5-minutes

DEATH CERTIFICATE

Counterfoil section – completed correctly with full patient details, signature and date
Death certificate section – completed correctly, signed and dated
Notice to informant – completed with patient's name; doctor's signature and date

As it is written – this death certificate could be issued

GLOBAL PROCEDURE MARK

A B C D E

Scenario 5: Reflection and Consolidation

History (From son – Mr Gerry Dennison)

The patient is Mr John Dennison a 78-year-old retired car factory worker. Of note he was previously a heavy drinker often drinking > 40 pints per week; lifelong smoker, smoking 30–40 cigarettes per day until about 2–3 years ago.
In the past five years he has had problems with hypertension, emphysema and prostatic symptoms, and has been denied a prostatectomy because of co-morbidities. Over the last two winters he has had several admissions for chest problems, one requiring him to have NIV.
He now presents with a one week history of diarrhoea and vomiting, leading to poor oral intake and anuria.

Initially he had only vomiting, lasting about 24–48 hours but this seems to have settled. No known haemetemesis.
The diarrhoea is yellow, fluid like and offensive and he has been opening his bowels at least 10–15 times per day. He is now incontinent of faeces.
Risk factors – he told his son he thought the vomiting may be due to a kebab he bought last Saturday evening. He has had no other contacts suffering with diarrhoea; no recent foreign travel.
He has been unable to eat or drink anything for the whole week and has been anuric for about 2–3 days
His son said he had not complained of any abdominal pain, jaundice or recent weight changes.
Over the last few days he has become increasingly confused and aggressive and has been biting people; his son also mentions he has been 'twitching'.

Examination

On examination this is a grossly unwell looking elderly patient; extremely dehydrated as evidence by – poor skin turgor, dry, cracked tongue, JVP not seen.
There were no signs of fluid overload and no signs of previous renal disease.
He had several features of uraemia including twitching of the limbs and asterixis; he is confused and agitated; AMTS = 2/10.
He was wearing a cardiac monitor and receiving oxygen via nasal prongs.
Vital observations include HR 132 bpm, BP = 85/58 mmHg, RR 24 bpm, O2 sats 84% on air, Temperature 39.5 °C ; CBG 6.4 mmol/l; urine output – none recorded at the present time.
Abdominal examination – soft, distended, unremarkable other than active/colitic bowel sounds.
DRE – liquid yellow stool; large smooth benign feeling prostate.
CV and RS examinations were likewise unremarkable with no features of heart failure or focal respiratory disease.

Data interpretation

His investigations confirm he is extremely unwell and has gone into multi-organ failure and DIC; there is evidence of

- Normocytic anaemia
- Neutrophilic leucocytosis
- Thrombocytopaenia and deranged clotting suggestive of DIC
- Severe renal impairment with hypernatraemia and hypokalaemia
- Hypoalbuminaemia
- Severe metabolic acidosis
- Type 2 respiratory failure

Management

This patient is seriously unwell and requires a high dependency care environment. He needs to be cared for in isolation with barrier nursing.

Therapeutic interventions should include:

- **Intravenous fluids** – he should receive Hartmans or saline to begin with and may benefit from an initial bolus of colloid; the volume and rate should be dictated by his response including HR, BP and urine output – targets should be HR < 100 bpm, BP > 100 mmHg systolic and U.O. > 0.5 ml/kg/hr
- **Intravenous antibiotics** – after discussion with a microbiologist
- **He will need oxygen at 2 l/min (target O_2 sats > 88%).**

An early decision should be made with the family around escalation of the therapy and resuscitation, balanced according to the patient's previous wishes, the family's wishes and the likely poor prognosis.

Further reading and web links

www.survivingsepsis.org/Pages/default.aspx
www.nc-hi.com/pdf%20files/certifiers_guidance_v2_tcm69-21289.pdf

Scenario 6: 'Washed out and totally drained'

Station 1

History *10-minute station*

You are the FY1 in a busy inner city GP practice. The next patient, Mrs Jenna Smith, has made an appointment to see the GP, and has kindly agreed to see you first.

- **Please take a comprehensive history with a view to making a diagnosis. You will be asked to present your history to the examiner at the end of the station.**

You will be assessed on the following areas, as well as the content and diagnostic reasoning of your history – take them into account in your presentation.

Professionalism

- Professional appearance (NHS dress code) – including general appearance, hair and jewellery
- Maintains patient and personal safety
- Polite introduction; identifies patient or interviewee correctly; confirms patient's date of birth from name band or other source
- Obtains informal consent; maintains patient's privacy
- Displays empathetic and caring attitudes and behaviours throughout.

Process

- Good organisation and structure; appropriate use of open and closed questions
- Appropriate fluency/rhythm/pace to the interview – this may change depending on environment and acute nature of the problem
- Appropriate time for the patient to respond/reply to questions
- Appropriate acknowledgement of difficult or emotional areas of the patient's history.

Communication skills

- Demonstrates caring and sympathetic attitude
- Asks open questions
- Invites patient to ask questions and answers them appropriately
- Addresses patient's ideas, concerns and expectations.

Station 2

Examination *10-minute station*

The GP agrees that Mrs Smith may have hypothyroidism and asks you to perform an appropriate clinical assessment.

- **Please examine this patient, including assessment of her:**
  Thyroid status
  Neck for any possible masses
  Any signs of autoimmune disease.

Equipment required for this examination: chair, glass of water, reflex hammer.

- **Once you have completed your assessment you should present the relevant findings (given within the station) to the GP in an appropriate manner for a busy GP surgery.**

You will be assessed on the following areas, as well as the content and skills of your examination – take them into account in your presentation.

Professionalism

- Professional appearance; maintains infection control standards, including hand cleaning and appropriate use of gloves and aprons
- Maintains patient and personal safety
- Polite introduction; identifies patient and confirms date of birth from name band or other source
- Obtains informal consent; maintains patient privacy and dignity
- Displays empathetic and caring attitudes and behaviours throughout.

Process

- Appropriate fluency/rhythm/pace to the examination – this may change depending on environment and acute nature of problem
- Good organisation and structure of examination; sensitive and empathetic approach
- Uses appropriate clinical techniques throughout
- Maintains privacy and dignity throughout.

Clinical communication

- Explains proposed examination/procedure; explains examination/procedure as it proceeds
- Offers information in a clear, structured and fluent manner, avoiding jargon
- Listens to patient and responds appropriately
- Demonstrates appropriate body language.

Please read the information below before presenting this case to the GP as if you were in a busy GP surgery.
[NB If you have a model do not read this section]

Clinical findings

- o Patient generally looking well but has a rather 'full' face and hair is dry and coarse; alert and orientated; of note she has vitiligo over her upper limbs and chest
- o Assessment of thyroid status – generally dry cool peripheries; no obvious tremor, palmar erythema or onycholysis; no thyroid acropachy; in the upper limbs there was marked vitiligo but no signs of proximal myopathy; no signs of thyroid eye disease; patient's voice is a little slow but has a normal quality to it
  Examination of lower limbs shows slow relaxing ankle reflexes; no sign of pre-tibial myxoedema;
  Assessment of neck is unremarkable with no obvious goitre, neck masses or lymphadenopathy; apart from the vitiligo, no other signs of autoimmune disease
- o In summary, this is a previously fit and well woman who now presents with signs consistent with hypothyroidism. This is most likely to be autoimmune in nature, as she has marked vitiligo.

Station 3

Data interpretation *10-minute station*

- The GP asks you to look at a number of thyroid function test (TFT) results that she has gathered from patients over the last few years. She asks you to match the various TFTs with the most likely diagnosis from the list below.

Diagnoses

Euthyroid
Hypopituitarism (secondary hypothyroidism)
Poor adherence to thyroxine therapy
Primary hypothyroidism
Primary thyrotoxicosis
Sick euthyroid syndrome
T3 thyrotoxicosis
TSH-secreting tumour (secondary thyrotoxicosis)

Patient	TSH (0.3–3.5 mU/l)	T_3 (1.2–3.1nmol/l)	$_fT_4$ (13–30 pmol/l)	Diagnosis
A	67.2	0.9	0.5	
B	0.05	39.1	14.5	
C	2.4	1.1	9.7	
D	4.0	12.6	54.2	
E	0.05	8.9	50.7	
F	2.4	2.9	24.6	
G	7.4	1.6	13.9	
H	0.21	2.0	11.8	

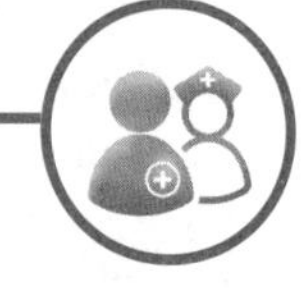

Station 4

Clinical communication skills *10-minute station*

Mrs Smith returns to the practice 10 days later to receive her results and to hear about any possible treatment. Her results are shown below:

TSH (0.3–3.5 mU/l)	49.8
T_3 (1.2–3.1 nmol/l)	0.84
$_fT_4$ (13–30 pmol/l)	3.9
a-TPO antibodies – highly positive	

- **The GP asks you to explain the results, her diagnosis, and the management of this condition to Mrs Smith.**

Station 5

Prescribing skills *10-minute station*

Part 1:

- **The Practice computer has 'gone down' and the GP asks you to write up an FP10 for Mrs Smith's loading course of thyroxine. Use the FP10 charts on page 368 and a copy of the BNF.**

Details

Mrs Jenna Smith; DOB: 11/07/1976; No known drug allergies

Part 2:

- While you are writing out the FP10 the GP sets you a quiz on medications and the thyroid gland. For each of the following questions, please indicate whether the statement is True or False.
  1. Another patient in the practice, Mrs JB, is on a 'block and replace' regime for her thyrotoxicosis. This regime includes steroids to dampen the autoimmune response.
  2. Propylthiouracil is used in the treatment of thyrotoxicosis. An important side-effect includes agranulocytosis.
  3. Patients taking the anti-arrhythmic amiodarone should be counselled about its effects on the thyroid gland. The main effects of amiodarone are related to it being composed of over one-third iodine.
  4. Common effects of amiodarone in the first few months of treatment include a suppression of TSH and T4, with an elevated T3 level.
  5. Patients taking lithium therapy should also be counselled about its effects on the thyroid. Lithium commonly blocks thyroid hormone release, causing hypothyroidism.
  6. The commonest effect of lithium on the thyroid is to induce a smooth, non-tender goitre.
  7. Patients taking thyroxine and H_2 antagonists should be warned that the absorption of thyroxine may be severely reduced if taken at the same time.
  8. Patients taking thyroxine and phenytoin are more likely to become thyrotoxic than those not taking phenytoin.

Remember: DRUG DRs **D**on't **F**orget **S**igning **O**ff (page 373)

Answers

Station 1 – History

Patient script

You are Mrs Jenna Smith (DOB 11 July 1976), a 35-year-old housewife, previously fit and well. Over the past 4–5 months you have felt increasingly 'tired, washed out, and totally drained'.

You were previously a very active and energetic person who gave up your full-time job as an insurance broker to start a family. You have spent the last 10 years or so bringing up three very lively children, now aged 5, 8 and 10 years. Recently things should have become a lot easier, because they are now all at school, and this is why you are a bit concerned. Although looking after the kids keeps you very busy, and can be very challenging, you are now able to have some time to yourself and have tried to start doing some exercise at the gym in the local sports centre. At first you thought the tiredness was simply a result of all the exercise but it just hasn't got any better.

You are married to 'a wonderful man, Doug' who is a chef for a large catering company and although things have been a bit tight recently, 'what with the economy and all', you are financially managing pretty well. You were hoping to go back to work in the coming few months but can't face it if you feel so tired.

You should not volunteer any of the following information unless directly asked. You have no respiratory or cardiovascular symptoms.

You have noticed that you are putting on 'quite a bit of weight' (maybe nearly a stone (6–7 kg) or so) and can't seem to shift it; you know this sounds a bit vain but 'my face looks podgy and horrible, like I'm letting myself go to pot ... when I'm definitely not'.
You have also noticed you've been a bit constipated, which is unusual for you. Your appetite is OK and you haven't had any other upper or lower GI problems.

You have no urinary symptoms, but your periods have been 'a bit all over the place' recently. Normally they would be very regular, 3–4/26–29, but recently they have been from 3 weeks to 2 months apart – the last started a few days ago. Doubt you are pregnant as you had a sterilisation after your third child, BUT you have also noticed that you're not very interested in sex lately and can't remember the last time you had intercourse.

You've had real problems concentrating over the last few months and seem to fall asleep at the drop of a hat. You enjoy doing the Guardian Saturday crossword but never seem to finish it ... and 'don't really care one way or the other'.

You are frustrated with the way you feel but are not low or sad. You deny any other features suggestive of depression and are looking forward to feeling better and perhaps going back to work.
PMH – sterilization, nothing else of note.
You are on no medications and have no known drug allergies.

Your mother had thyroid problems and your sister has pernicious anaemia; 'of course I got the vitiligo!'

You live in a three-bedroom house with your family; you previously smoked 10–20 cigarettes per day (aged 16–25) but gave up when you became pregnant with your first child. You enjoy a glass of white wine with your meals and probably drink a bottle or two per week (rarely any more); you don't take any illicit drugs.

Talking to your mum, you think you may have developed thyroid problems and are hoping that it's nothing more serious. Your mum told you that a simple blood test could prove whether the thyroid is OK or not, and you are hoping the GP can organise this as soon as possible.

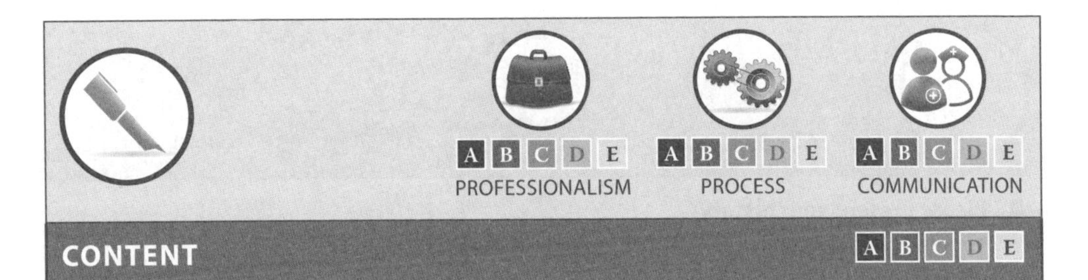

CONTENT

A B C D E

Identifies key information

- Very fit and well until 6 months ago with no significant previous medical history
- Insidious progression over the last 5–6 months
- General malaise and loss of energy – 'washed out and drained'.

Identifies important negatives, including systemic enquiry

- Weight gain
- Constipation
- Change in facial appearance
- Change in menstrual cycle
- Poor concentration
- Sleeping a lot and loss of energy
- Loss of libido
- Excludes biological and other features of depression – early morning waking, loss of appetite, loss of interest in family and friends, activities and hobbies.

Identifies key information from rest of the history

- Three children – keep her busy and are quite tiring
- Children all now in school, so 'life has become a lot easier'
- Hoping to go back to work – but feeling too tired.

Completing the patient history

- Drug and allergy history: nil
- Previous medical history – sterilisation after third child, nil else
- FHx – strongly positive for autoimmune disease; mother has thyroid problems
- Social and occupational history: lives with family; husband (Doug) is a chef for large catering company; ex-smoker (16–25 years); alcohol – a bottle or two of wine per week (about 14 units); no illicit drugs.

Summarises important areas of the history back to the patient

Invites patient to ask questions and is able to deal with them appropriately

Establishes patient's ideas, concerns and expectations

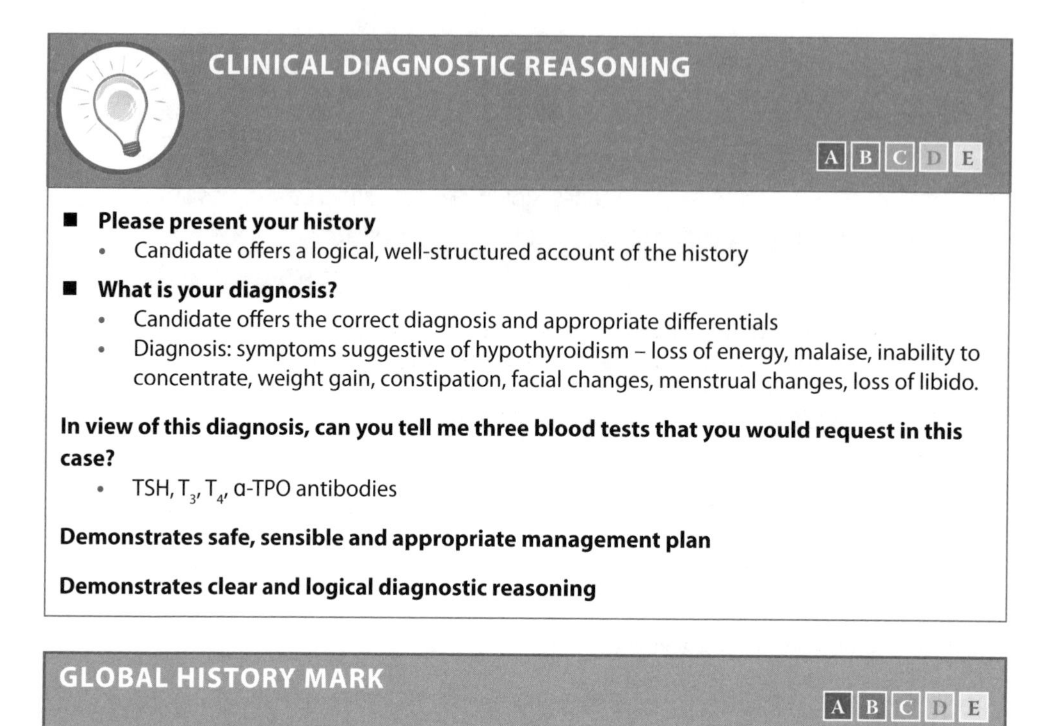

CLINICAL DIAGNOSTIC REASONING

A B C D E

- **Please present your history**
  - Candidate offers a logical, well-structured account of the history
- **What is your diagnosis?**
  - Candidate offers the correct diagnosis and appropriate differentials
  - Diagnosis: symptoms suggestive of hypothyroidism – loss of energy, malaise, inability to concentrate, weight gain, constipation, facial changes, menstrual changes, loss of libido.

In view of this diagnosis, can you tell me three blood tests that you would request in this case?

- TSH, T_3, T_4, α-TPO antibodies

Demonstrates safe, sensible and appropriate management plan

Demonstrates clear and logical diagnostic reasoning

GLOBAL HISTORY MARK

A B C D E

Station 2 – Examination

Patient script

If you are an actor/patient, read the patient history and physical signs fully – when the candidate comes to an abnormal site in their examination, act-out tenderness and/or volunteer the relevant physical sign.

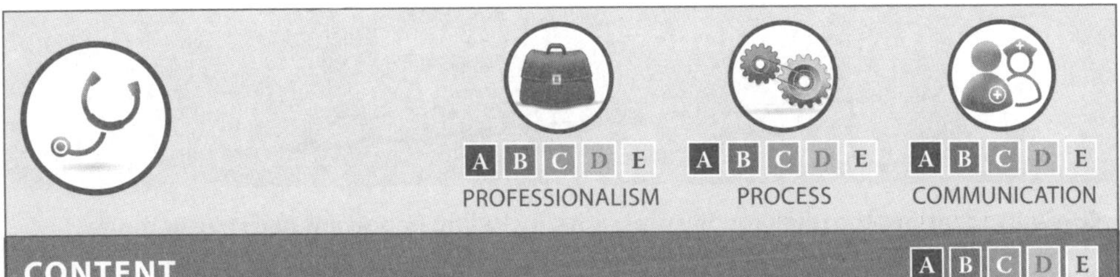

CONTENT

A B C D E

Exposes and positions patient correctly and maintains comfort

- Patient should be sat in a chair with neck fully exposed

Comments on wellbeing of patient, ie well or unwell

'Feet to face'

Observes and comments on patient and surroundings after taking a step back away from the seated patient

- Habitus – fat vs thin, hair and complexion, mood, concentration, obvious signs of thyroid dysfunction, goitre.

Performs and comments on relevant observations

- HR – bradycardia vs tachycardia
- BP – systolic hypertension (thyrotoxicosis)
- CBG (DM)
- Requests height and weight to calculate BMI (not presently known).

Assessment of thyroid status, signs of thyroid disease, signs of autoimmune disease

- Hands and upper limbs, including: vitiligo (dorsum of hands and upper limbs); nails – onycholysis, thyroid acropachy; hands cool and dry vs warm and sweaty; palms – palmar erythema, anaemia; fine tremor of outstretched hands; pulse – HR/regularity; proximal myopathy
- Face: thin and sweaty vs peaches and cream/toad-like facies; dry hair, loss of outer third of eyebrow; croaky voice
- Eyes: exophthalmos, proptosis, cranial nerve palsies, lid lag, injection of sclera
- Lower limbs: comments on presence/absence of pre-tibial myxoedema; ankle jerks – slow relaxing reflexes.

Formal assessment of the neck

- Observes neck anteriorally – comments on presence or absence of neck masses
- Asks patient to sip then swallow a mouthful of water – observing anterior neck
- Palpates neck from behind patient – systematic manner – excludes goitre, lymphadenopathy or other neck masses
- Auscultates over thyroid.

Looks for/comments on other signs of autoimmune disease – vitiligo, anaemia (PA), asks for CBG (DM)

Thanks patient, offers assistance, maintains patient's dignity and privacy until they are dressed

CLINICAL DIAGNOSTIC REASONING

A B C D E

Correctly identifies the relevant physical signs, including important negative findings

Is able to recount the three signs of autoimmune thyroid disease (Graves' triad)

- Thyroid acropachy
- Graves' eye signs
- Pre-tibial myxoedema.

Is able to recount the three differentiating clinical signs between hypo- and hyperthyroidism (see table below)

Thyroid status – clinical signs differentiating thyrotoxicosis from hypothyroidism		
	Thyrotoxicosis	**Hypothyroidism**
General appearance	Agitated, thin	Overweight, drowsy, poor concentration
Hands	Hot, sweaty, vasodilated	Cool, dry
	Fine tremor	
Palms	Palmar erythema	
Nails	Onycholysis	
Pulse	Tachycardia/irregular (AF)	Bradycardia
Upper limbs	Proximal myopathy	
	Systolic hypertension	
Hair		Coarse, dry hair
Face	Thin	Plump/overweight
		'Peaches and cream' complexion
Eyes	Lid lag	
Voice		Croaky quality
Goitre	Bruit	
Lower limbs		**Slow relaxing reflexes**

Signs of thyroid autoimmune disease – thyroid acropachy, Graves' orbitopathy, pre-tibial myxoedema, vitiligo

Demonstrates safe, sensible and appropriate management plan

Demonstrates clear and logical diagnostic reasoning

GLOBAL EXAMINATION MARK

A B C D E

Station 3 – Data interpretation

Patient	TSH (0.3–3.5 mU/l)	T_3 (1.2–3.1 nmol/l)	$_fT_4$ (13–30 pmol/l)	Diagnosis
A	67.2	0.9	0.5	Primary hypothroidism
B	0.05	39.1	14.5	T3 thyrotoxicosis
C	2.4	1.1	9.7	Sick euthyroid
D	4.0	12.6	54.2	TSH-secreting tumour
E	0.05	8.9	50.7	Primary thyrotoxicosis
F	2.4	2.9	24.6	Euthyroid
G	7.4	1.6	13.9	Poor adherence to thyroxine
H	0.21	2.0	11.8	Hypopituitarism

GLOBAL DATA INTERPRETATION MARK

A B C D E

Station 4 – Clinical communication skills

Patient script

You are Mrs Jenna Smith (DOB 11 July 1976), a 35-year-old housewife, previously fit and well. You have returned to the GP today for the results of your blood tests, which you had taken last week. You remember the young doctor and are happy to talk to him/her again.

The GP has pre-warned you that she agrees it may be your thyroid gland being 'underactive' and that you might need to take tablets to replace the thyroid hormones.

Ideas and concerns: you are convinced that you have developed 'thyroid problems' 'like my mum' but are slightly concerned it may all be 'nothing' and just down to your busy family life.

Expectations: you hope it will be easily treated with tablets, and you can get on with your plans to go back to work.

If asked you are happy to go on treatment.

SCENARIO 6

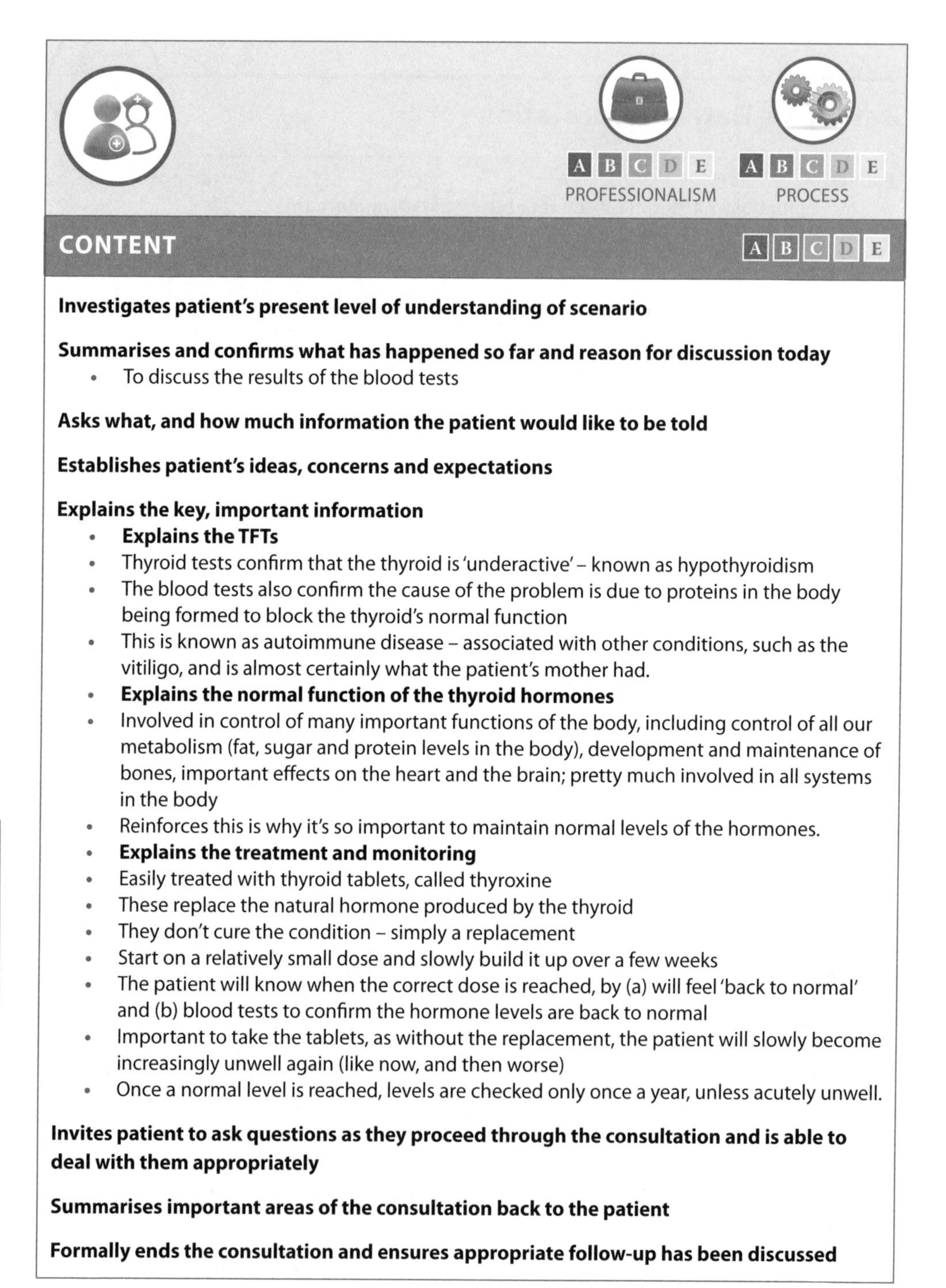

CONTENT

A B C D E

Investigates patient's present level of understanding of scenario

Summarises and confirms what has happened so far and reason for discussion today

- To discuss the results of the blood tests

Asks what, and how much information the patient would like to be told

Establishes patient's ideas, concerns and expectations

Explains the key, important information

- **Explains the TFTs**
- Thyroid tests confirm that the thyroid is 'underactive' – known as hypothyroidism
- The blood tests also confirm the cause of the problem is due to proteins in the body being formed to block the thyroid's normal function
- This is known as autoimmune disease – associated with other conditions, such as the vitiligo, and is almost certainly what the patient's mother had.
- **Explains the normal function of the thyroid hormones**
- Involved in control of many important functions of the body, including control of all our metabolism (fat, sugar and protein levels in the body), development and maintenance of bones, important effects on the heart and the brain; pretty much involved in all systems in the body
- Reinforces this is why it's so important to maintain normal levels of the hormones.
- **Explains the treatment and monitoring**
- Easily treated with thyroid tablets, called thyroxine
- These replace the natural hormone produced by the thyroid
- They don't cure the condition – simply a replacement
- Start on a relatively small dose and slowly build it up over a few weeks
- The patient will know when the correct dose is reached, by (a) will feel 'back to normal' and (b) blood tests to confirm the hormone levels are back to normal
- Important to take the tablets, as without the replacement, the patient will slowly become increasingly unwell again (like now, and then worse)
- Once a normal level is reached, levels are checked only once a year, unless acutely unwell.

Invites patient to ask questions as they proceed through the consultation and is able to deal with them appropriately

Summarises important areas of the consultation back to the patient

Formally ends the consultation and ensures appropriate follow-up has been discussed

CLINICAL DIAGNOSTIC REASONING

A B C D E

- **How long before the patient should expect to feel normal again?**
  - About 2 months or so (TSH usually within normal limits after 8–10 weeks)
- **Once she is OK, will she need any further blood tests?**
  - Not really as long as she feels well but a hormone level should be checked once a year to make sure she is not under- or over-treated

Demonstrates safe, sensible and appropriate management plan

Demonstrates clear and logical diagnostic reasoning

GLOBAL COMMUNICATION MARK

A B C D E

Station 5 – Prescribing skills

Check: DRUG DRs Don't Forget Signing Off (page 373)

Part 1:

Note: in young and healthy adults thyroxine replacement therapy may be started at a relatively high dose (50–75 µg) and titrated up over several weeks until an adequate dose (normally 125 µg) is reached. Most young healthy adults will tolerate an increased by 25 µg every 7–10 days. However, in the elderly or those with ischaemic heart disease, the starting dose is much lower, usually 25 µg, and the titration up towards 125 µg is a lot more cautious. An increase of 25 µg every 10 days to 2 weeks is sufficient. This cautious approach is to ensure that the heart is not stressed with rapid or large increase in thyroxine levels, leading to tachycardia and possible myocardial ischaemia.

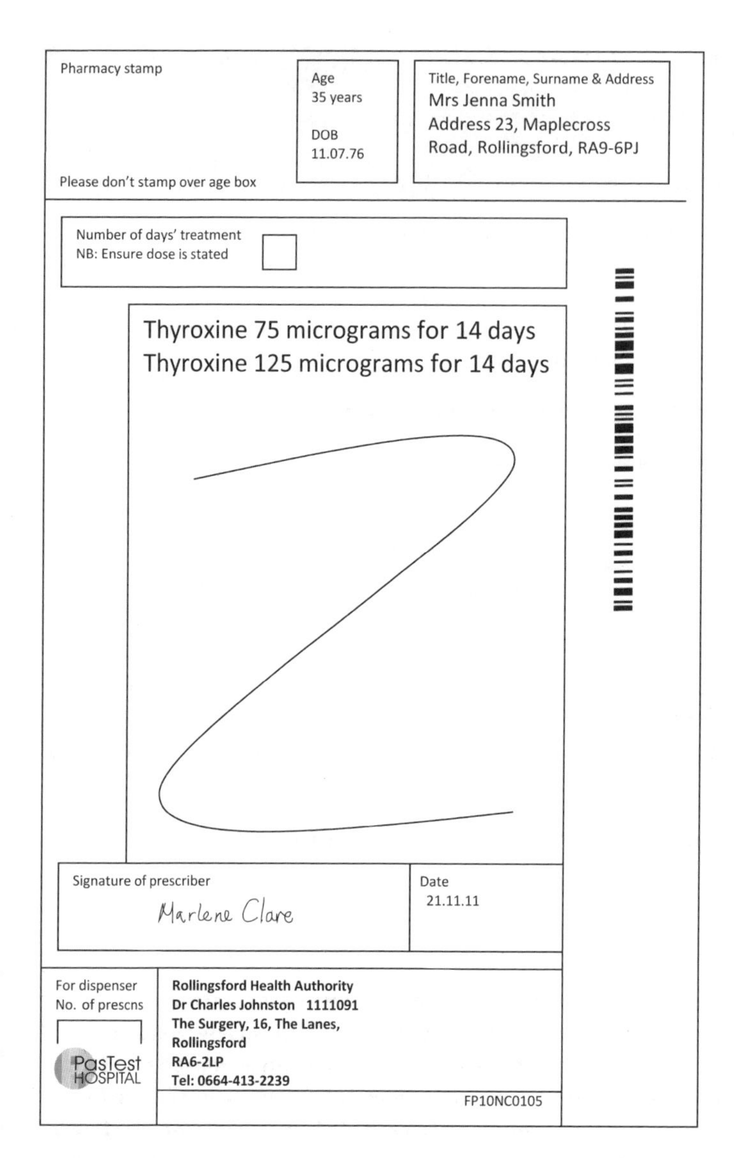

Pharmacy stamp

Please don't stamp over age box

Age
35 years

DOB
11.07.76

Title, Forename, Surname & Address
Mrs Jenna Smith
Address 23, Maplecross
Road, Rollingsford, RA9-6PJ

Number of days' treatment
NB: Ensure dose is stated

Thyroxine 75 micrograms for 14 days
Thyroxine 125 micrograms for 14 days

Signature of prescriber
Marlene Clare

Date
21.11.11

For dispenser
No. of prescns

PasTest HOSPITAL

Rollingsford Health Authority
Dr Charles Johnston 1111091
The Surgery, 16, The Lanes,
Rollingsford
RA6-2LP
Tel: 0664-413-2239

FP10NC0105

Part 2:

1. False – 'block and replace' involves giving an adequate dose of carbimazole to completely block the production of thyroid hormones, and then replacing these with exogenous thyroxine. This regime more readily dampens the autoimmune response against the thyroid, and studies suggest that it reduces the likelihood of relapse after the course of therapy has been completed (usually 18 months).

2. True – carbimazole and propylthiouracil, the commonest drugs used in the UK to treat thyrotoxicosis, both cause agranulocytosis. All patients taking these drugs should be told to seek medical assistance if they develop respiratory tract infections (or other sepsis), to check their white cell count.

3. True – amiodarone is composed of approximately 35–40% iodine. The drug leads to a massive rise in iodine levels in the body and may affect iodine metabolism, and thyroid hormone synthesis and secretion. It also exerts direct toxic effects on the thyroid. Patients commonly incur biochemical derangement in the early phases of treatment. Most commonly there is a rise in TSH, T4 and rT3, with suppression of T3, but these usually return to within normal limits after 4–6 months. Patients with underlying thyroid disease are more commonly affected than those with previously normal thyroid metabolism.

4. False – see answer 3.

5. True – lithium can have numerous effects on the hypothalamic–pituitary–thyroid axis, but most commonly it induces a smooth, non-tender goitre. It is thought its major effects are mediated by blocking the release of thyroid hormones.

6. True – see answer 5.

7. False – as with any patient being started on a new therapy, a comprehensive treatment history should be obtained for patients being started on thyroxine (see also answer 8). The absorption of thyroxine is reduced by concomitant administration of proton pump inhibitors, thus reducing its effect.

8. False – phenytoin is an enzyme inducer and will lower the effective dose of thyroxine. Thus if taken concomitantly patients taking thyroxine and phenytoin run the risk of under-treatment and thus hypothyroidism. Other enzyme inducers include carbamazepine, rifampicin, barbiturates, long-term alcohol excess, sulfonylureas (mnemonic PC BRAS):

GLOBAL PRESCRIBING MARK

A B C D E

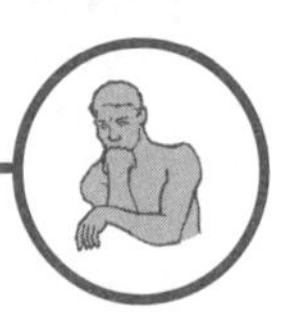

Scenario 6: Reflection and consolidation

History

This is Mrs Jenna Smith, a 35-year-old previously fit-and-well housewife. She describes herself as a previously energetic woman who has been bringing up three children and running a home. Her children are all now at school and she was looking forward to going back to work when she started to feel unwell. Over the past 4–5 months she has become increasingly tired and says she is 'washed out, and totally drained'.
Of note she has noticed significant weight gain that she estimates at about 6–7 kg; her face looks podgy and full, despite recent attempts to go to the gym. She has been constipated but has no other GI symptoms.
Her periods have been erratic and vary in duration between 3 weeks and 2 months. She has also noticed a loss of libido.
She has felt tired, falls asleep easily and is unable to concentrate, but has no unusual thought processes.
She has a strong family history of autoimmune disease – her mother had thyroid problems and her sister has pernicious anaemia; the patient has marked vitiligo.
She lives in a three-bedroom house with her husband and three children. She previously smoked 10–20 cigarettes per day (aged 16–25) but gave up when she became pregnant with her first child.
Alcohol – she enjoys a glass of white wine with meals and estimates she drinks a bottle or two per week (rarely any more); no illicit drugs.

Examination

On examination of this patient sitting in a chair, she was generally well looking but had a rather 'full' face and her hair was rather dry and coarse. She was noted to be alert and orientated. Of note she has vitiligo over her upper limbs and chest.
On assessment of her thyroid status, she had generally dry cool peripheries. There was no obvious tremor, palmar erythema or onycholysis. There was no thyroid acropachy.
In the upper limbs there was marked vitiligo but no signs of proximal myopathy.
Examination of her face showed her to have dry coarse hair with loss of the outer third of her eyebrow – her face was 'plump'.
There were no signs of thyroid eye disease.
Her voice was a little slow but had a normal quality to it.
Examination of her lower limbs showed slow relaxing ankle reflexes; there was no sign of pre-tibial myxoedema.
Assessment of her neck was unremarkable with no obvious goitre, neck masses or lymphadenopathy.
Apart from the vitiligo there were no other signs of autoimmune disease.
In summary this is a previously fit and well woman who now presents with signs consistent with hypothyroidism. This is most likely to be autoimmune in nature as she has marked vitiligo.

Data interpretation

She has a grossly elevated TSH with suppressed levels of fT4 and T3, and highly positive titres of auto-antibodies. She requires testing for other auto-antibodies.
Other blood tests that may become deranged in hypothyroidism include: FBC – macrocytosis; U&Es – hyponatraemia; raised AST and CK (myopathy).
This patient's blood tests confirm that she has primary autoimmune hypothyroidism.

Management

Thyroid replacement with thyroxine should be initiated as soon as possible. See note regarding thyroxine titration (page 111).

Further reading and web links

www.cks.nhs.uk/clinical_topics/by_clinical_specialty/endocrine_and_metabolic
www.bcguidelines.ca/pdf/thyroid.pdf

Scenario 7: 'Breathless patient'

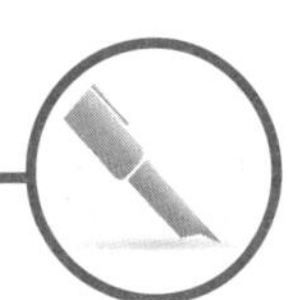

Station 1

History *10-minute station*

You are a FY1 doctor. Today you are on call for general medicine in the Medical Admissions Unit. Mrs Deirdre Hodge has been referred from the Emergency Department with a 2-week history of cough, shortness of breath and feeling generally unwell.

- **Please take a comprehensive history from Mrs Hodge with a view to making a diagnosis. You will be asked to present your history to the examiner at the end of the station.**

You will be assessed on the following areas, as well as the content and diagnostic reasoning of your history – take them into account in your presentation.

Professionalism

- Professional appearance (NHS dress code) – including general appearance, hair and jewellery
- Maintains patient and personal safety
- Polite introduction; identifies patient or interviewee correctly; confirms patient's date of birth from name band or other source
- Obtains informal consent; maintains patient's privacy
- Displays empathetic and caring attitudes and behaviours throughout.

Process

- Good organisation and structure; appropriate use of open and closed questions
- Appropriate fluency/rhythm/pace to the interview – this may change depending on environment and acute nature of the problem
- Appropriate time for the patient to respond/reply to questions
- Appropriate acknowledgement of difficult or emotional areas of the patient's history.

Communication skills

- Demonstrates caring and sympathetic attitude
- Asks open questions
- Invites patient to ask questions and answers them appropriately
- Addresses patient's ideas, concerns and expectations.

Station 2

Examination *10-minute station*

Mrs Hodge is tachypnoeic and very breathless during your history-taking. After you apply some oxygen (15 litres via a reservoir mask) you ask one of the nurses on the admissions unit monitored bay to complete a set of observations.

- **Please complete a general assessment of the patient with a focused respiratory examination.**
- **Once you have completed your assessment you should present the relevant findings (given within the station) to the ST3 Medical Registrar on call, who will then ask you about your initial management of this patient.**

You will be assessed on the following areas, as well as the content and skills of your examination – take them into account in your presentation.

Professionalism

- Professional appearance; maintains infection control standards, including hand cleaning and appropriate use of gloves and aprons
- Maintains patient and personal safety
- Polite introduction; identifies patient and confirms date of birth from name band or other source
- Obtains informal consent; maintains patient privacy and dignity
- Displays empathetic and caring attitudes and behaviours throughout.

Process

- Appropriate fluency/rhythm/pace to the examination – this may change depending on environment and acute nature of problem
- Good organisation and structure of examination; sensitive and empathetic approach
- Uses appropriate clinical techniques throughout
- Maintains privacy and dignity throughout.

Clinical communication

- Explains proposed examination/procedure; explains examination/procedure as it proceeds
- Offers information in a clear, structured and fluent manner, avoiding jargon
- Listens to patient and responds appropriately
- Demonstrates appropriate body language.

Please read the information below before presenting this case to the ST3 Medical Registrar as if you were on a busy medical take.
[NB If you have a model do not read this section]

Clinical findings

- o **Patient appears dyspnoeic as rest, using accessory muscles of respiration**
- o **Observations – HR 105 bpm, BP 112/75 mmHg, RR 30 bpm, O_2 sats 92% on air, 100% on 85% O_2, temperature 39.9 °C, GCS 15/15, peripheral capillary refill time <2 seconds, pulse regular in rhythm**
- o **RS examination – not cyanotic but able to complete only short sentences**
  Focused examination – no scars on thorax, reduced chest expansion on right side, decreased percussion note at right middle and upper zone
  On auscultation – reduced breath sounds in right upper and middle zones, reduced vocal resonance in right middle and upper zone
- o **CV examination – heart sounds easily heard, normal.**

Station 3

Procedural skills *10-minute station*

- **Your working diagnosis is that of pneumonia – using the equipment provided, take a peripheral blood culture before the administration of antibiotics.**

Equipment provided

- **Sterile cannulation pack with disposable tourniquet, dressing and gauze**
- **Cleaning swab for skin, such as ChloraPrep®**
- **Peripheral blood culture bottles – aerobic and anaerobic**
- **20 ml syringe**
- **22G needles ×3**
- **Alcohol swabs ×2**
- **Bedside sharps disposal bin.**

- **Using the equipment provided, insert an IV cannula in order to facilitate Mrs Hodge's resuscitation.**

Equipment provided

- **Sterile cannulation pack with disposable tourniquet, IV dressing and gauze**
- **Cleaning swab for skin, such as ChloraPrep®**
- **IV cannula of suitable gauge**
- **0.9% saline flush and connector.**

Station 4

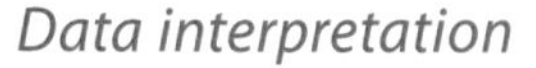

Data interpretation *10-minute station*

Mrs Hodge has had her basic investigations sent and her chest X-ray shows a right upper lobe consolidation. Her ABGs show type 1 respiratory failure with a PO_2 of 10.4 on high-flow oxygen. Her FBC shows a raised WCC with a lymphocytosis. Her biochemical profile demonstrates hyponatraemia of 127 mmol/l.

- **As a training exercise, your Registrar has collected abnormal blood results from a number of patients. She asks you to match the patient, diagnosis and biochemical abnormality from the table below.**

Patient	Biochemical abnormalities	Diagnosis
1 A 49-year-old man with dyspnoea, wheeze, flushing and diarrhoea	(A) Na^+ 145 mmol/l K^+ 2.1 mmol/l	(a) Liver metastases
2 A 50-year-old man with dry cough, fever and vomiting, and confusion	(B) AST 57 U/l ALP 567 U/l	(b) Ectopic ACTH
3 A 61-year-old man with confusion and seizures	(C) Urine 5-HIAA 55 mg/24 hr	(c) Ectopic PTH
4 A 68-year-old man with jaundice and 8 cm hepatomegaly	(D) Ca^{++} 4.07 mmol/l	(d) SIADH
5 A 47-year-old man with striae, hypertension, proximal myopathy and oedema	(E) Na 106 K 3.9 mmol/l	(e) Carcinoid syndrome

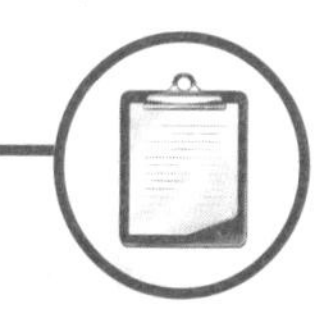

Station 5

Prescribing skills *10-minute station*

- **Mrs Hodge is being admitted to the hospital for treatment of her presumed pneumonia. You are been asked to prescribe her initial therapy on her inpatient drug chart. Using the charts on page 368 and the BNF provided please prescribe your initial therapy for Mrs Hodge, including:**

Oxygen
Thromboprophylaxis
Analgesia as required

Details

Mrs Deidre Hodge; DOB: 01/12/1961; No known drug allergies; Weight: 69 kg; Ward: MAU; Consultant: Dr Reilly

FBC: Hb 13.7 g/dl, MCV 89 fl, WCC 21.4 × 10^9/l, neutrophils 18.4 × 10^9/l, platelets 345 × 10^9/l

U&Es: Na^+ 126 mmol/l, K^+ 4.3 mmol/l, urea 12.4 mmol/l, creatinine 115 μmol/l

RBG: 6.2 mmol/l

CCa^{2+} 2.45 mol/l, PO_4^- 0.78 mmol/l, Mg 1.02 mmol/l

CRP 245

Clotting – INR 1.1

ECG – sinus tachycardia

CXR – right upper lobe consolidation.

Remember: DRUG DRs Don't Forget Signing Off (page 373)

Station 6

Clinical communication skills *10-minute station*

Mrs Hodge has been treated on the Medical Admissions Unit for the last 12 hours with antibiotics and high-flow oxygen. Her ABG shows that she is in type 1 respiratory failure with a pH 7.32, PO_2 7.9 and PCO_2 of 3.24. She appears tired but remains alert, with a GCS of 15. Your Registrar has decided to transfer her to the Medical High Dependency Unit to start non-invasive ventilatory support (continuous positive airway pressure, or CPAP).

- Please explain the situation to Mrs Hodge and her husband, who are both understandably very concerned about her condition. The information you must include is:
  - Mrs Hodge's current clinical status
  - Benefits of CPAP – to improve oxygenation
  - How CPAP is delivered – through a tight-fitting mask
  - Complications and problems with CPAP – discomfort, failure of treatment
  - If it fails, Mrs Hodge may need to be admitted to the ICU.

Answers

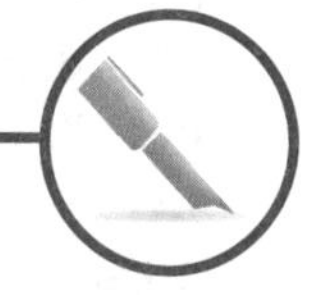

Station 1 – History

Patient script

You are a 50-year-old teacher, DOB 15 November 1961, who has been feeling very unwell for the last 4 days. Initially you felt you had a viral illness as you were feeling lethargic and achy and had a headache that would not improve with paracetamol.

However, over the last 2 days you have developed an extremely high fever and a dry cough. You can take a deep breath, but converse in short sentences. You have not been able to eat or drink anything for 24 hours. You have developed diarrhoea, and have had at least eight episodes today, which is very loose but of a normal colour. You were going to visit your GP today but you were too breathless to dress and leave the house. So your husband then called the ambulance service, who brought you to hospital.

Your medical history includes type 2 diabetes (diet-treated only), and hypercholesterolaemia. Your only regular medication is simvastatin, and you have no known drug allergies. You have never had anything like this before. You live with your husband in your own home and have no pets. You are a non-smoker and you enjoy drinking wine (approximately 10 units per week). You have two children of 14 and 17 and there is no family history of diabetes or other serious illnesses.

You are very active and love to travel. Indeed, you returned from a holiday in Greece only 5 days before you became unwell. You were well on this holiday and stayed in a small hotel; you do not know if anyone else from the hotel became unwell.

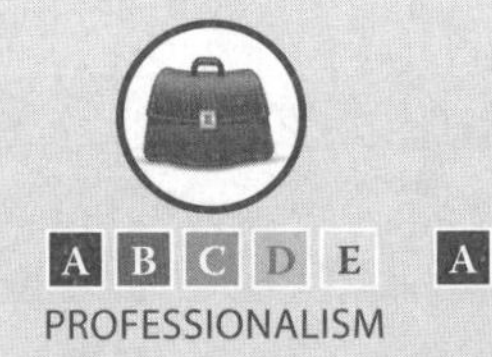

A B C D E PROFESSIONALISM

A B C D E PROCESS

A B C D E COMMUNICATION

CONTENT

A B C D E

Identifies key information

- Duration of illness including prodrome
- Presence of fever, shortness of breath and non-productive cough
- Presence of vomiting or diarrhoea

Includes important negatives, including systemic enquiry

- No chest pain or haemoptysis
- No confusion or decreasing consciousness
- No focal weakness

Identifies key information from rest of history

- Elicits travel history, including presence of hotel air-conditioning

Completing the patient history

- Relevant factors from employment, housing, social support
- Previous medical history: hypercholesterolaemia; type 2 diabetes – treated by diet
- Social and occupational history: non-smoker; alcohol intake of 10 units per week; no pets
- Drug and allergy history: simvastatin; no known drug allergies
- No relevant family history

Summarises important areas of the history back to the patient

Invites patient to ask questions and is able to deal with them appropriately

Establishes patient's ideas, concerns and expectations

CLINICAL DIAGNOSTIC REASONING

A B C D E

- **Please present your history**
  - Candidate offers a logical, well-structured account of the history.
- **What is your diagnosis?**
  - Candidate offers the correct diagnosis and appropriate differentials
  - The combination of systemic upset with headache, high-grade fever and progressive respiratory symptoms are suggestive of an atypical pneumonia but a sensible differential diagnosis would include influenza, community acquired pneumonia, or a viral lower respiratory tract infection.
- **What are the likely causative organisms?**
  - *Legionella pneumophila*: most likely, as gives a high-grade fever and gastrointestinal upset, and is also often contracted from environments with a source of stagnant water such as air-conditioning that is then aerosolised; this type of atypical pneumonia can be rapidly progressive and has a high mortality; it is a notifiable disease (www.hpa.org.uk)
  - *Mycoplasma pneumoniae*: pneumonia in younger patients, often with neurological symptoms and rashes such as erythema mulitforme
  - *Chlamydia pneumoniae*: milder form of atypical pneumonia with less severe symptoms; patients often confuse it with influenza.

GLOBAL HISTORY MARK

A B C D E

Station 2 – Examination

Patient script

If you are an actor/patient, read the patient history and physical signs fully – when the candidate comes to an abnormal site in their examination, act-out tenderness and/or volunteer the relevant physical sign.

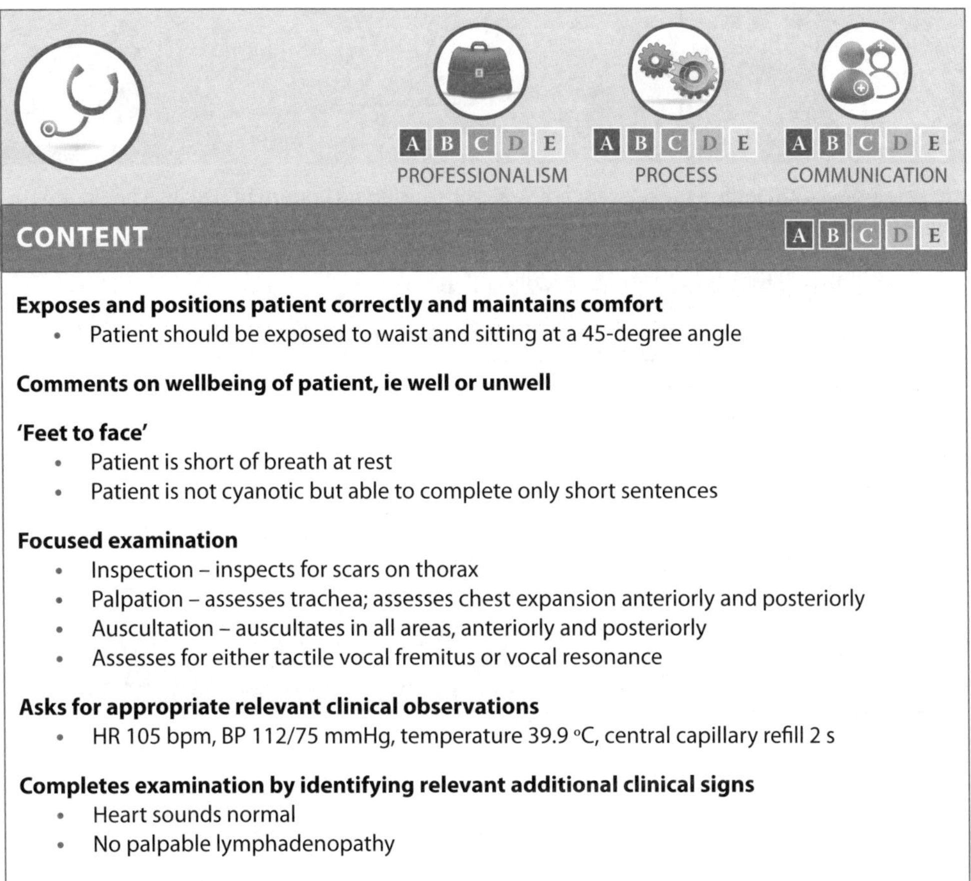

Exposes and positions patient correctly and maintains comfort

- Patient should be exposed to waist and sitting at a 45-degree angle

Comments on wellbeing of patient, ie well or unwell

'Feet to face'

- Patient is short of breath at rest
- Patient is not cyanotic but able to complete only short sentences

Focused examination

- Inspection – inspects for scars on thorax
- Palpation – assesses trachea; assesses chest expansion anteriorly and posteriorly
- Auscultation – auscultates in all areas, anteriorly and posteriorly
- Assesses for either tactile vocal fremitus or vocal resonance

Asks for appropriate relevant clinical observations

- HR 105 bpm, BP 112/75 mmHg, temperature 39.9 °C, central capillary refill 2 s

Completes examination by identifying relevant additional clinical signs

- Heart sounds normal
- No palpable lymphadenopathy

Thanks patient, offers assistance, maintains patient's dignity and privacy until they are dressed

CLINICAL DIAGNOSTIC REASONING

A B C D E

- Correctly identifies the relevant physical signs, including important negative findings
- Does not identify signs that are not present
- Pyrexia, tachypnoea and low oxygen saturations
- Decreased breath sounds right middle and upper zone

Demonstrates safe, sensible and appropriate management plan, including:

- Oxygen (high flow 15 l/min via a reservoir bag)
- IV access and blood tests
- Arterial blood gas analysis
- CXR
- Blood cultures and antibiotics
- Urinary antigen for *Legionella*

Demonstrates clear and logical diagnostic reasoning

GLOBAL EXAMINATION MARK

A B C D E

Station 3 – Procedural skills

Procedure A: Blood culture

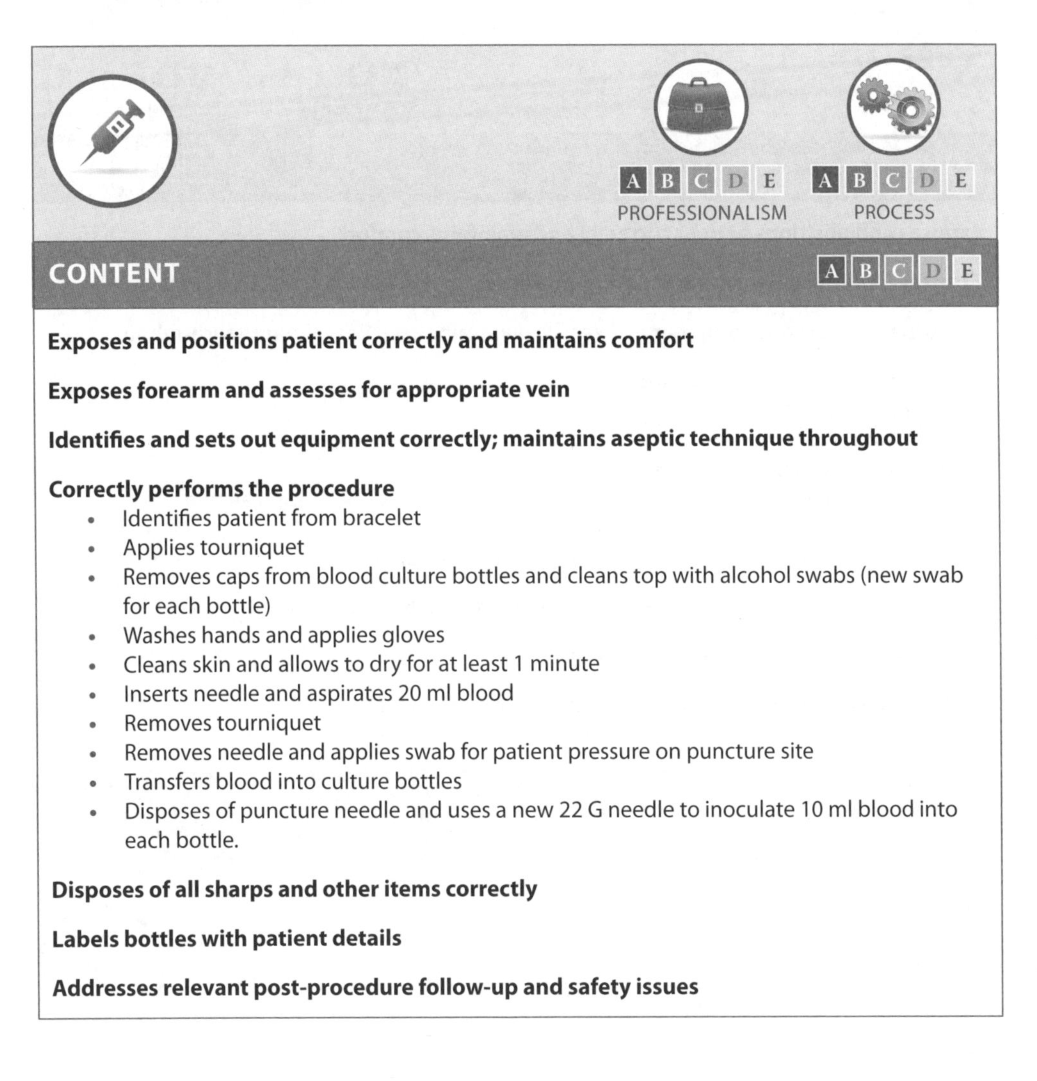

A B C D E
PROFESSIONALISM

A B C D E
PROCESS

CONTENT A B C D E

Exposes and positions patient correctly and maintains comfort

Exposes forearm and assesses for appropriate vein

Identifies and sets out equipment correctly; maintains aseptic technique throughout

Correctly performs the procedure

- Identifies patient from bracelet
- Applies tourniquet
- Removes caps from blood culture bottles and cleans top with alcohol swabs (new swab for each bottle)
- Washes hands and applies gloves
- Cleans skin and allows to dry for at least 1 minute
- Inserts needle and aspirates 20 ml blood
- Removes tourniquet
- Removes needle and applies swab for patient pressure on puncture site
- Transfers blood into culture bottles
- Disposes of puncture needle and uses a new 22 G needle to inoculate 10 ml blood into each bottle.

Disposes of all sharps and other items correctly

Labels bottles with patient details

Addresses relevant post-procedure follow-up and safety issues

Procedure B: Cannulation

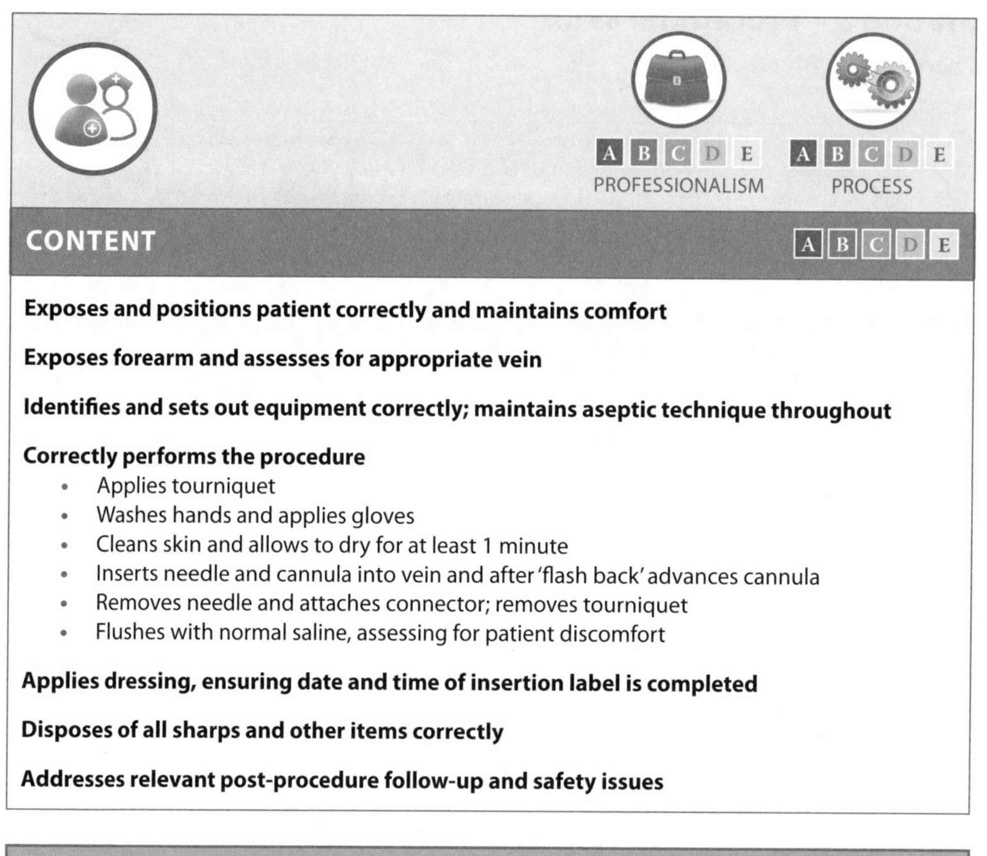

A B C D E
PROFESSIONALISM

A B C D E
PROCESS

CONTENT A B C D E

Exposes and positions patient correctly and maintains comfort

Exposes forearm and assesses for appropriate vein

Identifies and sets out equipment correctly; maintains aseptic technique throughout

Correctly performs the procedure

- Applies tourniquet
- Washes hands and applies gloves
- Cleans skin and allows to dry for at least 1 minute
- Inserts needle and cannula into vein and after 'flash back' advances cannula
- Removes needle and attaches connector; removes tourniquet
- Flushes with normal saline, assessing for patient discomfort

Applies dressing, ensuring date and time of insertion label is completed

Disposes of all sharps and other items correctly

Addresses relevant post-procedure follow-up and safety issues

GLOBAL PROCEDURE MARK A B C D E

Station 4 – Data interpretation

1 (C) (e)

The carcinoid syndrome is more commonly associated with gastrointestinal tumours but is well recognised with pulmonary lesions. The tumours produce 5HT, which causes wheeze and diarrhoea. The flushing is caused by various mediators, including substance P, kallikrein and bradykinins.

2 (D) (c)

Hypercalcaemia associated with lung tumours may be caused by ectopic parathyroid hormone, bony metastases, cyclic-AMP-stimulating factor or prostaglandin. Ectopic

parathyroid hormone is most commonly expressed by squamous cell carcinomas. Initial therapy should include intravenous rehydration and the use of intravenous bisphosphonates followed by oral maintenance therapy.

3 (E) (d)

The SIADH is caused by *Legionella* spp. pneumonia. SIADH is proven by a paired urinary and plasma osmolality, where the urinary osmolality is raised relative to the plasma osmolality. The urinary sodium may be normal or raised but the plasma sodium is always low. Other criteria for diagnosing SIADH include normal renal and adrenal function and the absence of hypotension, hypovolaemia and oedema.

4 (B) (a)

Lung tumours metastasise to lymph nodes, brain, liver and bone. The enlarged liver feels hard and 'craggy' and may present with jaundice or deranged LFTs.

5 (A) (b)

Small cell tumours and bronchial carcinoid may both produce ectopic ACTH. The patient presents with the familiar clinical features of Cushing's syndrome but is characterised by severe malaise and hypokalaemic metabolic alkalosis.

GLOBAL DATA INTERPRETATION MARK A B C D E

Station 5 – Prescribing skills

Check: DRUG DRs Don't Forget Signing Off (page 373)

Allergies, sensitivities and adverse drug reactions					Patient details/addressograph
No known allergies ✓		Initials LIL	Gender M / (F)		NHS/ Hospital No: 7017334
Not possible to ascertain ☐		Date 13.01	Weight (kg)	Date	
Medicine/substance	Reaction & Severity	Initials & Date	69	13.01	Surname: HODGE
			Height		First name: DEIRDRE
			1.62m		
Alerts			Surface area (m²)		Date of birth: 01.12.61

IN-PATIENT MEDICATION PRESCRIPTION AND ADMINISTRATION RECORD

PasTest HOSPITAL

Consultant	Trainee Dr. Name and Bleep no.	Date of admission	Date chart reboarded	Estimated date of discharge
REILLY	LILIS 164	13.01.12		
This chart is no. 1 of 1	Transcribing Check by Pharmacy Sign .... Date	Ward 1. MAU 2.		

SCENARIO 7

As required medications				
Medication PARACETAMOL				Date
Indication				Time
Dose 1g	Route PO	Maximum frequency / dose 6 hour	Start date 21/11	Dose
			Stop date	Route
Signature LIL 164			Bleep no. 601	Given
Additional instructions:				Pharmacy

Thromboprophylaxis please prescribe treatment regimens in the regular medications section						
Choice of mechanical prophylaxis and leg(s) to be applied to						Enter Time / Enter details below
Graduated elastic compression stockings	Intermittend pneumatic compression device (IPC)		Leg			
			Left	Right	Both	
13.01 Start Date:	End Date:	Signature and Bleep No.	☐	☐	☑	
Start Date:	End Date:	Signature and Bleep No.	☐	☐	☐	

Medication		Dose	Dose Change	Enter Time / Enter details below
CLEXANE		40mg		
Please ensure you have completed the VTE risk assessment form	Date	13.01.12		
	Route	SC		
	Signature	LIL		Instructions / Pharmacy
	Bleep no.	164		

Oxygen			
Target Saturation	88-92% ☐	94/98% ☑	If oxygen saturation falls below target range on prescribed oxygen, patient needs urgent clinical review. If oxygen saturation is above targent range on prescribed oxygen, ask for review.
Other specify)			*Device: N= nasal cannula, SM = simple face mask, V = venturi, H = humidified, RM = reservoir mask, OTHER = other eg. NCPAP/NIPPV / Pharmacy
Target Saturation not applicable			

	Date Started	Date Changed	Date Changed	Enter Time / Enter details below
	13.01			
* Device	NON-RE-BREATHE			
% or L/min (Specify a range eg 1-12 L/min)	15L/MIN			
Signature and Bleep No.	LIL	164		

The candidate may also wish to add antibiotics and comment on Simvastatin

GLOBAL PRESCRIPTION MARK

A B C D E

Station 6 – Clinical communication skills

Patient script

You are very anxious about this new treatment. You are uncertain about how an 'oxygen mask' will help you recover: you think you are getting better without it. When the information about this treatment is given to you in a clear way you are amenable to a trial of this treatment.

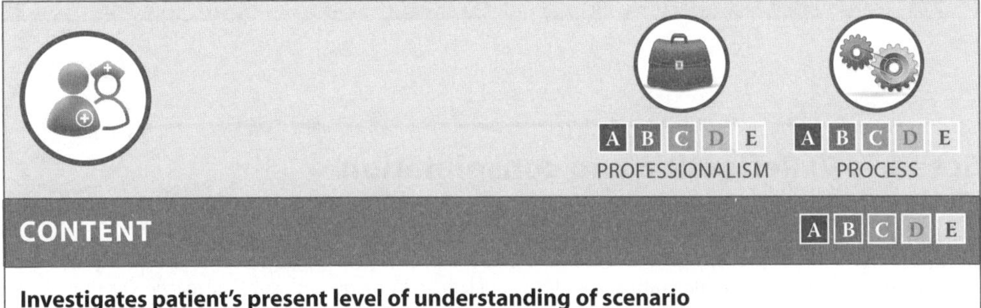

Investigates patient's present level of understanding of scenario

Summarises and confirms what has happened so far

- Mrs Hodge is not improving on her current treatment for her pneumonia (oxygen and antibiotics)
- Explains need for escalation of treatment in clear and concise way.

Asks what, and how much information the patient would like to be told

Establishes patient's ideas, concerns and expectations

- Mrs Hodge does not feel that she has deteriorated on current treatment so is unsure what CPAP will do to help.

Explains the key, important information

- Explains NIPPV including:
- Benefits of improving oxygenation
- Mechanics of CPAP – a tight-fitting mask, high-pressure oxygen flow, need for regular blood gas monitoring
- Complications and problems – discomfort and failure of treatment.

Invites patient to ask questions as they proceed through the consultation and is able to deal with them appropriately

Explains that if treatment is not successful referral and assessment by intensive-care doctors may be required

Summarises important areas of the consultation back to the patient

Formally ends the consultation and ensures appropriate follow-up has been discussed

GLOBAL COMMUNICATION MARK

A B C D E

Scenario 7: Reflection and consolidation

History

Mrs Hodge is a 50-year-old woman with a 4-day history of lethargy, myalgia and global headache. Over the last 48 hours she has developed high-grade fever, a non-productive cough and progressive dyspnoea, leading to her husband calling an ambulance. She denies leg swelling, chest pain or haemoptysis. She has developed profuse diarrhoea, which is of normal colour and is not blood stained. She has recently returned from a holiday in Greece 5 days before the start of this illness. She is unaware of anyone becoming unwell. She has a past medical history of diet-treated type 2 diabetes and hypercholesterolaemia. She takes regular simvastatin, has no allergies and is a non-smoker with a good exercise tolerance. She lives with her husband and has no pets.

Examination

On examination Mrs Hodge is breathless at rest with a raised respiratory rate of 30 and low oxygen saturations on room air. She is pyrexial at 39.9, tachycardic at 105 with a normal BP and normal central capillary refill time. On examination of her chest she has decreased breath sounds at the right mid and upper zones with normal chest expansion, dull percussion note and reduced vocal resonance.
Mrs Hodge has the classical signs of a right upper lobe pneumonia with decreased breath sounds, a dull percussion note and reduced vocal resonance. However, it is often the case that atypical pneumonias present without a lobar consolidation. Many patients with severe atypical pneumonias have relatively normal chest X-ray appearance and respiratory examination.

Investigations

The pathogens that cause the atypical pneumonias are 'atypical' in that they do not grow in the tradition culture media; so specific investigation must be sent when there is a suspicion of an atypical pathogen. This is often referred to a as an atypical screen and should include:

- Urinary antigen for *Legionella*
- Serology for *Mycoplasma* and *Chlamydia pneumoniae*
- Molecular diagnosis by PCR from respiratory swab (*Mycoplasma pneumonia*).

Management

Non-invasive positive pressure ventilation (NIPPV) is a method of supporting the ventilatory effort of conscious patients with respiratory failure. It can be used in the acute hospital setting for conditions such as pneumonia, pulmonary oedema or exacerbations of COPD, and in the community for treatment of chronic conditions such as sleep apnoea. It can either be continuous (CPAP) or bi-level positive airway pressure (BiPAP).

It is applied using a tight-fitting mask and a machine that can generate positive airway pressure. It requires the patient to be alert and able to tolerate the mask. Regular arterial blood gas measurement is vital to monitor the efficacy and to tailor the pressure settings on the machine.

Contraindications to use of NIV are:

- The presence of a pneumothorax without a chest drain
- Low systolic BP as the increase in the intra-thoracic pressure caused by the machine can decrease venous return to the heart and in turn cause a cardiac arrest
- NIV is not appropriate if a patient as a decreased conscious level (high-risk of aspiration of gastric contents)
- Patients with claustrophobia often do not tolerate this therapy, as NIV is delivered via a very tight-fitting mask.

If NIV fails to improve oxygenation, then intubation and invasive positive pressure ventilation (IPPV) may be required in liaison with the intensive-care physicians.

Further reading and web links

Treatment of community-acquired pneumonia:
www.brit-thoracic.org.uk/Portals/0/Clinical%20Information/Pneumonia/Guidelines/CAPQuickRefGuide-web.pdf

Use of NIPPV in acute respiratory failure:
www.brit-thoracic.org.uk/guidelines/nippv-%E2%80%93-niv-in-acute-respiratory-failure-guideline.aspx

Scenario 8: 'Cold feet'

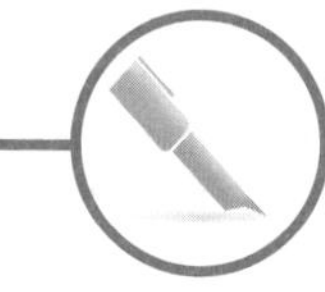

Station 1

History *10-minute station*

You are a final year medical student on attachment at a GP surgery. Your supervising GP has asked you to take a history from a patient, Mr Jim Harrop, who presents with pain in his legs.

- **Please take a full history, which you should then present to the GP, who will ask you some questions about the patient.**

You will be assessed on the following areas, as well as the content and diagnostic reasoning of your history – take them into account in your presentation.

Professionalism

- Professional appearance (NHS dress code) – including general appearance, hair and jewellery
- Maintains patient and personal safety
- Polite introduction; identifies patient or interviewee correctly; confirms patient's date of birth from name band or other source
- Obtains informal consent; maintains patient's privacy
- Displays empathetic and caring attitudes and behaviours throughout.

Process

- Good organisation and structure; appropriate use of open and closed questions
- Appropriate fluency/rhythm/pace to the interview – this may change depending on environment and acute nature of the problem
- Appropriate time for the patient to respond/reply to questions
- Appropriate acknowledgement of difficult or emotional areas of the patient's history.

Communication skills

- Demonstrates caring and sympathetic attitude
- Asks open questions
- Invites patient to ask questions and answers them appropriately
- Addresses patient's ideas, concerns and expectations.

Station 2

Examination *10-minute station*

After discussion with your GP you agree that this gentleman is likely to be suffering from symptoms of peripheral vascular disease.

- **You are now asked to examine Mr Harrop's vascular system. The Practice Nurse has performed a full set of observations, which you may ask for. You will not be required to perform ankle-brachial pressure index measurement.**
- **After you have examined the patient you should turn the page for a summary of the examination findings, which you should read (within the station). You will then be asked to present the examination and answer some questions.**

You will be assessed on the following areas, as well as the content and skills of your examination – take them into account in your presentation.

Professionalism

- Professional appearance; maintains infection control standards, including hand cleaning and appropriate use of gloves and aprons
- Maintains patient and personal safety
- Polite introduction; identifies patient and confirms date of birth from name band or other source
- Obtains informal consent; maintains patient privacy and dignity
- Displays empathetic and caring attitudes and behaviours throughout.

Process

- Appropriate fluency/rhythm/pace to the examination – this may change depending on environment and acute nature of problem
- Good organisation and structure of examination; sensitive and empathetic approach
- Uses appropriate clinical techniques throughout
- Maintains privacy and dignity throughout.

Communication skills

- Explains proposed examination/procedure; explains examination/procedure as it proceeds
- Offers information in a clear, structured and fluent manner, avoiding jargon
- Listens to patient and responds appropriately
- Demonstrates appropriate body language.

Please read the information below before presenting the examination findings. ***[NB If you have a model do not read this section]***

Clinical findings

- General examination – overweight, tar staining to fingers, corneal arcus
- Observations – HR 84 bpm, BP 148/92 mmHg, RR 18 bpm, O_2 sats 96% on air, temperature 36.7 °C, CBG 10.9 mmol/l
- Height 1.75 m, weight 104 kg, BMI $104/(1.75)^2 = 34.0$
- CV examination – normal upper limb pulses, normal carotid pulses and no carotid bruits heard, no abdominal aortic aneurysm identified
- Focused examination – right leg cool relative to left, slightly pale at foot, with flaking atrophic skin at toes; femoral pulses palpated both sides, equal pulse volume; popliteal pulse palpated on left, absent on right; dorsalis pedis and posterior tibialis pulses not palpated at either foot; Buerger's angle 15° right leg, 45° left leg; reactive hyperaemia noted at both legs when hung over edge of examination couch.

Station 3

Clinical communication skills *10-minute station*

The GP agrees that Mr Harrop's symptoms are due to intermittent claudication, secondary to atherosclerotic vascular disease. He wishes to observe while you continue the consultation with Mr Harrop.

- Please explain the diagnosis to Mr Harrop, advise him about management options and answer any questions that he may have.

Station 4

Prescribing skills *10-minute station*

Part 1:

Twelve months later you are working as an FY1 in surgery. During the middle of your night shift, the Vascular Registrar bleeps you to inform you that he has admitted a lady with critical ischaemia of the leg secondary to peripheral arterial occlusion. She has been booked for an emergency bypass operation as soon as the case in the operating theatre is finished (this may be several hours).

- In the meantime you are asked to prescribe a heparin infusion for the patient. Use the heparin infusion chart provided and a copy of the BNF to aid you in this.

Part 2:
The heparin infusion is continued intra-operatively, and your consultant, Mr Sanderson, would like to continue the infusion for a further 24 hours. The APTT ratio has been checked post-operatively, and is entered on the chart.

- **Please use the tables to calculate the adjustment and compete the heparin prescription.**

Details

Mrs Sara Bucknall; Hospital No. 732789; DOB: 10/10/1936; No known drug allergies; No regular medication; Weight: 72 kg; Ward: Maple Ward; Consultant: Mr Sanderson; Clotting screen: INR 1.1, PTT 11.9, APTT 24 s, APTT ratio 1.0

Unfractionated heparin infusion chart

Name:
Date of birth: Weight:
Hospital Number:
Ward:
Consultant:

Loading dose

Date	Time	Drug/ dose	Route	Dose	Rate	Doctor's signature	Nurse's signature
					5 minutes		

Maintenance dose

Heparin infusion prepared as 20 000 units diluted with 0.9% sodium chloride for injection, giving a total volume of 40 ml (heparin concentration of 500 units/ml).

- **Start infusion at 18 units/kg/h. Maximum initial infusion rate 3.6 ml/h.**
  Monitor the APTT ratio 6 hours after starting the infusion and adjust the infusion rate according to the table below.
  Adjust the rate of infusion only, not the concentration of the infusion.

SCENARIO 8

Infusion rate prescription and APTT ratio monitoring record

Date and time of result	APTT ratio	Bolus dose	Infusion rate	Doctor's signature	Nurse's signature	Date and time of change
(Post-op)	1.36					

APTT ratio: this should be performed every 24 hours when in range and 6 hours after any dose change.

- **Adjust doses according to the guidance below. Maximum bolus dose for heparin is 5000 units.**

APTT ratio	Rate adjustment	Timing of APTT monitoring
<1.20	80 units/kg bolus and increase by 4 unit/kg/h	6 hours
1.20–1.49	40 units/kg bolus and increase by 2 units/kg/h	6 hours
1.50–2.50	No change	24 hours
2.51–3.00	Reduce by 2 units/kg/h	6 hours
3.01–4.00	Stop 1 hour, reduce by 3 units/kg/h	6 hours
>4.00	Stop 2 hours, reduce by 4 units/kg/h	6 hours

Heparin dose change	Additional infusion rate
100 units	0.2 ml
200 units	0.4 ml
300 units	0.6 ml
400 units	0.8 ml

Remember: DRUG DRs Don't Forget Signing Off (page 373)

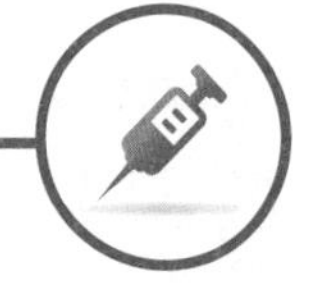

Station 5

Procedural skills *10-minute station*

Procedure

The Ward Sister suggests she observe you setting up the heparin infusion pump as a DOPS assessment for your training portfolio. For the purpose of the station you should draw up saline as your infusion drug, but you should demonstrate awareness of safety checks required for the administration of all medications.

- **Using the following equipment, please set up and commence the infusion at a rate of 2.6 ml/h.**

Equipment provided

- **Graseby (or equivalent) infusion pump**
- **IV administration set**
- **IV fluid for administration (use saline in this station)**
- **Normal saline flush**
- **Labels for fluids and tubing**
- **Gloves**

Station 6

Data interpretation *10-minute station*

After the weekly multidisciplinary team meeting between the Vascular Surgical Team and the Interventional Radiology Team your Registrar decides to show you some angiogram studies.

- **You are asked to match the labels A–H to the anatomical structures identified in the pictures below.**

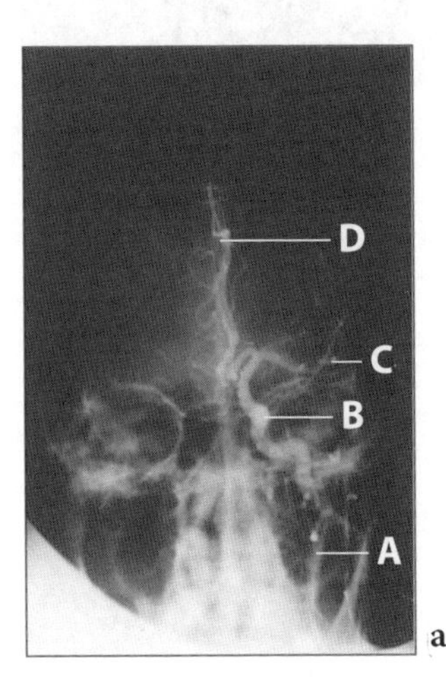

a

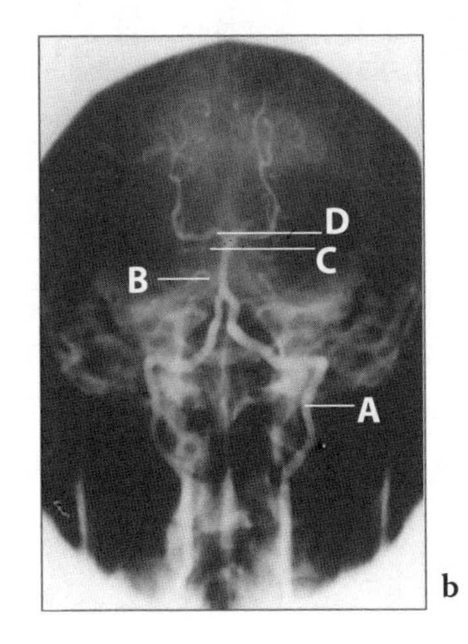

b

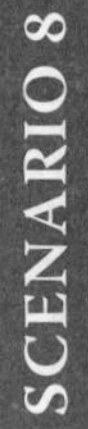

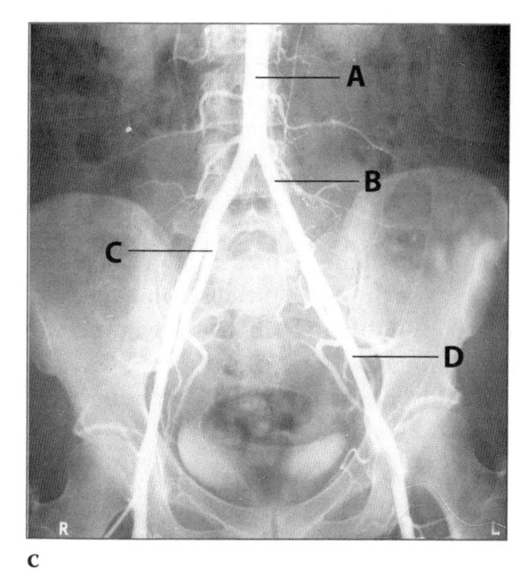

c

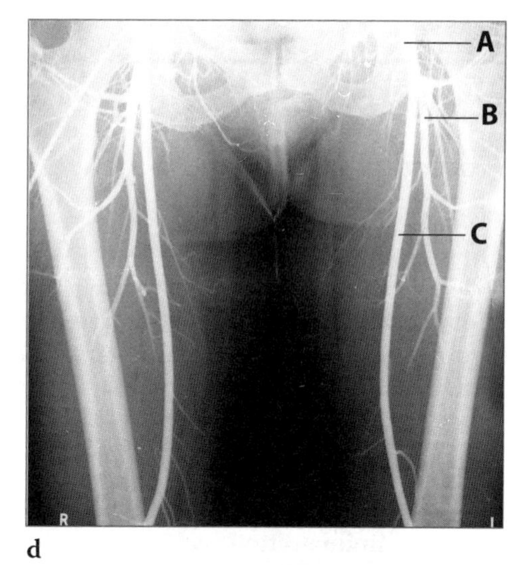

d

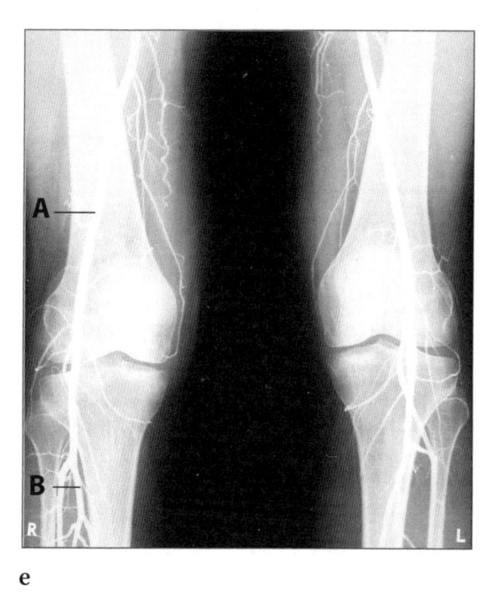

e

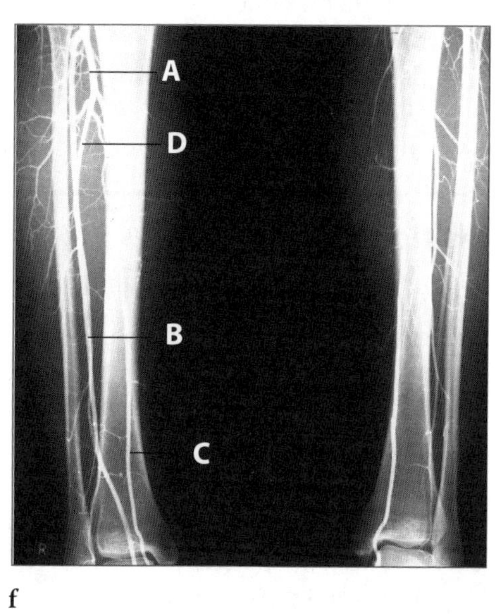

f

Answers

Station 1 – History

Patient script

Your name is Jim Harrop and you are 62 years old (DOB 1 August 1949). You are a retired taxi driver. You have made this appointment as you have been having pain in your right leg for the past few months and are increasingly concerned about it.

The pain affects the calf area of the right leg and feels like a terrible cramp. It comes and goes, and particularly comes on when you are out walking. It now comes on even when you are only popping to the local shops, which are less than 200 m from your home. When the pain comes, you find that it eases after a couple of minutes of rest, and so you find that you are often needing to sit down on a bench for a while when you are out and about. The pain is only in the calf area, and does not affect the foot, upper leg or buttock. You have never had the pain at night, or when you are at rest.

On one or two occasions you have also had a similar pain to the left calf but this happens far less frequently.

You have had no history of injury to the leg or back.

You have poor health generally. You had a heart attack 6 years ago and had to have two stents placed. You were diagnosed with diabetes last year, and were told that improvements to your diet were strongly advised. You found this very difficult, and have now been started on metformin and gliclazide. You also know that you have high blood pressure and high cholesterol. Twenty years or so ago you once had a painful toe, and were told that you had gout.

You are overweight. You drink one or two beers most evenings in the pub, and plenty more on darts night. You smoke a few roll-ups every day (5–10/day), but used to smoke a lot more before the smoking ban. You live in a maisonette with your wife and your dog.

Besides the metformin and gliclazide, you also take simvastatin, bisoprolol, ramipril and allopurinol. You are allergic to aspirin, although you are not sure what sort of reaction you have.

Your father died at the age of 61 from a heart attack, and your mother in her 80s from breast cancer. You have a brother who recently had a stroke, but otherwise you don't know of any other family health problems.

Ideas and concerns: you suspect that you have poor circulation although you also wonder if the pain in your leg is due to wear and tear or arthritis because of your weight.

Expectations: you are really finding that the pain is limiting what you are able to do and would appreciate any help in improving it. You aren't expecting to need tests or specific treatment as such, but hope some medicine could be prescribed to help with the symptoms. You know that smoking and drinking can't be helping, together with being overweight, and are open to help with these health issues.

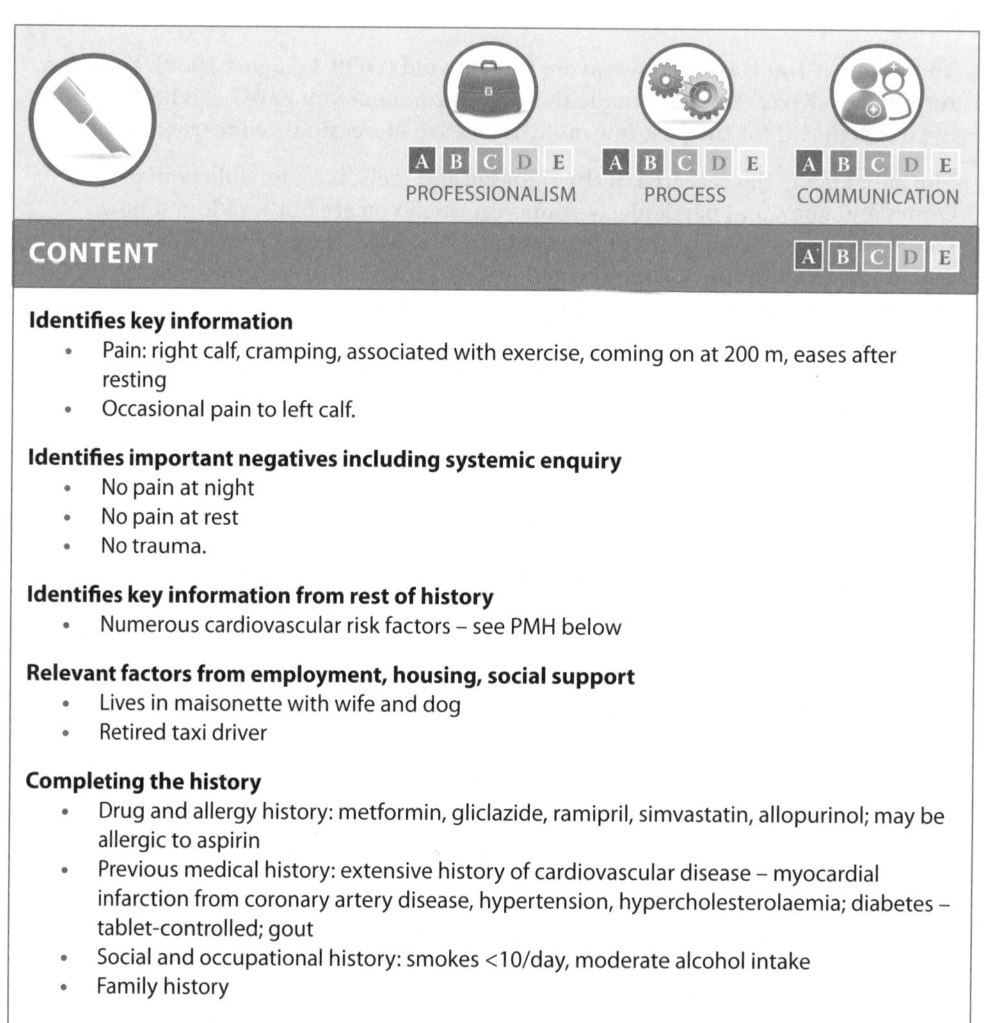

A B C D E
PROFESSIONALISM

A B C D E
PROCESS

A B C D E
COMMUNICATION

CONTENT

A B C D E

Identifies key information

- Pain: right calf, cramping, associated with exercise, coming on at 200 m, eases after resting
- Occasional pain to left calf.

Identifies important negatives including systemic enquiry

- No pain at night
- No pain at rest
- No trauma.

Identifies key information from rest of history

- Numerous cardiovascular risk factors – see PMH below

Relevant factors from employment, housing, social support

- Lives in maisonette with wife and dog
- Retired taxi driver

Completing the history

- Drug and allergy history: metformin, gliclazide, ramipril, simvastatin, allopurinol; may be allergic to aspirin
- Previous medical history: extensive history of cardiovascular disease – myocardial infarction from coronary artery disease, hypertension, hypercholesterolaemia; diabetes – tablet-controlled; gout
- Social and occupational history: smokes <10/day, moderate alcohol intake
- Family history

Summarises important areas of the history back to the patient

Invites patient to ask questions and is able to deal with them appropriately

Establishes patient's ideas, concerns and expectations

CLINICAL DIAGNOSTIC REASONING

A B C D E

- **Please present your history**
  - Candidate offers a logical, well-structured account of the history
- **What is your diagnosis?**
  - Candidate offers the correct diagnosis and appropriate differentials
  - Diagnosis: symptoms of intermittent claudication secondary to peripheral vascular disease
- **In view of this diagnosis, are there any specific tests that you would want to perform?**
  - Examination of vascular system to include abdominal aorta and assessment of peripheral pulses
  - Ankle-brachial pressure index (ABPI)
  - Buerger's test.

GLOBAL HISTORY MARK

A B C D E

Station 2 – Examination

Patient script

If you are an actor/patient, read the patient history and physical signs fully – when the candidate comes to an abnormal site in their examination, act-out tenderness and/or volunteer the relevant physical sign.

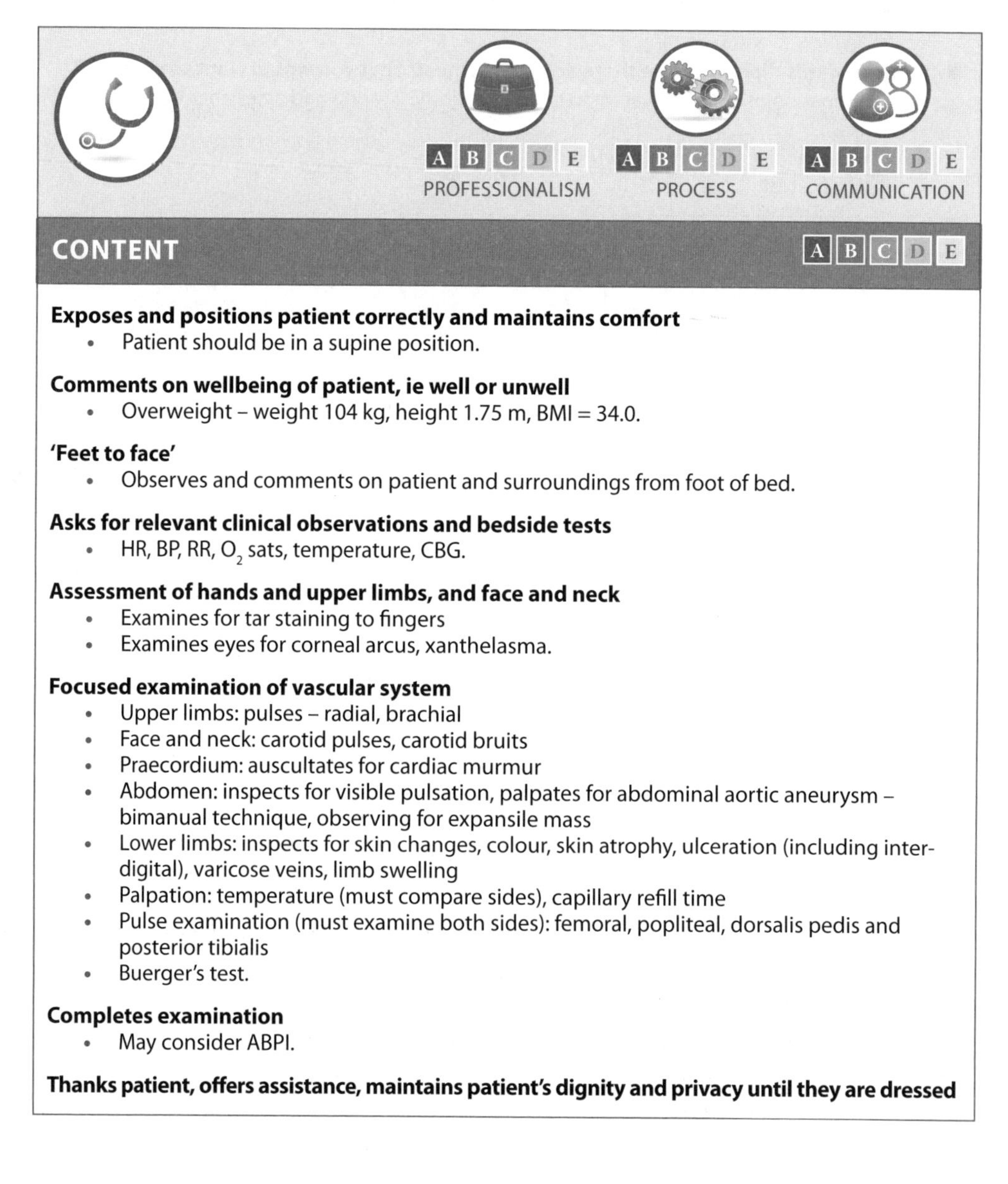

CONTENT A B C D E

Exposes and positions patient correctly and maintains comfort
- Patient should be in a supine position.

Comments on wellbeing of patient, ie well or unwell
- Overweight – weight 104 kg, height 1.75 m, BMI = 34.0.

'Feet to face'
- Observes and comments on patient and surroundings from foot of bed.

Asks for relevant clinical observations and bedside tests
- HR, BP, RR, O_2 sats, temperature, CBG.

Assessment of hands and upper limbs, and face and neck
- Examines for tar staining to fingers
- Examines eyes for corneal arcus, xanthelasma.

Focused examination of vascular system
- Upper limbs: pulses – radial, brachial
- Face and neck: carotid pulses, carotid bruits
- Praecordium: auscultates for cardiac murmur
- Abdomen: inspects for visible pulsation, palpates for abdominal aortic aneurysm – bimanual technique, observing for expansile mass
- Lower limbs: inspects for skin changes, colour, skin atrophy, ulceration (including inter-digital), varicose veins, limb swelling
- Palpation: temperature (must compare sides), capillary refill time
- Pulse examination (must examine both sides): femoral, popliteal, dorsalis pedis and posterior tibialis
- Buerger's test.

Completes examination
- May consider ABPI.

Thanks patient, offers assistance, maintains patient's dignity and privacy until they are dressed

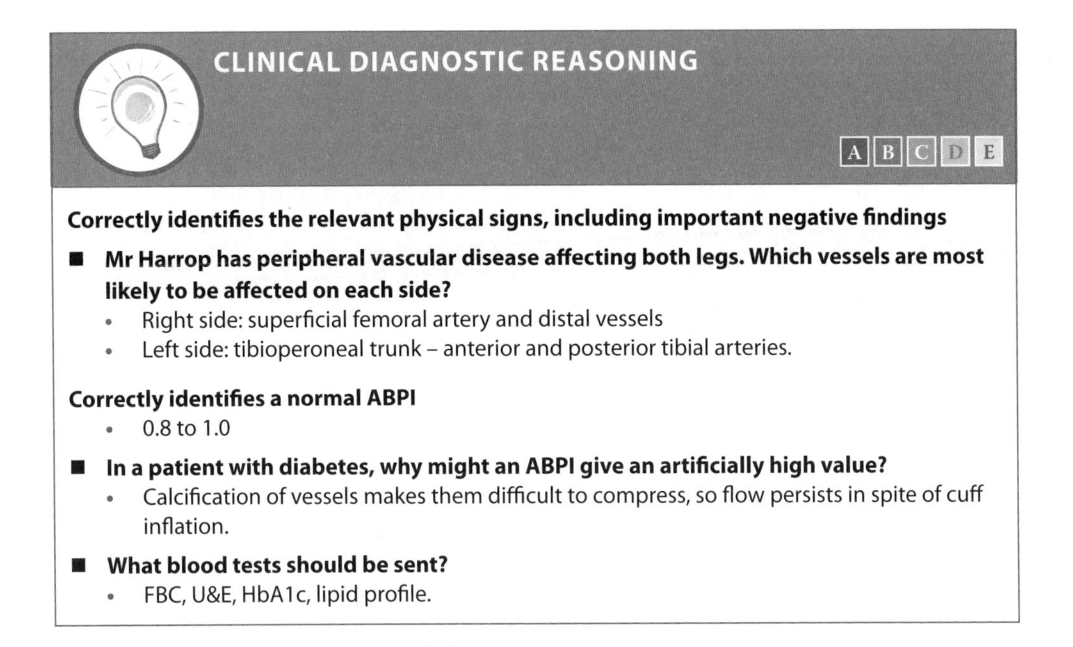

CLINICAL DIAGNOSTIC REASONING

A B C D E

Correctly identifies the relevant physical signs, including important negative findings

- **Mr Harrop has peripheral vascular disease affecting both legs. Which vessels are most likely to be affected on each side?**
  - Right side: superficial femoral artery and distal vessels
  - Left side: tibioperoneal trunk – anterior and posterior tibial arteries.

Correctly identifies a normal ABPI

- 0.8 to 1.0

- **In a patient with diabetes, why might an ABPI give an artificially high value?**
  - Calcification of vessels makes them difficult to compress, so flow persists in spite of cuff inflation.
- **What blood tests should be sent?**
  - FBC, U&E, HbA1c, lipid profile.

GLOBAL EXAMINATION MARK

A B C D E

Station 3 – Clinical communication skills

Patient script

You already suspect that your circulation is poor because your feet feel colder than they used to. You had not realised that the pains you have been getting were because of circulation problems as well.

You are worried in particular because you need to be able to get out and about to walk your dog and do the shopping, and you are finding this very difficult now. You expected you could be given some medications to help take the pain away. You are not aware that the problem can get much worse and are surprised when this is explained.

You understand that stopping smoking may help, but you think this will be incredibly difficult because you have smoked all your life and spend a lot of time with your friends who also smoke.

If invited, you have several questions:
1 Are there any tests that can confirm how the blockage is?
2 Is there any medicine that I can take which might help?
3 Will surgery be needed?

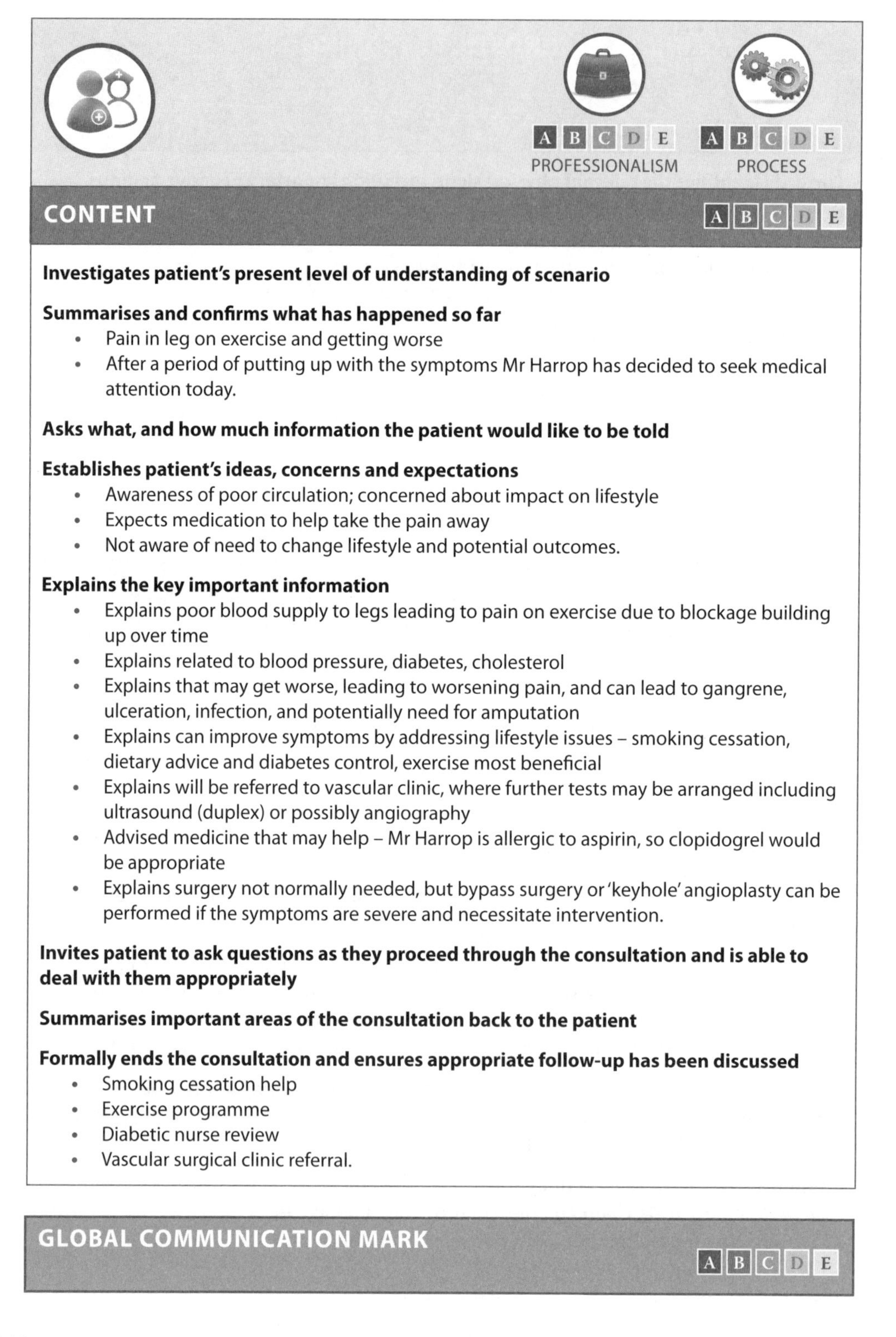

CONTENT

A B C D E

Investigates patient's present level of understanding of scenario

Summarises and confirms what has happened so far

- Pain in leg on exercise and getting worse
- After a period of putting up with the symptoms Mr Harrop has decided to seek medical attention today.

Asks what, and how much information the patient would like to be told

Establishes patient's ideas, concerns and expectations

- Awareness of poor circulation; concerned about impact on lifestyle
- Expects medication to help take the pain away
- Not aware of need to change lifestyle and potential outcomes.

Explains the key important information

- Explains poor blood supply to legs leading to pain on exercise due to blockage building up over time
- Explains related to blood pressure, diabetes, cholesterol
- Explains that may get worse, leading to worsening pain, and can lead to gangrene, ulceration, infection, and potentially need for amputation
- Explains can improve symptoms by addressing lifestyle issues – smoking cessation, dietary advice and diabetes control, exercise most beneficial
- Explains will be referred to vascular clinic, where further tests may be arranged including ultrasound (duplex) or possibly angiography
- Advised medicine that may help – Mr Harrop is allergic to aspirin, so clopidogrel would be appropriate
- Explains surgery not normally needed, but bypass surgery or 'keyhole' angioplasty can be performed if the symptoms are severe and necessitate intervention.

Invites patient to ask questions as they proceed through the consultation and is able to deal with them appropriately

Summarises important areas of the consultation back to the patient

Formally ends the consultation and ensures appropriate follow-up has been discussed

- Smoking cessation help
- Exercise programme
- Diabetic nurse review
- Vascular surgical clinic referral.

GLOBAL COMMUNICATION MARK

A B C D E

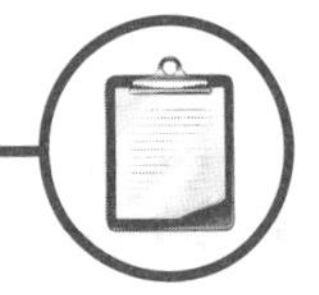

Station 4 – Prescribing skills

Check: DRUG DRs Don't Forget Signing Off (page 373)

Unfractionated heparin infusion chart
Name: Sara Bucknall
Date of birth: 10/10/1936 **Weight: 65 kg**
Hospital Number: 732789
Ward: Maple
Consultant: Mr Sanderson

Loading Dose

Date	Time	Drug/ dose	Route	Dose	Rate	Doctor's signature	Nurse's signature
-/-/--	--:--	Heparin	IV	5000 U	5 minutes		

Infusion rate prescription and APTT ratio monitoring record

Date and time of result	APTT ratio	Bolus dose	Infusion rate	Doctor's signature	Nurse's signature	Date and time of change
–/–/––	1.00	-	2.6 ml/h	Dr Smart		
(Post-op) –/–/––	1.36	5.76 ml	2.9 ml/h	Dr Smart		

APTT ratio: this should be performed every 24 hours when in range and 6 hours after any dose change. Adjust doses according to the guidance below. Maximum bolus dose for heparin is 5000 units.

Station 5 – Procedural skills

Setting up an infusion pump

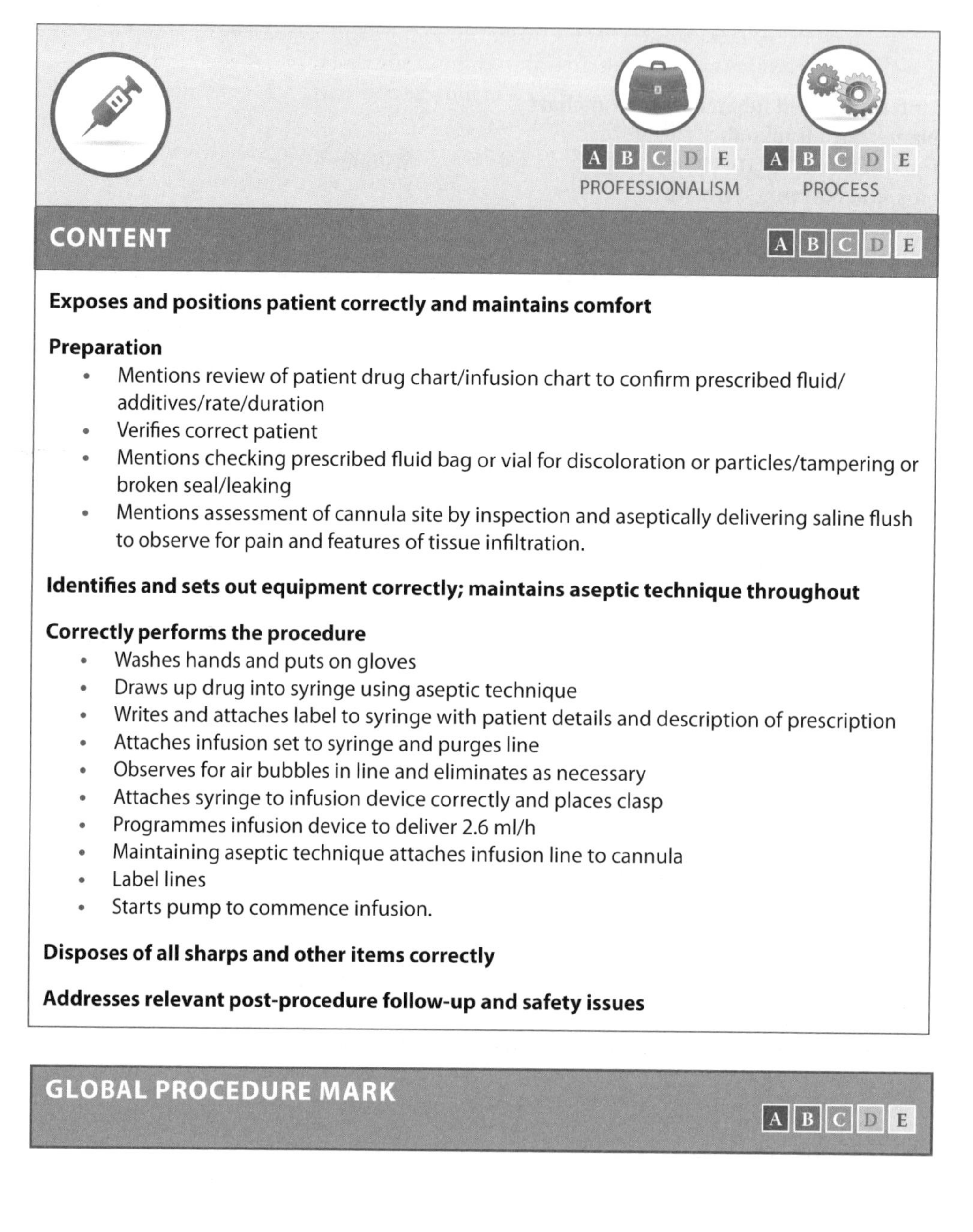

Exposes and positions patient correctly and maintains comfort

Preparation

- Mentions review of patient drug chart/infusion chart to confirm prescribed fluid/additives/rate/duration
- Verifies correct patient
- Mentions checking prescribed fluid bag or vial for discoloration or particles/tampering or broken seal/leaking
- Mentions assessment of cannula site by inspection and aseptically delivering saline flush to observe for pain and features of tissue infiltration.

Identifies and sets out equipment correctly; maintains aseptic technique throughout

Correctly performs the procedure

- Washes hands and puts on gloves
- Draws up drug into syringe using aseptic technique
- Writes and attaches label to syringe with patient details and description of prescription
- Attaches infusion set to syringe and purges line
- Observes for air bubbles in line and eliminates as necessary
- Attaches syringe to infusion device correctly and places clasp
- Programmes infusion device to deliver 2.6 ml/h
- Maintaining aseptic technique attaches infusion line to cannula
- Label lines
- Starts pump to commence infusion.

Disposes of all sharps and other items correctly

Addresses relevant post-procedure follow-up and safety issues

GLOBAL PROCEDURE MARK A B C D E

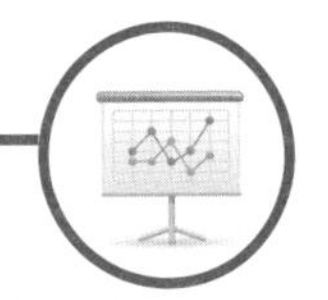

Station 6–Data interpretation

a. **Left Carotid arteriogram (antero-posterior view): A Left internal carotid artery in neck; B Internal carotid artery curving upwards within the cavernous sinus; C Branches of middle cerebral artery; D Overlapping anterior cerebral arteries (the right anterior cerebral artery is filled through the anterior communicating artery).**

b. **Vertebral arteriogram (antero-posterior view): A Vertebral artery; B Basilar artery; C Superior cerebellar artery; D Posterior cerebral artery.**

c-f Lower limb arteriogram

c. **A Abdominal aorta; B Common iliac artery; C Internal iliac artery; D External iliac artery.**

d. **A Common femoral artery; B Profunda femoris (deep femoral) artery; C Superficial femoral artery.**

e. **A Popliteal artery; B Tibioperoneal trunk.**

f. **A Tibioperoneal trunk; B Anterior tibial artery; C Posterior tibial artery; D Peroneal artery.**

GLOBAL DATA INTERPRETATION MARK

A B C D E

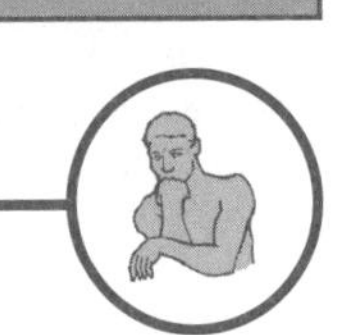

Scenario 8: Reflection and consolidation

History

Mr Harrop is a 62-year-old retired taxi driver who is attending today complaining of pain at his right leg for the past few months. The pain is cramp-like in nature and affects the calf area without radiation elsewhere. It is brought on by walking less than 200 m, and settles after approximately 2 minutes of rest. He has not noticed pain coming on when he is at rest, or during the night. He has also noticed the pain at the left calf on one or two occasions but this is very infrequent.

He has numerous cardiovascular risk factors, including previous myocardial infarction, tablet-controlled diabetes, hypertension and hypercholesterolaemia. He is also overweight, is a life-long smoker of at least 10/day, and has an excessive alcohol intake of approximately 40 to 50 units per week. His only other previous medical history is gout.

His medications consists of metformin, gliclazide, simvastatin, bisoprolol, ramipril and allopurinol. He reports being allergic to aspirin.

Mr Harrop is married and lives with his wife and dog in a maisonette.

Examination

This 62-year-old gentleman, who is overweight with a BMI of 34, appears comfortable at rest. His observations are all within normal limits except for a raised blood pressure at 148/92 mmHg. His CBG is 10.9. Examination of his hands demonstrates tar staining to his fingertips, and examination of his eyes shows corneal arcus. Examination of his upper limb pulses is normal. He has no carotid bruit and his heart sounds are normal. Examination of his abdomen does not demonstrate the presence of an abdominal aortic aneurysm.

Examination of his legs reveals that his right leg is slightly pale at the foot, and there is evidence of skin atrophy at the toes. There is no ulceration seen. The right leg feels cool in comparison with the left, which is of a normal temperature. Femoral pulses are present bilaterally. On the left side the popliteal pulse is present, but the pedal pulses cannot be palpated, and Buerger's angle is 45°. On the right side, the popliteal and pedal pulses are not palpable, with Buerger's angle of 15°.

Management of peripheral vascular disease

The initial management of a patient like this involves addressing of the various important lifestyle issues: smoking and alcohol cessation, enrolment in exercise programmes, careful blood pressure and glycaemic control (diabetic specialist nurse clinic). Other medical management includes anti-platelet therapy with aspirin, clopidogrel or modified-release dipyidamole.

Further radiographical investigations would normally be initiated in the vascular outpatient setting, starting with duplex ultrasound to 'map' the patency and flow dynamics in the peripheral circulation. If further intervention is required, angiography and/or angioplasty can be performed, although this is not without risk and so is generally reserved for patients in whom bypass surgery will be advocated if interventional radiological procedures are not successful.

Procedure – infusion devices

Although infusion devices are traditionally the realm of nurses, anaesthetists and intensive-care doctors, it is important to be familiar with their use and function. They are commonly found in ward environments and are frequently used for delivery of 'sliding-scale' insulin, heparin, patient-controlled analgesia (PCA) and opiates such as diamorphine in palliative and end-of-life care. As with any infusion drug it is particularly important to carefully check the prescription and calculate the dose and concentration of the preparation. It is mandatory to double-check this with a colleague. All infusion lines must be clearly labelled and formularies or preparation guides consulted if a line is being used simultaneously for more than one drug infusion at a time (as is often the case on the ITU).

Prescribing IV heparin

Owing to the necessity of monitoring APTT closely and a variety of potentially severe complications, heparin has largely become redundant in favour of a variety of subcutaneously administered 'low-molecular weight heparin' preparations such as tinzaparin, enoxaparin and dalteparin. However, in patients where accurate antithrombotic therapy is essential, such as in surgical patients whose regular warfarin has been stopped, or those awaiting vascular salvage procedures such as in this scenario, heparin still has its place.

Further reading and web links

www.sign.ac.uk/pdf/sign89.pdf

www.patient.co.uk/health/Peripheral-Arterial-Disease-in-Legs.htm

Scenario 9: 'Feeling awful!'

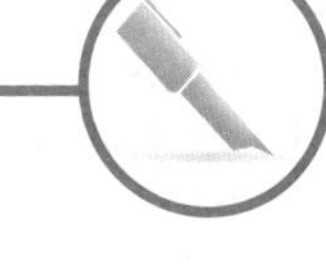

Station 1

History *10-minute station*

You are a final year medical student attached to the Emergency Department. The Supervising Consultant would like to observe you assessing a patient and would like you to start off by taking a focused history from a patient called Annie Morgan.

- **Please take a full history for Mrs Morgan, which you should then present in an appropriate manner for a busy Emergency Department and answer any questions you may be asked.**

You will be assessed on the following areas, as well as the content and diagnostic reasoning of your history – take them into account in your presentation.

Professionalism

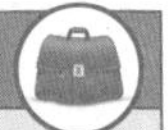

- Professional appearance (NHS dress code) – including general appearance, hair and jewellery
- Maintains patient and personal safety
- Polite introduction; identifies patient or interviewee correctly; confirms patient's date of birth from name band or other source
- Obtains informal consent; maintains patient's privacy
- Displays empathetic and caring attitudes and behaviours throughout.

Process

- Good organisation and structure; appropriate use of open and closed questions
- Appropriate fluency/rhythm/pace to the interview – this may change depending on environment and acute nature of problem
- Appropriate time for the patient to respond/reply to questions
- Appropriate acknowledgement of difficult or emotional areas of the patient's history.

Communication skills

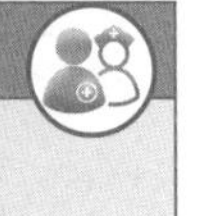

- Demonstrates caring and sympathetic attitude
- Asks open questions
- Invites patient to ask questions and answers them appropriately
- Addresses patient's ideas, concerns and expectations.

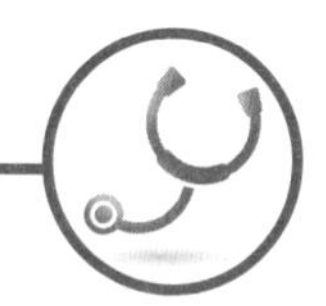

Station 2

Examination *10-minute station*

After discussion with the Consultant in the Emergency Department, you agree that Mrs Morgan could be presenting with a significant upper gastrointestinal bleed (UGIB).

- **You are now asked to examine her, focusing your examination in line with the features that she has presented with. A nurse in the Emergency Department has performed a full set of observations, which you may ask for.**
- **After you have examined the patient you should turn the page for a summary of the examination findings, which you should read (within the station). You will then be asked to present the examination and answer some questions.**

You will be assessed on the following areas, as well as the content and skills of your examination – take them into account in your presentation.

Professionalism

- Professional appearance; maintains infection control standards, including hand cleaning and appropriate use of gloves and aprons
- Maintains patient and personal safety
- Polite introduction; identifies patient and confirms date of birth from name band or other source
- Obtains informal consent; maintains patient privacy and dignity
- Displays empathetic and caring attitudes and behaviours throughout.

Process

- Appropriate fluency/rhythm/pace to the examination – this may change depending on environment and acute nature of problem
- Good organisation and structure of examination; sensitive and empathetic approach
- Uses appropriate clinical techniques throughout
- Maintains privacy and dignity throughout.

Clinical communication

- Explains proposed examination/procedure: explains examination/procedure as it proceeds
- Offers information in a clear, structured and fluent manner, avoiding jargon
- Listens to patient and responds appropriately
- Demonstrates appropriate body language.

Please read the information below before presenting the examination findings. ***[NB If you have a model do not read this section]***

Clinical findings

- **Patient appears unwell and in moderate pain**
- **Observations – HR 114 bpm, BP 102/68 mmHg, RR 20 bpm, CRT 2 s, O_2 sats 99% on air, temperature 35.9 °C**
- **General examination – pale, slightly clammy and cool peripheries, dark vomit stains around face and on chest**
- **Focused examination – abdomen tender ++ at epigastrium with guarding, rebound tenderness and rigidity, bowel sounds present but infrequent**
- **DRE – must be requested to confirm presence of malaena.**

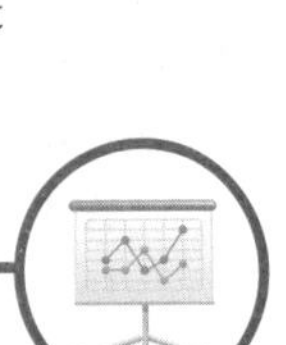

Station 3

Data interpretation *5-minute station*

Part 1:

A Barrett's oesophagus
B Gastric carcinoma
C Peptic ulcer
D Duodenal ulcer
E Crohn's disease
F Gastroenteritis
G Oesophageal variceal disease
H Mallory–Weiss syndrome
I Aortoenteric fistula
J Peutz–Jeghers syndrome

- **For each of the following clinical scenarios, select the most appropriate cause, A–J, for their haematemesis. Each option may be used more than once.**

1. **A 27-year-old stockbroker presents with haematemesis after a prolonged alcohol binge and several episodes of vomiting.**
2. **A 69-year-old retired schoolteacher presents with weight loss and dyspepsia, and occasional mild haematemesis. Her medical history includes vitamin B_{12} deficiency.**
3. **A 39-year-old alcoholic man presents with haematemesis and malaena. On examination he is found to have several spider naevi and has moderate ascites.**
4. **A 46-year-old psychiatrist presents after vomiting moderate amounts of blood. He reports several weeks of epigastric pain, which seems to be worse at night and is eased by eating.**
5. **A 53-year-old woman presents with infrequent haematemesis on a background of heartburn for 2 years. Oesophagogastroduodenoscopy demonstrates columnar epitheliar metaplasia at the distal oesophagus.**

Part 2:

A Intravenous hydrocortisone
B Oesophagogastroduodenoscopy (OGD)
C Ranitidine
D Naproxen
E Lansoprazole
F Oral prednisolone
G Intravenous fluids
H Mebeverine
I Laparotomy
J Triple therapy: clarithromycin, amoxicillin, lansoprazole

■ For each of the following clinical scenarios, select the most appropriate management plan, A–J. Each option may be used once, more than once, or not at all.

1 A 49-year-old banker presents with a 1-day history of severe epigastric pain. On examination he is tachycardic and pyrexial, and has features of peritonism. An erect chest X-ray demonstrates subdiaphragmatic free air.
2 A 29-year-old man with Crohn's disease presents with abdominal pain, increased frequency of stool and occasional rectal bleeding. On examination his observations demonstrate a tachycardia at 129 bpm and a temperature of 38.4 °C. His abdomen is soft with generalised tenderness. Blood tests reveal: WCC 16 $\times 10^9$/l, CRP 189 mg/l, ESR 59 mm/h.
3 A 35-year-old woman with irritable bowel syndrome presents with cramping abdominal pain and bloating. On examination she appears well and her abdomen is soft with mild discomfort on palpation. Investigations, including pregnancy test, are unremarkable.
4 A 60-year-old chronic alcoholic man with known cirrhotic liver disease presents with malaena.
5 A 46-year-old woman with symptoms of acid-reflux undergoes an OGD, which demonstrates severe oesophagitis.

Station 4

Prescribing skills *10-minute station*

The blood tests that are performed demonstrate a normocytic anaemia (Hb 7.1 g/dl) suggestive of acute blood loss. The consultant has arranged a blood transfusion (which is now ready to commence) and would like to assess your prescribing skills.

- **Please prescribe two units of blood and any other appropriate medications for the management of upper gastrointestinal bleeding. Use the drug chart and infusion chart provided on page 368 for this.**

Details

Mrs Annie Morgan; Hospital No. 7114543; DOB: 13/12/1958; Ward: Lilac Ward; Consultant: Dr Church

Remember: DRUG DRs **D**on't **F**orget **S**igning **O**ff (page 373)

Station 5

Procedural skills *10-minute station*

Procedure

The Gastroenterology Registrar on call was called by the Emergency Department Consultant, and an urgent endoscopy has been arranged. As part of the ongoing resuscitation you are now asked to insert a urinary catheter.

- **Using the following equipment, please perform this procedure.**

Equipment provided

- **'Catheter pack' including sterile gloves, drape, sterile pots, gauze swabs, yellow disposal bag**
- **16 Fr catheter and 10 ml pre-filled water syringe**
- **Topical anaesthetic gel**
- **Collecting bag**

Answers

Station 1 – History

Patient script

Your name is Annie Morgan, and you are 53 years old (DOB 13 December 1958). You are feeling very unwell! For the past 2 days you have had a terrible burning pain in the upper part of your abdomen that has got a lot worse today. You have never had such a severe pain. You feel very weak and tired. The pain does not radiate and is not alleviated or exacerbated by anything.

This morning you have vomited four or five times. The vomit was very black in colour 'like coffee-grounds'. You still feel very sick.

If asked about your bowels – you have noticed that the colour of your stool has been very dark for the past 48 hours and particularly foul-smelling.

You have not had a fever that you are aware of.

You have had burning 'acid-like' pains in the same place for quite some months now. You find that generally the pain goes away when you have a glass of milk or something to eat and so it hasn't troubled you too much. You find that your sleep is often interrupted now as you notice the pain is particularly bad at night.

You don't have any medical history except that about a year ago you hurt your back lifting some heavy books, and even though it got a lot better, you still have some back pain most days and often take ibuprofen and paracetamol to help. You don't take any other regular medications. You have no allergies.

You work as a teacher, and don't drink alcohol or smoke, although you worry that you probably drink too much coffee. You are married, and live at home with your husband, you have no children. No relevant family history.

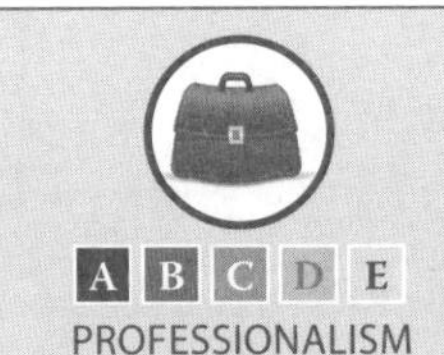

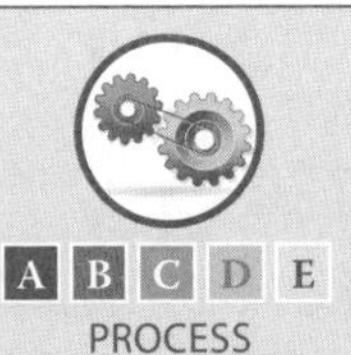

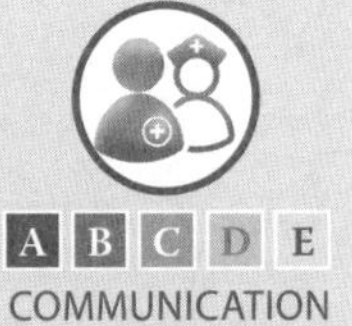

CONTENT

A B C D E

Identifies key information

- Severe abdominal pain for 48 hours, burning character
- No radiation, no exacerbating or alleviating factors
- Associated with 'coffee-ground' vomiting
- Associated with foul-smelling black stools.

Identifies important negatives, including systemic enquiry

- No fever.

Identifies key information from rest of history

- 'Acid-like' pains for many months
- Alleviated by milk/eating, worse at night (lying flat)
- Taking regular NSAID ibuprofen for back pain.

Completing the history

- Drug and allergy history: paracetamol and Ibuprofen PRN, no known drug allergies
- Previous medical history: back pain – NSAID use, no other PMH
- Social history: non-smoker, does not drink alcohol, heavy caffeine intake
- Family history.

Summarises important areas of the history back to the patient

Invites patient to ask questions and is able to deal with them appropriately

Establishes patient's ideas, concerns and expectations

CLINICAL DIAGNOSTIC REASONING

A B C D E

- **Please present your history**
  - Candidate offers a logical, well-structured account of the history
- **What is your diagnosis?**
  - Candidate offers the correct diagnosis and appropriate differentials
  - Diagnosis: abdominal pain associated with haematemesis and malaena suggestive of upper gastrointestinal tract bleeding secondary to a bleeding or perforated ulcer
  - Differential diagnosis includes acute pancreatitis, acute cholecystitis, acute myocardial infarction (atypical).
- **In view of this diagnosis, can you name two common causes of upper GI bleeding, and the principal risk factors for each?**
  - Ulcers: gastric or duodenal – risk factors are *Heliobacter pylori* infection, NSAIDs, Zollinger–Ellison syndrome
  - Oesophageal varices – risk factors are portal hypertension, usually secondary to cirrhotic liver disease as a result of excessive chronic alcohol use.

GLOBAL HISTORY MARK

A B C D E

Station 2 – Examination

Patient script

If you are an actor/patient, read the patient history and physical signs fully – when the candidate comes to an abnormal site in their examination, act-out tenderness and/or volunteer the relevant physical sign.

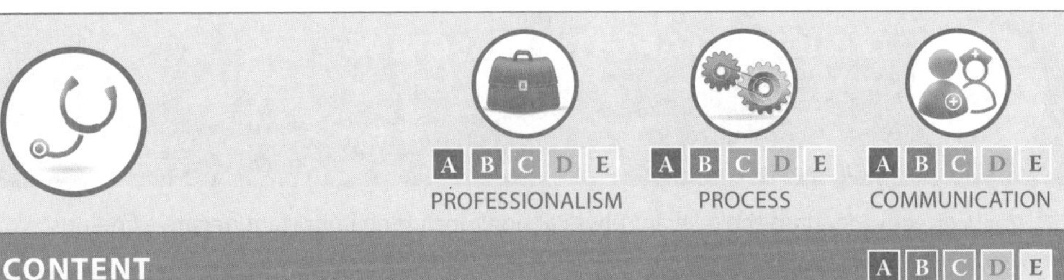

CONTENT

A B C D E

Exposes and positions patient correctly and maintains comfort

- Patient should be in a supine position, with abdomen exposed and modesty preserved.

Comments on wellbeing of patient, ie well or unwell

- Unwell and in moderate pain.

'Feet to face'

- Observes and comments on patient and surroundings from foot of bed
- Pale, some staining of dark vomit around patient's mouth and chest.

Asks for relevant clinical observations and bedside tests

- HR, BP, RR, O_2 sats, temperature, CRT.

Assessment of hands and upper limbs, and face and neck

- Pulse, capillary refill time 2 s
- Inspects for features of anaemia or jaundice.

Focused abdominal examination

- Inspection: inspects for scars and masses
- Palpation: identifies area of maximal tenderness – starts away from this site; superficial and deep palpation in systematic manner; comments on areas of guarding or rigidity, and attempts to elicit rebound tenderness in epigastrium
- Auscultation: presence and quality of bowel sounds.

Completes examination

- Digital rectal examination for presence of malaena.

Thanks patient, offers assistance, maintains patient's dignity and privacy until they are dressed

CLINICAL DIAGNOSTIC REASONING

A B C D E

- Correctly identifies the relevant physical signs, including important negative findings
- This 53-year-old lady is clearly unwell and in moderate pain
- She has evidence of blood-stained vomit around her mouth
- Her observations demonstrate a tachycardia and hypotension, and her capillary refill time is borderline at 2 s
- She is pale and clammy
- She has marked epigastric tenderness with features of peritonism
- Digital rectal examination confirms the presence of malaena.

■ **Please advise your initial management plan**

- Transfer patient to resus room if not already there – close observation and full monitoring
- IVI × 2 with fluid/blood resuscitation
- NGT
- Catheterise (measurement of urinary output)
- Antibiotics (broad spectrum)
- IV PPI eg omeprazole
- Analgesia and anti-emetic
- NIL BY MOUTH.

■ **What blood tests should be sent?**

- FBC, U&E, amylase, LFTs, Group & Save & Crossmatch 4–6 units, clotting screen.

■ **What X-rays should be requested?**

- Erect chest X-ray to look for air under the diaphragm may help confirm diagnosis of perforation, but the absence of sub-diaphragmatic air does not rule out the diagnosis.

■ **If a different patient with known cirrhotic liver disease and oesophaegeal varices presented in the same way as Mrs Morgan has, is there any other pharmacological treatment that you would consider?**

- Terlipressin (synthetic analogue of vasopressin (ADH)) or octreotide (or somatostatin analogue) reduce variceal bleeding due to vasoconstrictive action on the splanchnic circulation, and can be administered ahead of endoscopic intervention.

GLOBAL EXAMINATION MARK

A B C D E

Station 3 – Data interpretation

Part 1:	Part 2:
1 H	1 I
2 B	2 A
3 G	3 H
4 D	4 B
5 A	5 E

GLOBAL DATA INTERPRETATION MARK A B C D E

Station 4 – Prescribing skills

Check: DRUG DRs Don't Forget Signing Off (page 373)

Allergies, sensitivities and adverse drug reactions					Patient details/addressograph
No known allergies ✓		Initials LIL	Gender M / (F)		NHS/ Hospital No: 7114543
Not possible to ascertain ☐		Date 13.01	Weight (kg)	Date	
Medicine/substance	Reaction & Severity	Initials & Date	78	13.01	Surname: MORGAN
			Height		First name: ANNIE
			1.64m		
Alerts			Surface area (m²)		Date of birth: 13.12.58

IN-PATIENT MEDICATION PRESCRIPTION AND ADMINISTRATION RECORD — PasTest HOSPITAL

Consultant	Trainee Dr. Name and Bleep no.	Date of admission	Date chart reboarded	Estimated date of discharge
REILLY	LILIS 164	13.01.12		
This chart is no. 1 of 1	Transcribing Check by Pharmacy Sign .... Date	Ward 1. MAU 2.		

As required prescriptions			Date	Time	Dose	Route	Date	Time	Dose	Route	Date	Time	Dose	Route	Date	Time	Dose	Route
Drug PARACETAMOL	Allergies Checked	Dose 1g																
Frequency	Max Dose/24 hrs 4g	Route PO/ PR																
Indication																		
Signature LIL 164	Pharmacy	Start 13.01																

As required prescriptions

			Date	Time	Dose	Route	Date	Time	Dose	Route	Date	Time	Dose	Route	Date	Time	Dose	Route
Drug METOCLOPRAMIDE	Allergies Checked	Dose 10mg																
Frequency	Max Dose/24 hrs	Route S/C IM/IV																
Indication																		
Signature LIL 164	Pharmacy	Start 13.01																

As required prescriptions

			Date	Time	Dose	Route	Date	Time	Dose	Route	Date	Time	Dose	Route	Date	Time	Dose	Route
Drug CYCLIZINE	Allergies Checked	Dose 50mg																
Frequency	Max Dose/24 hrs	Route S/C IM/IV																
Indication																		
Signature LIL 164	Pharmacy	Start 13.01																

As required prescriptions

			Date	Time	Dose	Route	Date	Time	Dose	Route	Date	Time	Dose	Route	Date	Time	Dose	Route
Drug CODEINE PHOSPHATE	Allergies Checked	Dose 30-60 mg																
Frequency 6 HOURLY	Max Dose/24 hrs 60mg	Route PO																
Indication																		
Signature LIL 164	Pharmacy	Start 13.01																

As required prescriptions

			Date	Time	Dose	Route	Date	Time	Dose	Route	Date	Time	Dose	Route	Date	Time	Dose	Route
Drug MORPHINE	Allergies Checked	Dose 2.5-5 mg																
Frequency	Max Dose/24 hrs	Route IM/IV																
Indication																		
Signature LIL 164	Pharmacy	Start 13.01																

Infusion prescriptions continued — SC = subcutaneous; IVC = intravenous central, IVP = intravenous peripheral

Date & time	Route	Infusion Fluid: Name & strength	Infusion Fluid: Volume	Medication: Approved name with expiry / unit number	Medication: Dose	Duration	Rate	Prescriber's signature & bleep no.	Date given	Given by / Added by	Check by	Start time	Finish time	Pharmacy
13/01	IV	0.9% SALINE Exp: Batch/unit no:	500ml run until blood is available				4 hourly	LIL 164						
13/01	IV	Packed Cells Exp: Batch/unit no:					30-60 mins	LIL 164						
13/01	IV	Packed Cells Exp: Batch/unit no:					30-60 mins	LIL 164						
13/01	IV	0.9% SALINE Exp: Batch/unit no:	500ml run after 2nd unit of blood				4 hourly	LIL 164						

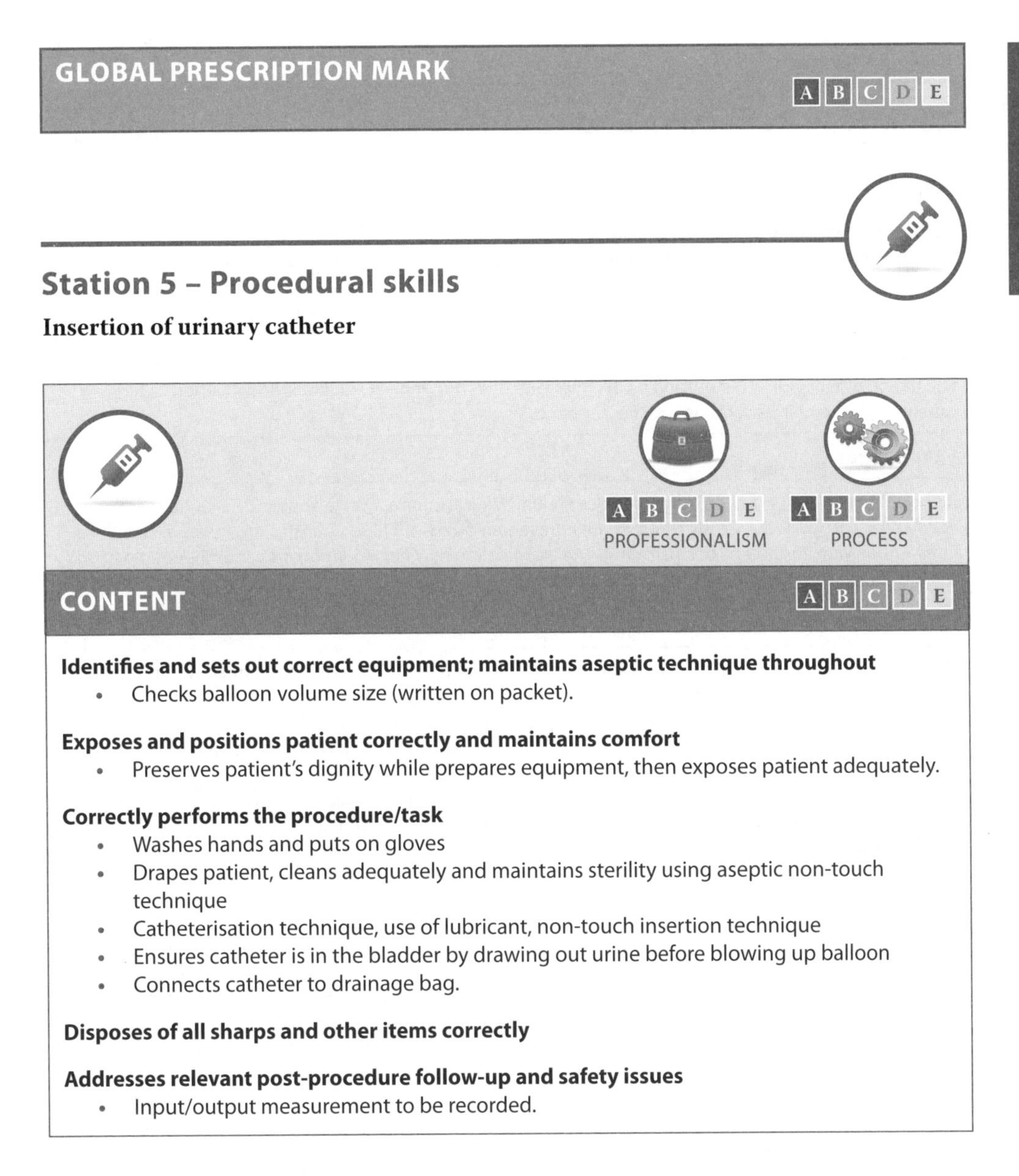

GLOBAL PRESCRIPTION MARK

A B C D E

Station 5 – Procedural skills

Insertion of urinary catheter

A B C D E
PROFESSIONALISM

A B C D E
PROCESS

CONTENT

A B C D E

Identifies and sets out correct equipment; maintains aseptic technique throughout

- Checks balloon volume size (written on packet).

Exposes and positions patient correctly and maintains comfort

- Preserves patient's dignity while prepares equipment, then exposes patient adequately.

Correctly performs the procedure/task

- Washes hands and puts on gloves
- Drapes patient, cleans adequately and maintains sterility using aseptic non-touch technique
- Catheterisation technique, use of lubricant, non-touch insertion technique
- Ensures catheter is in the bladder by drawing out urine before blowing up balloon
- Connects catheter to drainage bag.

Disposes of all sharps and other items correctly

Addresses relevant post-procedure follow-up and safety issues

- Input/output measurement to be recorded.

GLOBAL PROCEDURE MARK

A B C D E

Scenario 9: Reflection and consolidation

History

This patient, Mrs Annie Morgan, is 53 years old and presents with five episodes of coffee-ground vomiting and malaena. She developed a severe burning epigastric pain 2 days ago, which worsened today. She feels generally unwell, in that she is weak and tired, and has ongoing nausea. She does not report any fever. She has been having some dyspeptic symptoms for several months, which have been worse at night and eased by eating, or drinking milk.

Of note, she suffered a back injury a year ago and has been frequently using ibuprofen to help with the pain. She has no other medical history and no allergies. She does not drink or smoke, although reports a high caffeine intake, and lives at home with her husband.

Examination

In the emergency setting, the history provides enough clinical information to appreciate that this patient is very unwell and will require resuscitation with intravenous fluids and blood transfusion, as well as definitive intervention with endoscopy or laparotomy. The examination may help identify clues as to the aetiology of the bleeding, particularly in patients with features of chronic liver disease suggesting oesophageal varices.

Investigations

This patient demonstrates features of hypovolaemic shock, and this is likely to be confirmed with a low haemoglobin and low haematocrit. It may take several hours for these values, however – this is because there is a decreased circulating volume immediately after an acute bleed; as the volume normalises, haemodilution occurs and accurate levels become evident. The most important investigation in the emergency setting is early group and crossmatch so that patient-appropriate blood products can be prepared urgently. A clotting screen should be performed, especially in patients with chronic liver disease, in whom clotting derangement may be expected. U&E may demonstrate a raised urea with a normal creatinine suggestive of a significant bleed, as a consequence of the protein load in the GI tract.

An erect CXR should be performed to look for free subdiaphragmatic air, as may be seen after perforation of an intra-abdominal viscus.

Management

In most cases of upper GI bleeding an OGD will be performed. The endoscopist will normally be able to visualise the site of bleeding and treat with injection of adrenaline (potent vasoconstrictor), sclerotherapy or banding. The procedure is normally well tolerated with only topical anaesthetic spray to the oropharynx, but light sedation may be required.

Owing to the success of modern endoscopy, surgery is not often required in the management of acute haematemesis. However, laparotomy and resection of the affected area may be performed in cases of uncontrollable bleeding.

Further reading and web links

Management of UGIB:
www.sign.ac.uk/pdf/sign105.pdf
www.patient.co.uk/doctor/Upper-Gastrointestinal-Bleeding.htm
Transfusion guidelines and hazards information:
www.shotuk.org
www.transfusionguidelines.org.uk

Scenario 10: 'Tingle in my fingers'

Station 1

History *10-minute station*

You are a FY1 doctor completing a 4-month placement in the Neurology Department. A young woman, Miss Sarah Tennant, has been referred to Neurology Outpatients by her GP with a 1-month history of abnormal sensation in her hands and feet.

- **Please take a full history from this patient and then present it to your Consultant with a differential diagnosis.**

You will be assessed on the following areas, as well as the content and diagnostic reasoning of your history – take them into account in your presentation.

Professionalism

- Professional appearance (NHS dress code) – including general appearance, hair and jewellery
- Maintains patient and personal safety
- Polite introduction; identifies patient or interviewee correctly; confirms patient's date of birth from name band or other source
- Obtains informal consent; maintains patient's privacy
- Displays empathetic and caring attitudes and behaviours throughout.

Process

- Good organisation and structure; appropriate use of open and closed questions
- Appropriate fluency/rhythm/pace to the interview – this may change depending on environment and acute nature of problem
- Appropriate time for the patient to respond/reply to questions
- Appropriate acknowledgement of difficult or emotional areas of the patient's history.

Communication skills

- Demonstrates caring and sympathetic attitude
- Asks open questions
- Invites patient to ask questions and answers them appropriately
- Addresses patient's ideas, concerns and expectations.

Station 2

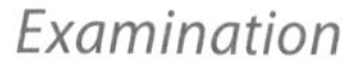

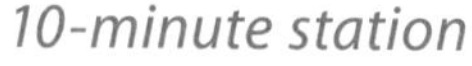

After presenting your patient's history to the Consultant in clinic you are asked to perform a full examination of the neurological system of Miss Tennant's arms and legs in front of your Consultant.

- **Examine the patient, present your clinical findings (within the station) and answer the following questions from your Consultant:**
  - **What are the most common causes of this presentation?**
  - **What additional examinations would you like to perform?**
  - **What initial investigations would you request?**

You will be assessed on the following areas, as well as the content and skills of your examination – take them into account in your presentation.

Professionalism

- Professional appearance; maintains infection control standards, including hand cleaning and appropriate use of gloves and aprons
- Maintains patient and personal safety
- Polite introduction; identifies patient and confirms date of birth from name band or other source
- Obtains informal consent; maintains patient privacy and dignity
- Displays empathetic and caring attitudes and behaviours throughout.

Process

- Appropriate fluency/rhythm/pace to the examination – this may change depending on environment and acute nature of problem
- Good organisation and structure of examination; sensitive and empathetic approach
- Uses appropriate clinical techniques throughout
- Maintains privacy and dignity throughout.

Clinical communication

- Explains proposed examination/procedure: explains examination/procedure as it proceeds
- Offers information in a clear, structured and fluent manner, avoiding jargon
- Listens to patient and responds appropriately
- Demonstrates appropriate body language.

Please read the information below before presenting the examination findings. ***[NB If you have a model do not read this section]***

Clinical findings

- o Patient appears comfortable at rest
- o No wasting, tremor or fasciculations present
- o Upper limbs: normal tone, power and reflexes; reduced light touch sensation in right hand and forearm but not of a dermatomal distribution; normal on the left; reduced proprioception up to the elbow on the right, normal on the left; normal pinprick and temperature sensation bilaterally; normal upper limb co-ordination.
- o Lower limbs: normal tone, power and reflexes; reduced light touch sensation in the right foot and calf but not of a dermatomal distribution; normal on the left; reduced proprioception in the right foot, normal on the left; normal pinprick and temperature sensation bilaterally; normal lower limb co-ordination
- o Romberg's test positive; gait normal.

Station 3

Procedural skills *10-minute station*

Procedure A

Your Consultant has asked you to take some samples of blood from Miss Tennant in order to check her inflammatory markers, as well as her baseline full blood count, renal and liver function.

- **Using the following equipment, please perform venepuncture on this arm and explain what you are doing to your patient.**

Equipment provided

- Model arm for venepuncture
- Vacutainer venepuncture system – needle, vacutainer
- Bedside sharps bin
- Alcohol swab for skin
- Gauze
- Blood bottles for the samples taken
- Blood request forms

Procedure B

Your Consultant has asked you to also perform a random blood glucose test via a glucometer to ensure that Miss Tennant does not have undiagnosed diabetes, causing a peripheral neuropathy.

- **Using the following equipment, please perform this procedure.**

Equipment provided

- **Gloves**
- **An alcohol wipe**
- **A glucose monitor**
- **Test strips**
- **Spring-loaded lancet**
- **Cotton wool**

Station 4

Data interpretation *10-minute station*

Part 1:

Miss Tennant has been electively admitted for a diagnostic lumbar puncture. Your Consultant also has a number of other lumbar puncture results for his other patients.

- **As a training exercise he would like you to look at the following CSF analysis results and match them to the likely diagnosis and clinical scenario.**

Patient history	CSF	Diagnosis
1 A 29-year-old woman with painful blurring of vision and numbness in the hands	(A) Xanthochromia	(a) Meningococcal meningitis
2 A neonate with diarrhoea and vomiting, 'off feeds' and extremely irritable	(B) High red cell count in all three CSF bottles	(b) Tertiary syphilis
3 A 12-year-old schoolgirl with purpura, DIC and severe headache, photophobia and neck stiffness	(C) Positive for VDRL, TPHA, FTA	(c) Subarachnoid haemorrhage
4 A 78-year-old man with recurrent falls and confusion	(D) Raised protein, low glucose, Gram-negative coccobacillus	(d) Multiple sclerosis
5 A 27-year-old woman with sudden onset of headache and coma	(E) Raised protein, low glucose, Gram-negative diplococci	(e) Subdural haemorrhage
6 A 61-year-old woman with increasing confusion and a previous history of pelvic inflammatory disease	(F) Oligoclonal bands	(f) *Haemophilus influenzae* Meningitis

Part 2:

A Methylprednisolone
B Baclofen
C Paroxetine
D Natalizumab
E Gabapentin
F Broad-spectrum antibiotics
G Physiotherapy
H Glatiramer acetate
I Sildenafil

- For each of the following clinical scenarios, select the most appropriate therapy, A–J, each option may be used once, more than once or not at all.
  1. A 35-year-old woman with secondary progressive multiple sclerosis (MS) presents with a worsening of her left side hemiparesis and increased lethargy. Her temperature is 38.5 °C on admission, with urine dip positive for leucocytes and nitrates.
  2. A 42-year-old woman with relapsing remitting MS is referred by her GP to Neurology Outpatients with severe shooting pain in her left leg after an episode of paresthesia 6 months ago.
  3. A 42-year-old man with primary progressive MS, who is now bedbound, has pain due to increased spasticity of both his lower limbs.
  4. A 23-year-old woman presents with an episode of left eye pain, blurred vision and reduced colour vision. Her MRI scan is normal and her blood CSF demonstrate oligoclonal bands.
  5. A 47-year-old man with three previous relapses from his MS presents with a 6-month history of erectile dysfunction.

Station 5

Clinical communication skills *10-minute station*

Miss Tennant has returned to clinic following her recent investigations. Unfortunately the MRI shows lesions strongly suggestive of demyelination in the spine and brain, and her CSF analysis shows oligoclonal bands (no serum oligoclonal bands). This meets the diagnostic criteria for MS. Your Consultant has asked you break this news to Miss Tennant as you have met her on a number of occasions. She will observe you in this consultation.

- Please speak to Miss Tenant, concentrating on conveying the diagnosis and ensuring understanding. Complex discussions about treatment and prognosis are beyond the scope of this consultation. Address any questions that Miss Tennant may raise.

Answers

SCENARIO 10

Station 1 – History

Patient script

Your name is Sarah Tennant and you are 29 years old and otherwise fit and well. One month ago you noticed tingling in your right hand associated with numbness, which has got worse over the weeks. You also feel quite clumsy, and this has been causing difficulty with your work as a graphic designer. Over the last week you have also felt unsteady on your feet, with similar tingling in your right foot and toes. You have not fallen but felt as though you might, especially when walking in the dark.

You have not had any weakness in your arms or legs. You have not had any headaches, blackouts or fits. You have had no bladder or bowel dysfunction. You have started no new medications and have not had any infections recently. You have no other medical history. You are on no regular medications and have no known allergies. You are a smoker of 10 per day and drink more than you know you should – approximately three bottles of wine most weekends.

You are unsure of any medical history as you were adopted as a baby.

You are very concerned that you might have had a type of stroke as you have been reading about your symptoms on the internet.

On direct questioning:

1. You do recall having an episode of blurred vision and headaches last year, but it resolved after 3 weeks so you did not seek any medical help.

2. The abnormal sensation in your arm and leg do get worse after a hot bath.

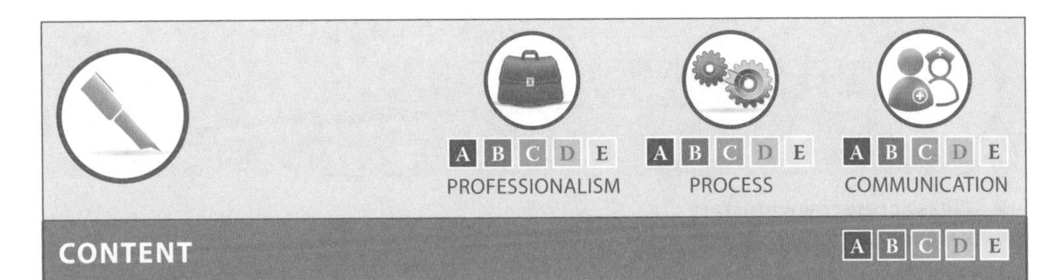

CONTENT

A B C D E

Identifies key information

- Unilateral paresthesia, numbness, dyspraxia
- Gait ataxia
- Uhthoff's phenomenon
- Previous episode of visual disturbance – probably optic neuritis
- No motor symptoms.

Identifies important negatives, including systemic enquiry

- No headache, LOC, seizures or back pain
- No bladder or bowel dysfunction
- No bulbar symptoms
- No mood change.

Completing the history

- Drug and allergy history: nil
- Previous medical history: nil known
- Social and occupational history: graphic designer, smoker 10 per day, excess alcohol – 30 units per week
- Family history: nil known as adopted

Summarises important areas of the history back to the patient

Invites patient to ask questions and is able to deal with them appropriately

Establishes patient's ideas, concerns and expectations

- Establishes patient concern that she has had a stroke

CLINICAL DIAGNOSTIC REASONING

A B C D E

- **Please present your history**
  - Candidate offers a logical, well-structured account of the history
- **What is your diagnosis?**
  - Candidate offers the correct diagnosis and appropriate differentials
  - The differential diagnosis of the combination of both peripheral and central neurological symptoms separated in time and place is small, as this is the hallmark of demyelinating disease.
- **(If demyelinating disease is offered as a diagnosis): What patterns of disease do you know in multiple sclerosis?**
  - Relapsing remitting
  - Secondary progressive
  - Primary progressive
  - Progressive relapsing.

GLOBAL HISTORY MARK

A B C D E

Station 2 – Examination

Patient script

If you are an actor/patient, read the patient history and physical signs fully – when the candidate comes to an abnormal site in their examination, act-out tenderness and/or volunteer the relevant physical sign.

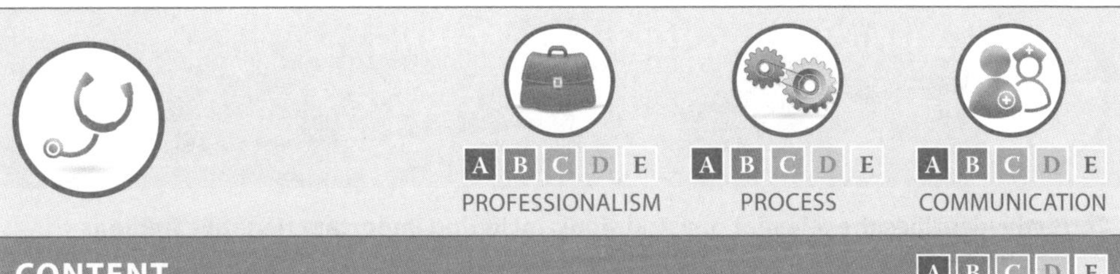

CONTENT

A B C D E

Exposes and positions patient correctly and maintains comfort

Comments on wellbeing of patient, ie well or unwell

- No fasciculation or wasting.

'Feet to face'

Asks for appropriate relevant clinical observations

Upper limb assessment

- Tone
- Power – shoulder (ab- and adduction), elbow (flex and extend), wrist (flex and extend, supinate and pronate), fingers (ab- and adduction)
- Reflexes – biceps, triceps and supinator
- Sensation – light touch, pinprick and joint position sense in all dermatomes
- Co-ordination – past pointing and assessment for dysdiadachokinesis.

Lower limb assessment

- Tone – including assessment for clonus
- Power – hip (flex and extend, ab- and adduction), knee (flex and extend), ankle (inversion, eversion, plantar and dorsiflexion)
- Reflexes – knee jerk, ankle jerk and plantars
- Sensation – light touch, pinprick and joint position sense in all dermatomes
- Co-ordination – heel shin co-ordination
- Completes examination with assessment for Romberg's test and gait.

CLINICAL DIAGNOSTIC REASONING

A B C D E

Correctly identifies the relevant physical signs, including important negative findings

- Does not identify signs that are not present.

Correctly identifies the most common causes of peripheral sensory neuropathy

- Diabetes mellitus
- Vitamin deficiency, particularly B_{12} and folate
- Toxins such as alcohol, drugs such as vincristine, and heavy metals
- Autoimmune diseases
- Demyelinating disease.

Correctly identifies relevant further examinations

- Fundoscopy to exclude other causes of visual problems and establish the presence of optic atrophy due to possible previous optic neuritis
- Cranial nerve examination.

Correctly identifies relevant initial investigations

- Lumbar puncture to confirm the presence of oligoclonal bands in the CSF
- MRI of the brainstem and cervical cord – to establish the presence of areas of demyelination (plaques)
- Visual evoked responses.

Demonstrates clear and logical diagnostic reasoning

GLOBAL EXAMINATION MARK

A B C D E

Station 3 – Procedural skills

Procedure A: Venepuncture

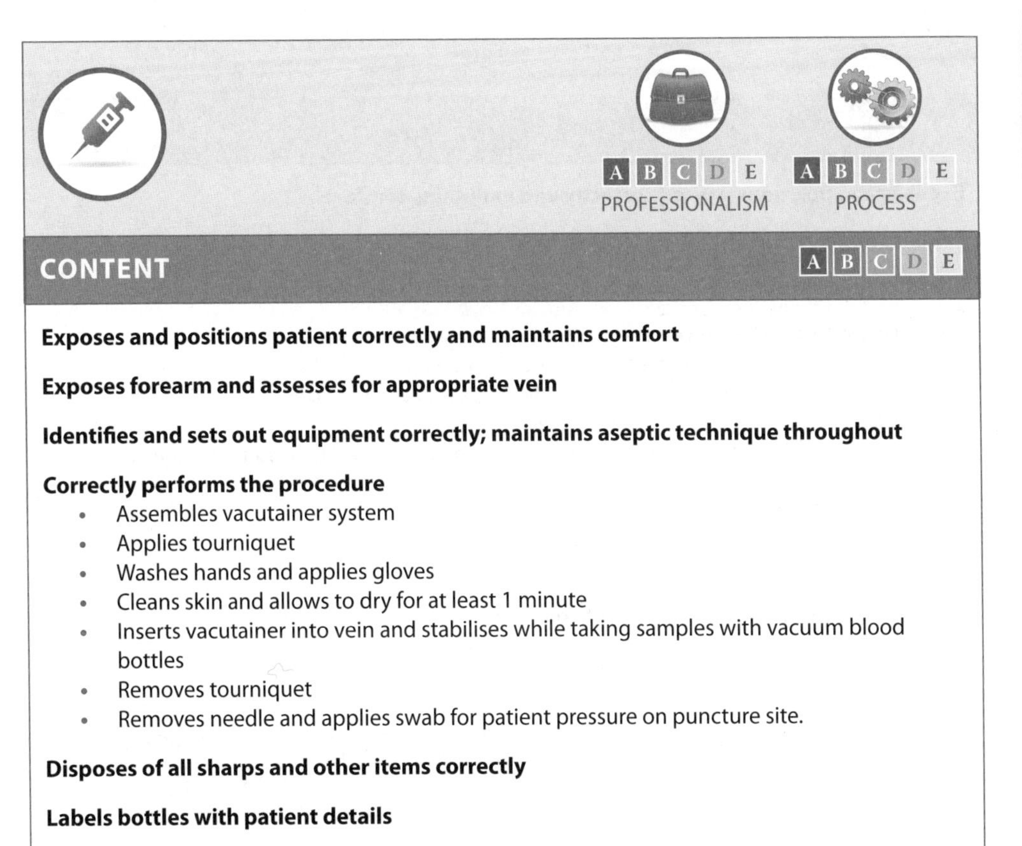

A B C D E
PROFESSIONALISM

A B C D E
PROCESS

CONTENT A B C D E

Exposes and positions patient correctly and maintains comfort

Exposes forearm and assesses for appropriate vein

Identifies and sets out equipment correctly; maintains aseptic technique throughout

Correctly performs the procedure

- Assembles vacutainer system
- Applies tourniquet
- Washes hands and applies gloves
- Cleans skin and allows to dry for at least 1 minute
- Inserts vacutainer into vein and stabilises while taking samples with vacuum blood bottles
- Removes tourniquet
- Removes needle and applies swab for patient pressure on puncture site.

Disposes of all sharps and other items correctly

Labels bottles with patient details

Addresses relevant post-procedure follow-up and safety issues

Procedure B: Blood glucose testing

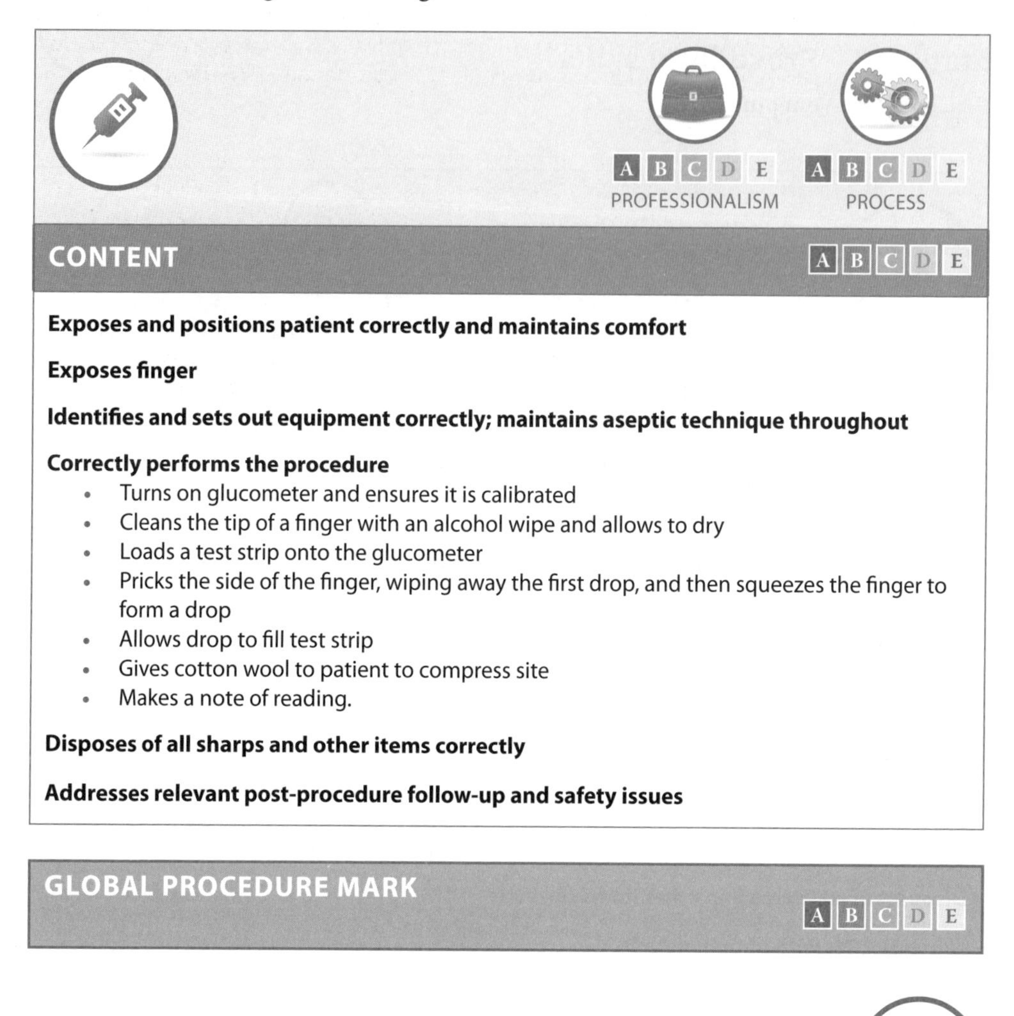

A B C D E PROFESSIONALISM

A B C D E PROCESS

CONTENT A B C D E

Exposes and positions patient correctly and maintains comfort

Exposes finger

Identifies and sets out equipment correctly; maintains aseptic technique throughout

Correctly performs the procedure

- Turns on glucometer and ensures it is calibrated
- Cleans the tip of a finger with an alcohol wipe and allows to dry
- Loads a test strip onto the glucometer
- Pricks the side of the finger, wiping away the first drop, and then squeezes the finger to form a drop
- Allows drop to fill test strip
- Gives cotton wool to patient to compress site
- Makes a note of reading.

Disposes of all sharps and other items correctly

Addresses relevant post-procedure follow-up and safety issues

GLOBAL PROCEDURE MARK A B C D E

Station 4 – Data interpretation

Part 1:

1 (F) (d)

Oligoclonal bands, shown by protein electrophoresis, are present in the CSF in over 80% of cases of multiple sclerosis. They are formed by IgG within the CSF but the antigen they are directed against as yet remains unclear. Oligoclonal bands may also be found in the CSF of patients with sarcoidosis, SLE, Behçet's syndrome, neurosyphilis and viral encephalitis.

2 (D) (f)

This neonate has *Haemophilus influenzae* **meningitis, which is more common in this age group. As with other bacterial meningitides, there is a high protein content and a low glucose concentration. A Gram stain gives the microbiological diagnosis.**

3 (E) (a)

This history is highly suggestive of meningococcal meningitis with secondary DIC. The patient should be treated empirically with high doses of benzylpenicillin and contact tracing should be arranged. All close contacts should receive prophylactic treatment with rifampicin.

4 (A) (e)

This patient gives a classical history of a subdural haemorrhage, but over 50% of patients give no history of trauma. Subdural haemorrhages are usually represented by a hyperdense concave rim around the cerebrum on CT head scan. However, at 10 days they appear as an isodense rim and therefore may be overlooked.

5 (B) (c)

A sudden severe headache with an associated decreased level of consciousness must be treated as a subarachnoid haemorrhage until proven otherwise. The CSF samples are blood stained in the first 24 to 48 hours but samples taken 48 to 72 hours after the onset of symptoms appear discoloured due to altered blood, termed xanthochromia.

6 (C) (b)

Patients presenting with insidious worsening of a dementing type illness should have a dementia screen to exclude treatable causes. This should include VDRL, TPHA and TPA, TFTs and B_{12}. If syphilis serology is positive, the patient should have a lumbar puncture to exclude tertiary syphilis. As in this case, the patient should receive a course of benzylpenicillin after 24 hours cover with steroids. This is to reduce the risk of a Jarisch–Herxheimer reaction.

Part 2:

1 F 2 E 3 B 4 A 5 I

GLOBAL DATA INTERPRETATION MARK

A B C D E

Station 5 – Clinical communication skills

Patient script

You are optimistic about your diagnosis, as your symptoms are nearly entirely resolved since your last appointment. 'It can't be that bad if it's got better already.'

You live alone in a flat and work as a graphic designer. You have a close relationship with your adopted mother, who lives close to you.

You are very shocked by the diagnosis of multiple sclerosis, as a friend of your mother had that diagnosis and ended up in a wheelchair within a couple of years of her diagnosis. You are very concerned this is inevitable.

You know that multiple sclerosis is not curable and feel hopeless, as there will be 'no treatment' of your disease.

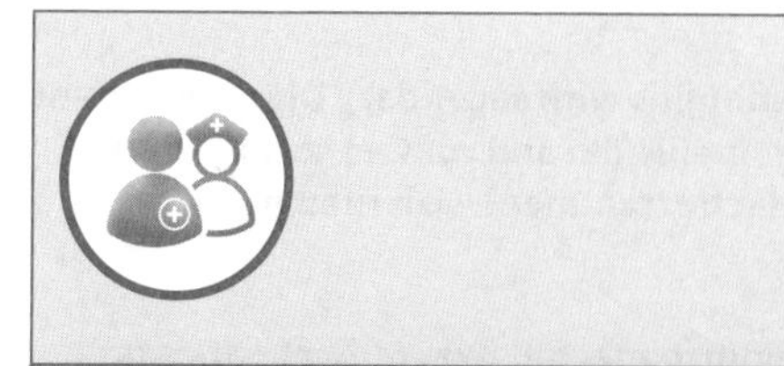

A B C D E
PROFESSIONALISM

A B C D E
PROCESS

CONTENT

A B C D E

Investigates patient's present level of understanding of scenario

Summarises and confirms what has happened so far
- Summarises history of peripheral neuropathy and probable optic neuritis
- Explains results of lumbar puncture and MRI.

Asks what, and how much information the patient would like to be told

Establishes patient's ideas, concerns and expectations
- Patient has had resolution of symptoms and feels that she is 'better'.

Explains the key important information
- Clearly explains diagnosis of MS as an autoimmune disease, in which nerves throughout body are attacked
- Explains the relapsing remitting nature of episodes separated in time and throughout the nervous system
- Explains that MS can have different courses and that some people do not have any further episodes
- Affects many systems and there is a possibility of significant disability
- There are many agents to suppress the immune system and decrease the severity and frequency of flares
- Explains that it is not curable but there are many treatments to alleviate symptoms/ disability due to the disease.

Invites patient to ask questions as they proceed through the consultation and is able to deal with them appropriately

Summarises important areas of the consultation back to the patient

Formally ends the consultation and ensures appropriate follow-up has been discussed
- Support available with MS society and nurse specialists
- Arranges for follow-up with MS nurse and further clinic appointment.

GLOBAL COMMUNICATION MARK

A B C D E

Scenario 10: Reflection and consolidation

History

Miss Tennant is a 29-year-old woman who presents with a month-long episode of paresthesia and numbness of the hands and feet with associated dyspraxia. She has no focal weakness, although she does have some gait ataxia. She has no symptoms of raised intracranial pressure, seizures or current visual disturbance. She has no bladder or bowel dysfunction. She also describes an episode of visual disturbance 1 year ago with associated headache, which resolved spontaneously. She has no previous medical history, no drug history or allergies. She has no known family history, as she was adopted. She also describes Uhthoff's phenomena, as her symptoms appear to be worse after a hot bath.

The most likely diagnosis of these neurological symptoms that are separated in time and location is demyelinating disease, multiple sclerosis.

Examination

On examination of the neurological system of Miss Tennant's upper and lower limbs there is no wasting or fasciculation at rest. There is normal tone, power and reflexes throughout. There is reduced light touch sensation in the right lower limb and right hand but no area of absent sensation and the area does not correspond to any dermatomal distribution. This is associated with reduced proprioception in the right hand and foot. Pinprick sensation and temperature sensation are preserved. Co-ordination is preserved in heel shine and finger nose testing bilaterally. Gait appears normal but Romberg's test is positive.

As well as the symptoms seen in our patient here, it is important to remember that MS is a multisystem disorder and any history or examination should assess the systems that MS commonly affects:

Visual and gaze assessment

- Optic neuritis is a common presentation and an assessment of acuity, colour vision and fundoscopy should be performed (repeated episodes of neuritis lead to optic atrophy)
- Gaze abnormalities are also common, leading to diplopia and nystagmus, intra-nuclear opthalmoplegia is an interesting and challenging diagnosis to make (see below).

Cranial nerve palsies

- Facial nerve palsies can occur and trigeminal neuralgia is not uncommon
- Cranial nerve eight demyelination can lead to hearing loss and unsteadiness.

Cognitive and psychological symptoms

- Decreased concentration, impaired memory and even rarely psychotic symptoms
- Depression is a common problem.

Unpleasant sensations

- Impaired taste and smell should be specifically asked about
- Loss of thermal and pain sensation can be a distressing symptom.

Autonomic symptoms

- Bladder symptoms
- Sexual problems
- Loss of thermoregulation: excess sweating, pyrexia or hypothermia.

Management

Management of MS as a chronic disease requires a multidisciplinary approach:
Acute attacks – intravenous steroids (usually methylprednisolone)
Disease-modifying agents (immunomodulators) to decrease the frequency of relapses and try to minimise disability

- Interferon beta
- Monoclonal antibodies
- Glatiramer.

Management of effects of the disease

- Physiotherapy and neurorehabilitation
- Occupational therapy to maintain independence
- Drug therapy for specific problems – baclofen for spasticity, medication for bladder instability, antidepressants for mood disturbance
- Specialist nurse advice and input.

Further reading and web links

Management of multiple sclerosis in primary and secondary care:
www.nice.org.uk/CG8
Ophthalmological manifestations of multiple sclerosis:
emedicine.medscape.com/article/1214270-overview
Multiple Sclerosis Society:
www.mssociety.org.uk

Scenario 11: 'A confused young man'

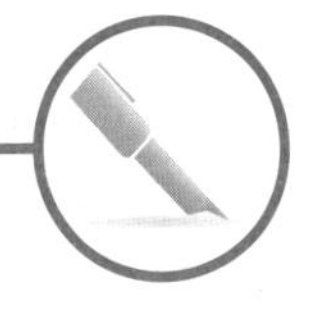

Station 1

History *10-minute station*

You are the FY1 on call with the Acute Medical Team. The ST4 on call has asked you to take a corroborative history from the girlfriend of a 23-year-old man, Mr Jack Da Costa, who has recently been brought into the Emergency Department with a high fever and confusion.

- **Please take a comprehensive history with a view to making a diagnosis. You will be asked to present your history to the examiner at the end of the station.**

You will be assessed on the following areas, as well as the content and diagnostic reasoning of your history – take them into account in your presentation.

Professionalism

- Professional appearance (NHS dress code) – including general appearance, hair and jewellery
- Maintains patient and personal safety
- Polite introduction; identifies patient or interviewee correctly; confirms patient's date of birth from name band or other source
- Obtains informal consent; maintains patient's privacy
- Displays empathetic and caring attitudes and behaviours throughout.

Process

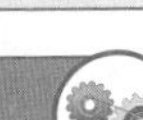

- Good organisation and structure; appropriate use of open and closed questions
- Appropriate fluency/rhythm/pace to the interview – this may change depending on environment and acute nature of the problem
- Appropriate time for the patient to respond/reply to questions
- Appropriate acknowledgement of difficult or emotional areas of the patient's history.

Clinical communication

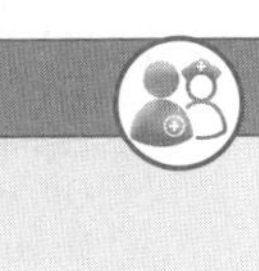

- Demonstrates caring and sympathetic attitude
- Asks open questions
- Invites patient to ask questions and answers them appropriately
- Addresses patient's ideas, concerns and expectations.

Station 2

Examination *10-minute station*

Given the history, the ST4 asks you to perform a focused, diagnostic assessment of the patient.

- **Please examine Mr Da Costa to assess for:**
  - **General wellbeing of the patient**
  - **Diabetic ketoacidosis and complications**
  - **Chest infection.**
- **Once you have completed your assessment (from information within the station), please present the relevant findings to the ST4 in an appropriate manner for a busy Emergency Department.**

You will be assessed on the following areas, as well as the content and skills of your examination – take them into account in your presentation.

Professionalism

- Professional appearance; maintains infection control standards, including hand cleaning and appropriate use of gloves and aprons
- Maintains patient and personal safety
- Polite introduction; identifies patient and confirms date of birth from name band or other source
- Obtains informal consent; maintains patient privacy and dignity
- Displays empathetic and caring attitudes and behaviours throughout.

Process

- Appropriate fluency/rhythm/pace to the examination – this may change depending on environment and acute nature of problem
- Good organisation and structure of examination; sensitive and empathetic approach
- Uses appropriate clinical techniques throughout
- Maintains privacy and dignity throughout.

Clinical communication

- Explains proposed examination/procedure; explains examination/procedure as it proceeds
- Offers information in a clear, structured and fluent manner, avoiding jargon
- Listens to patient and responds appropriately
- Demonstrates appropriate body language.

Please read the information below before presenting this case to the ST4 as if you were in a busy Emergency department.
[NB If you have a model do not read this section]

Clinical findings

- o **Acutely unwell, confused and agitated young man**
- o **Observations – HR 120 bpm, BP 82/54 mmHg; regular, low volume; RR >30 bpm; O_2 sats 98% on air; temperature 39.6 °C; CBG > 48 mmol/l**
- o **General examination – cold and clammy to the touch, drenched in sweat, since arrival no measured urine output, clinically very dehydrated, marked oral candidiasis**
- o **Focused examination of chest – trachea in the midline, percussion reduced in right lower zone associated with coarse crackles, TVF normal throughout**
- o **No signs of meningism, abdomen soft and non-tender and he has no signs of skin sepsis (the toe web spaces are normal)**
- o **In summary, this is a previously fit and well young man who now presents with signs consistent of hyperglycaemic pre-coma, most likely DKA, and a right lower zone chest infection. He is severely dehydrated and overtly septic.**

Station 3

Data interpretation *10-minute station*

Part 1:

Mr Da Costa's investigation results become available and the ST4 asks you to write them in the notes. She then sets you a series of questions to answer shown below.

- **Please write up the following results in the patient's notes.**

  FBC: Hb 14.3 g/dl, MCV 84 fl, WCC 29.6 × 10^9/l, (neutrophils 23.9 × 10^9/l), platelets 61 × 10^9/l
  U&Es: Na^+ 153 mmol/l, K^+ 4.9 mmol/l, chloride 105 mmol/l, bicarbonate 7.9 mmol/l, urea 23.6 mmol/l, creatinine 154 μmol/l
  RBG: 53.1 mmol/l
  Serum ketones (normal <0.6 mmol/l) 16.9 mmol/l
  Coagulation: INR 1.6, APTT 44 s, FDP 65 μg/ml, D-dimer 3.9 iu/l
  Blood cultures sent

- **For each of the questions below, please indicate whether it is TRUE (T) or FALSE (F).**
  1. **The white cell and differential are suggestive of an atypical pneumonia.**
  2. **The thrombocytopenia is consistent with haemolysis.**
  3. **The urea:creatinine ratio confirms pre-renal impairment.**
  4. **The calculated serum osmolality is 392.5 mOsmo/l.**
  5. **Given this patient's serum sodium, he should receive dextrose rather than saline solution.**
  6. **Given this patient's serum potassium, he should receive 20 mmol/l of potassium supplementation.**
  7. **The anion gap is 26 mmol/l.**
  8. **The coagulation screen is consistent with disseminated intravascular coagulopathy.**
  9. **Given these results this patient should be given VTE prophylaxis with low molecular weight heparin.**
  10. **The results are consistent with hyperglycaemic, hyperosmolar non-ketotic syndrome.**

Part 2:
While you are in the Emergency Department one of the middle grades shows you a series of interesting ABGs from other patients who have passed through the department that day.

- **For each of the following patient scenarios, select the correct ABG result from the table below.**
  1. **A 43-year-old woman with known mental health problems and type2 diabetes mellitus presents to the Emergency Department after being found unconscious by her mother at home. She looked to have taken a large number of her metformin tablets.**
  2. **A 69-year-old man with 'chronic indigestion' and increasing dysphagia to solids presents to the Emergency Department with a 2-week history of projectile vomiting after meals.**
  3. **A 68-year-old man with a chronic 'smoker's cough' and increasing wheeze presents in the Emergency Department with a 5-day history of cough productive of greenish sputum and increasing shortness of breath at rest. On examination he has an audible wheeze throughout his chest and coarse crackles at the left base.**
  4. **A 71-year-old man with known COPD is seen in the local chest clinic after being started on LTOT 3 weeks previously by the Respiratory Consultant. He reports feeling 'really well' and has been able to play with his grandchildren for the first time in years.**

5 A 15-year-old boy with known 'brittle' asthma is brought to the Emergency Department with severe shortness of breath. His observations show BP 90/60 mmHg, HR 66 bpm, RR < 10 bpm, temperature 38.2 °C. On examination he is unable to speak and on auscultation his chest is quiet throughout.

6 A 23-year-old woman presents in the Emergency Department with 'hyperventilation'. Of note she is on the oral contraceptive pill and has just returned from California, where she has been visiting her boyfriend. Her initial observations show BP 90/60 mmHg, HR 123 bpm, RR 32 bpm, temperature 37.2 °C. Examination of her chest reveals a 'squeaky' extra sound in the right axilla but there is nothing else of note.

	pH	PaO_2 (kPa)	Sats (%)	$PaCO_2$ (kPa)	HCO_3^- (mmol/l)	Base excess (mmol/l)	Lactate (mmol/l)	% Inspired O_2
Normal values	7.35–7.45	10.6–13.6	92–98	4.6–6.4	22–28	0±2.0	0.5–2.0	Room air (R/A)
Patient A	6.92	14.6	99	1.1	4.2	–24.3	12.8	Nasal 2 l/min
Patient B	7.14	6.9	73	11.7	20.0	–4.9	5.7	28% venturi mask
Patient C	7.35	9.9	91	2.9	20.6	–2.9	2.6	R/A
Patient D	7.43	10.1	90	6.9	35.8	+14.6	1.1	Nasal 2 l/min
Patient E	7.51	15.7	100	2.9	25.4	+0.8	0.7	R/A
Patient F	7.64	13.9	97	4.1	60.8	+23.4	0.6	R/A
Patient G	7.22	9.9	89	7.2	15.8	–8.6	8.8	15 l/min Non-rebreathe mask

Station 4

Procedural skills *10-minute station*

Procedure A

The ST4 asks you to repeat Mr Da Costa's ABGs 1 hour after the start of his treatment. Mr Da Costa remains confused and drowsy but is otherwise improving.

- Using the manikin arm and the rest of the equipment listed below, please take an ABG sample. You should talk to the examiner as if they are the patient.

Details

Mr Jack Da Costa; Hospital No. 236543; DOB: 15/01/1988; Allergies: penicillin – severe rash

Equipment provided

- Manikin arm for ABG sampling
- Hospital bracelet on arm with correct patient details
- ABG syringe and needle
- Alcohol solution and gauze
- Gauze to press over puncture wound
- Gloves
- Sharps bin

Procedure B

While you are taking the ABGs the nursing staff on the ward ask if you could insert an NG tube for Mr Da Costa, as he has been retching.

■ Using the manikin and the rest of the equipment listed below, please insert an appropriate NG tube. You should talk to the examiner as if they are the patient.

Equipment:

- Manikin for insertion of NG tube
- Hospital bracelet near manikin with correct patient details
- Gloves
- A choice of different NG tubes
- Sticky tape to secure NG tube
- Water-based gel
- Gauze

Station 5

Prescribing skills *10-minute station*

You have been asked to write up Mr Da Costa's drug and fluid charts.

■ Using the BNF and charts provided, please write up the following interventions:

A fixed-rate intravenous insulin infusion (FRIVII)

24-hours of intravenous fluids (he has had a single litre of 0.9% saline so far and is written up for a second over the next hour)

Appropriate intravenous antibiotics

Appropriate medications on the 'as required' side of the chart.

Details

Mr Jack Da Costa; Hospital No. 236543; DOB: 15/01/1988; Allergies: penicillin – severe rash; Weight: about 70 kg; Height: 1.76 m; Ward HDU; Consultant: Dr Richards

Observations: BP 98/74 mmHg, HR 110 bpm, RR 24 bpm, UO: 12 ml in the last hour, O_2 sats 98% on 2 l/min, rousable but drowsy and confused.

Remember: DRUG DRs Don't Forget Signing Off (page 373)

Station 6

Clinical communication skills *10-minute station*

Over the next 48 hours Mr Da Costa makes a good recovery and is discharged to Ward C, under the care of your team – the Diabetes and Endocrine Team.

- **The Diabetes Specialist Nurse (DSN) asks you to come to see the patient with her as a Mini-CEX. She asks you to:**
  - **Explain the new diagnosis to the patient**
  - **Explain his new treatment – the DSN has recommended he be started on Levemir® 14 Units once nightly and NovoRapid® 8 Units with meals**
  - **Give the patient some general education about the new diagnosis.**

Answers

Station 1 – History

Patient script

You are Dianne Robinson, a 21-year-old secretary working for a large record company. You are the long-term girlfriend (you've been going out for over 3 years) of the patient Mr Jack Da Costa. He was brought in to the Emergency Department this afternoon by ambulance after you called the GP at lunchtime. Jack had become increasingly confused and unwell over the last few days.

Jack is a trainee carpenter and is normally very fit and well. He has had no major illnesses as far as you know, and is on no regular medications. He is very healthy and keeps very fit as he takes part in competitive taekwando. He has been hospitalised twice in the last 3 years, once due to a broken right arm, needing an operation to fix it, and once due to concussion – both suffered in taekwando competitions. He is very fit and 'I must say has a lovely body!'

Jack told you that 'he's been feeling weird' over the last month or so, may be 6–8 weeks. You remember because it was just after his last major competition 2 months ago. He has been very thirsty, 'always has a cold drink in his hand', and in his own words is 'drinking and weeing for England'. He gets up all through the night and is 'continually disappearing to pee during the day'.

In the last few weeks he has also complained of blurring of his vision, especially (on the rare occasions) that he sits down and watches TV. He has also mentioned that he's been finding it very difficult to maintain his fighting weight, despite eating more and training less (he's felt tired and washed out).

Over the last 36 hours he's become increasingly confused, 'he didn't recognise me this morning' 'he was mumbling jibberish under his breath and was really quite frightening ... that's when I called the GP'. 'He was burning up and sweating profusely ... he looked terrible'. During this time he's had a terrible chesty cough. He's coughing up thick greenish spit. He's been mildly wheezy and short of breath but you haven't noticed if he's coughed any blood.

PMH: nil of note.

Meds: nil; occasional 'painkillers' after fights.

Allergies: he can't take penicillin – makes him 'come out in a really horrible rash'.

Family history: father – well, no known illnesses; mother died in car accident; two younger sisters both well.

You live together in a ground-floor, rented flat; he is a trainee carpenter – doing really well on his apprenticeship. He has never smoked and takes no illicit drugs. He drinks alcohol very rarely because of his training.

Ideas and concerns: you don't know what is wrong with him but you were really worried about him today. He has lost lots of weight and 'I'm just worried he might have cancer or something serious like that'.

Expectations – you are hoping that he will be admitted to the hospital at least overnight and can be sorted out. 'I really hope he hasn't got anything serious'.

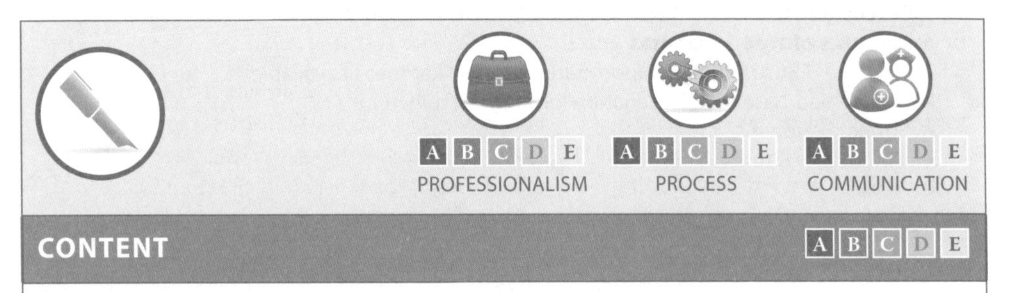

CONTENT

A B C D E

Establishes relationship to patient

Identifies key information

- Very fit and well until recent illness
- Competitive taekwando/martial arts expert.
- Insidious progression over the last 2 months
- Polyuria, polydypsia, blurred vision, weight loss
- General malaise and loss of energy – unable to train for fights
- Chest symptoms – cough, sputum, pyrexia, unwell, confusion.

Completing the history

- Drug and allergy history: nil meds, allergy to penicillin – severe rash
- Previous medical history: vascular risk, FHx
- Social and occupational history: lives with girlfriend, apprentice carpenter, non-smoker, no illicit drugs, alcohol rarely.

Summarises important areas of the history back to the girlfriend

Invites the girlfriend to ask questions and is able to deal with them appropriately

Establishes the girlfriend's ideas, concerns and expectations

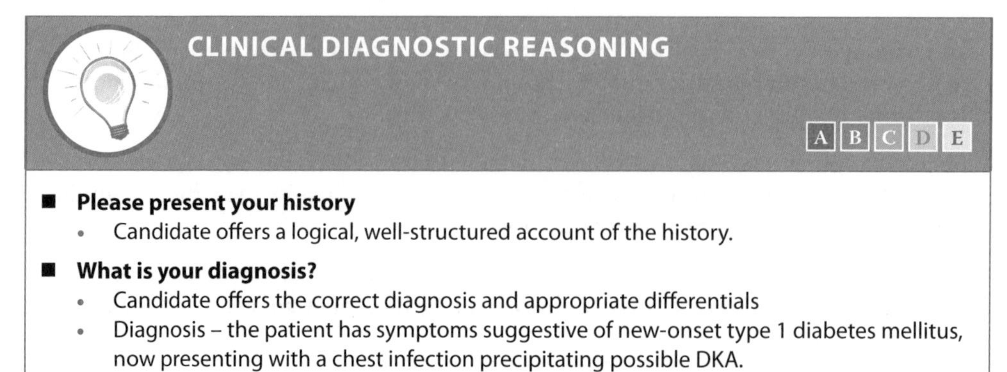

- **Please present your history**
  - Candidate offers a logical, well-structured account of the history.
- **What is your diagnosis?**
  - Candidate offers the correct diagnosis and appropriate differentials
  - Diagnosis – the patient has symptoms suggestive of new-onset type 1 diabetes mellitus, now presenting with a chest infection precipitating possible DKA.
- **Correctly identifies five essential investigations that should be ordered immediately on a diagnosis of type 1 diabetes**
  - Bloods – FBC, U&Es, RBG, blood cultures, blood ketones (if available)
  - ABG – acid/base and oxygenation (given chest infection)
  - Urine – ketones
  - Sputum – cultures
  - CXR.

GLOBAL HISTORY MARK

A B C D E

Station 2 – Examination

Patient script

If you are an actor/patient, read the patient history and physical signs fully – when the candidate comes to an abnormal site in their examination, act-out tenderness and/or volunteer the relevant physical sign.

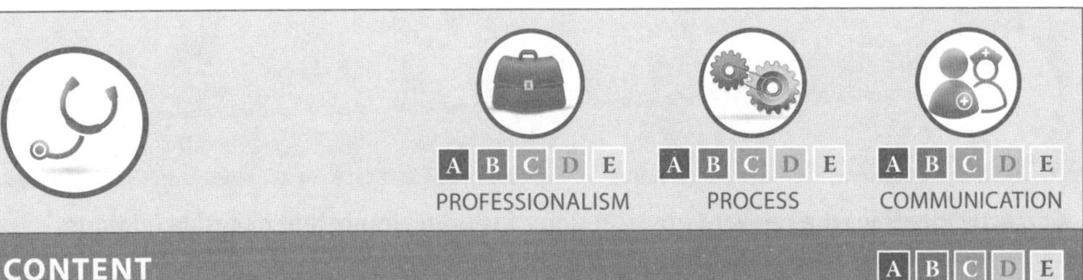

CONTENT

A B C D E

Exposes and positions patient correctly and maintains comfort

Comments on wellbeing of patient, ie well or unwell

Acknowledges patient is confused and tailors assessment accordingly

'Feet to face'

- Observes, and comments on patient and surroundings from foot of bed – confused, agitated, monitor leads, IV access.

Asks for relevant clinical observations and bedside tests

- HR, BP, RR,O_2 sats, temperature, RBG
- Asks specifically about urine output/urinary catheter.

Assessment of hands and upper limbs, and face and neck

- Perfusion of hands and signs of sepsis – hot, sweaty, vasodilated or cool and clammy
- LNs, hydration, signs of oral candidiasis, fluid status – JVP

Focused assessment of anterior and posterior chest

- Tracheal position
- Chest expansion – patient may not be able to co-operate
- Percussion – assesses right and left one side vs other; specifically percusses in right axilla
- TVF/VF – assesses right and left one side vs other; specifically palpates of auscultates in right axilla
- Auscultation – assesses right and left one side vs other; specifically auscultates in right axilla

Completes examination

- Specifically excludes other signs of sepsis:
- Meningism – examines to exclude neck stiffness and photophobia
- Abdomen – soft, non-tender
- Skin – no obvious infections – toe webs, cellulitis.

Thanks patient, offers assistance, maintains patient's dignity and privacy until they are dressed

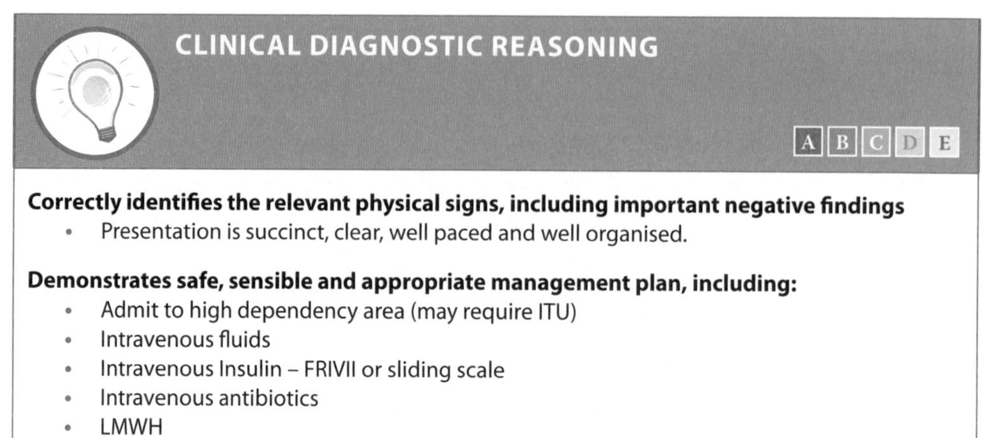

CLINICAL DIAGNOSTIC REASONING

A B C D E

Correctly identifies the relevant physical signs, including important negative findings

- Presentation is succinct, clear, well paced and well organised.

Demonstrates safe, sensible and appropriate management plan, including:

- Admit to high dependency area (may require ITU)
- Intravenous fluids
- Intravenous Insulin – FRIVII or sliding scale
- Intravenous antibiotics
- LMWH
- Consider an NG tube
- Monitor HR, BP, temperature, RR and O_2 sats; hourly blood ketones, pH and bicarbonate, UO.

Demonstrates clear and logical diagnostic reasoning

GLOBAL EXAMINATION MARK

A B C D E

Station 3 – Data interpretation

Part 1:

1. **False – There is a neutrophilic leucocytosis suggestive of a 'regular' bacterial infection such as streptococcal pneumonia. The white cell count in atypical pneumonias may be normal or even low, with relative abnormalities within the differential count.**
2. **False – Haemolysis is signified by anaemia, macrocytosis, reticulocytosis and does not cause thrombocytopenia per se.**
3. **True – The urea has risen approximately 4- to 5-fold but the creatinine has risen only 1.5- to 2-fold. Thus the ratio is 5:2, confirming marked pre-renal impairment.**
4. **True – The calculated serum osmolality = 2 [Na^+ + K^+] + urea + glucose = 2 [153 + 4.9] + 23.6 + 53.1 = 392.5 mOsmo/l. This is grossly elevated, normal serum osmolality being 285–295 mOsmo/l.**
5. **False – His hypernatraemia is of importance here but will slowly correct with dilution by added 'water'. In severely ill patients Hartmann's solution may be preferred because of the reduced chloride it contains compared with saline solutions. Dextrose should not be used until (a) his blood glucose is under control (normally accepted to be <15 mmol/l), and (b) his sodium is normalised. Dextrose contains no sodium and will rapidly drop the serum sodium and thus the osmolality. This rapid change may induce cerebral oedema and other CNS effects.**

6. **True – Patients may become rapidly potassium-depleted and supplementation is recommended once serum potassium is within normal or subnormal limits.**

   K^+ >5.5 mmol/l – no additional K^+ is required

   K^+ 3.5–5.5 mmol/l – add 20 mmol K^+ per litre of fluid given

   K^+ <3.5 mmol/l – add 40 mmol K^+ per litre of fluid given (after first or second 'stat' litres).

7. **False – DKA would be expected to produce a high anion gap due to presence of ketones and lactate. The anion gap = [Na^+ + K^+] – [chloride + bicarbonate] = [153 + 4.9] – [105 + 7.9] = 157.9 – 112.9 = 45 mmol/l.**

8. **True – The coagulation screen has all the features of disseminated intravascular coagulopathy (DIC), including thrombocytopenia, elevated INR and APTT, and elevated FDPs and D-dimer (as a result of the intravascular coagulation). As the patient is auto-anticoagulating, this contraindicates any VTE prophylaxis with heparin – thus proving one occasionally has to overrule guidelines and recommendations.**

9. **False – See answer to question 8.**

10. **False – this patient does have hyperglycaemia and is hyperosmolar but (a) he has evidence of marked ketosis (very elevated blood ketones), and (b) the hyperglycaemia and hyperosmolality seen with HHN-K syndrome are often grossly elevated with sodium levels above 160–170 mmol/l and blood glucose over 70–80 mmol/l.**

Part 2:

Patient	Blood gas set (Patient A–F)	Likely underlying diagnosis
1	A	Severe metabolic acidosis consistent with metformin-induced lactic acidosis.
2	F	Metabolic alkalosis secondary to gastric outflow tract obstruction secondary to a gastric malignancy.
3	B	Mixed respiratory/metabolic acidosis, with type 2 respiratory failure consistent with an acute exacerbation of COPD.
4	D	Compensated respiratory acidosis, consistent with a well COPD patient. His LTOT is maintaining acceptable levels of oxygen and oxygen saturations.
5	G	This patient has several features of life-threatening asthma and will almost certainly require intubation and ventilation. The ABGs reveal a mixed respiratory/metabolic acidosis, with type 2 respiratory failure consistent with an asthmatic patient who is about to have a respiratory arrest.
6	C	This patient has had a pulmonary embolism and should be treated as such. She is hypoxic and has early stages of a lactic acidosis consistent with a PE, and NOT hysterical behaviour.

GLOBAL DATA INTERPRETATION MARK

A B C D E

Station 4 – Procedural skills

Procedure A: Arterial blood gas sample

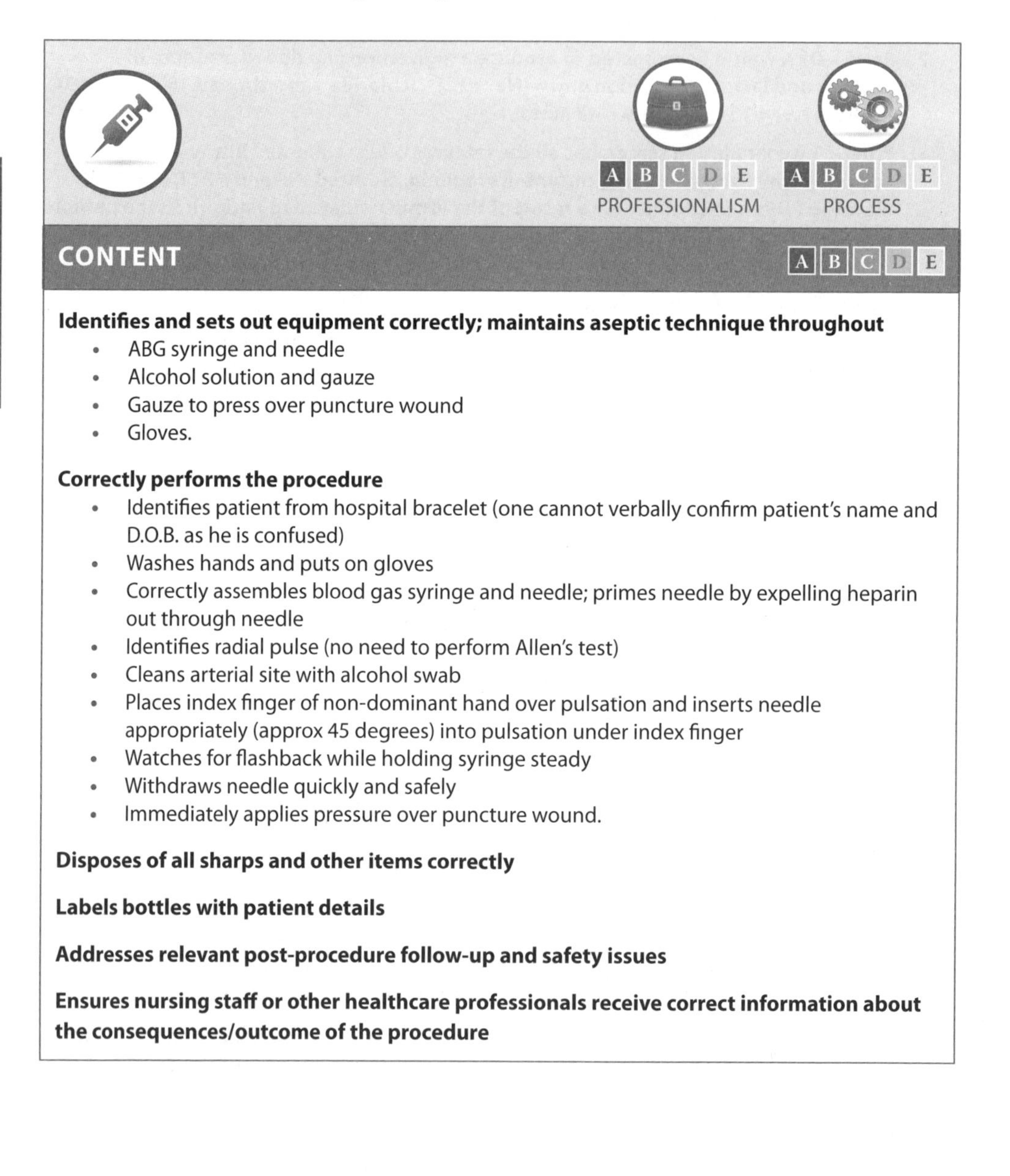

A B C D E
PROFESSIONALISM

A B C D E
PROCESS

CONTENT A B C D E

Identifies and sets out equipment correctly; maintains aseptic technique throughout

- ABG syringe and needle
- Alcohol solution and gauze
- Gauze to press over puncture wound
- Gloves.

Correctly performs the procedure

- Identifies patient from hospital bracelet (one cannot verbally confirm patient's name and D.O.B. as he is confused)
- Washes hands and puts on gloves
- Correctly assembles blood gas syringe and needle; primes needle by expelling heparin out through needle
- Identifies radial pulse (no need to perform Allen's test)
- Cleans arterial site with alcohol swab
- Places index finger of non-dominant hand over pulsation and inserts needle appropriately (approx 45 degrees) into pulsation under index finger
- Watches for flashback while holding syringe steady
- Withdraws needle quickly and safely
- Immediately applies pressure over puncture wound.

Disposes of all sharps and other items correctly

Labels bottles with patient details

Addresses relevant post-procedure follow-up and safety issues

Ensures nursing staff or other healthcare professionals receive correct information about the consequences/outcome of the procedure

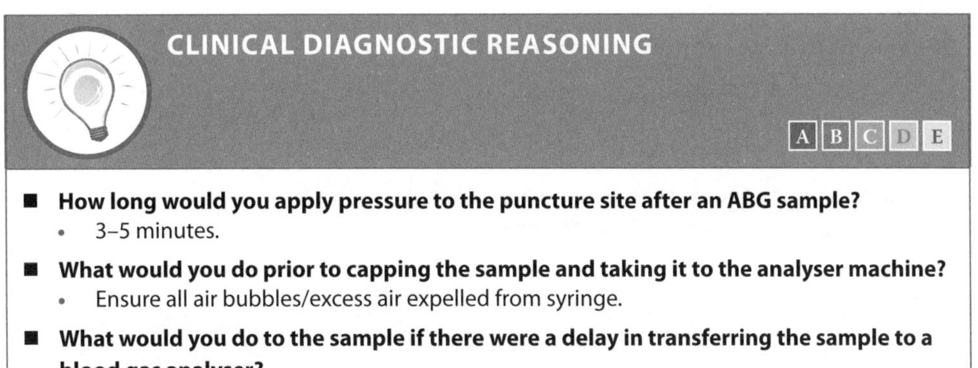

CLINICAL DIAGNOSTIC REASONING

- **How long would you apply pressure to the puncture site after an ABG sample?**
  - 3–5 minutes.
- **What would you do prior to capping the sample and taking it to the analyser machine?**
  - Ensure all air bubbles/excess air expelled from syringe.
- **What would you do to the sample if there were a delay in transferring the sample to a blood gas analyser?**
  - Place the sealed sample in a cup or bag of ice.

Demonstrates clear and logical diagnostic reasoning

Procedure B: Insertion of naso-gastric tube

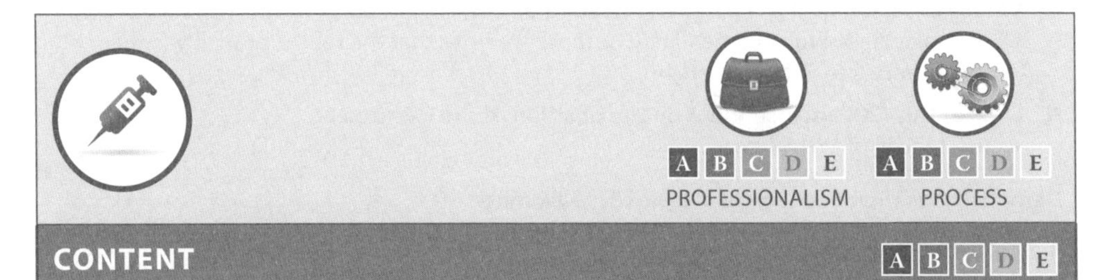

CONTENT

A B C D E

Identifies and sets out equipment correctly; maintains aseptic technique throughout

- Gloves
- Choice of different NG tubes
- Sticky tape to secure NG tube
- Water-based gel
- Gauze.

Correctly performs the procedure

- Identifies patient from hospital bracelet (one cannot verbally confirm patient's name and D.O.B. as he is confused)
- Washes hands and puts on gloves
- Chooses appropriate NG tube from selection
- Assesses patency of nares; chooses most appropriate according to findings
- Measures and marks length of NGT to be inserted using a standardised method, eg measures from tip of nose to earlobe and then to tip of xiphisternum; marked with piece of tape
- Sits patient up with neck in extension
- Lubricates 3–5 cm of NGT to be inserted with water-based gel
- Inserts/pushes tube gently back towards naso and oro-pharynx
- Checks tube is not coiling in mouth by opening patient's mouth
- Continues to advance tube until desired length is achieved
- Secures NGT to face using tape.

Disposes of all sharps and other items correctly

Ensures patient is comfortable

Addresses relevant post-procedure follow-up and safety issues

Ensures nursing staff or other healthcare professionals receive correct information about the consequences/outcome of the procedure

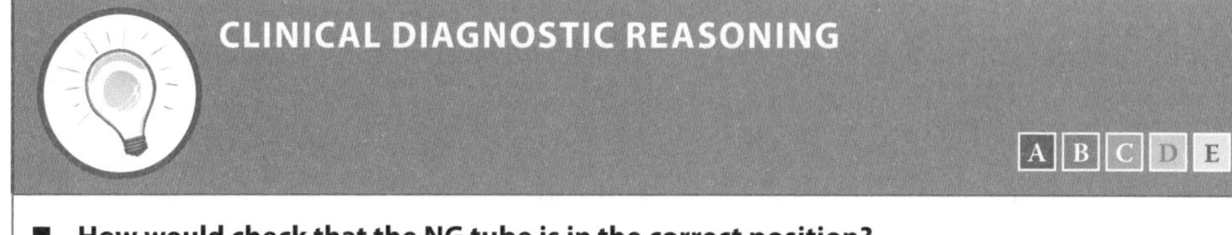

- **How would check that the NG tube is in the correct position?**
  - Either: check the position on CXR (one should be able to see the tube below the diaphragm), or aspirate the fluid and check its acidic with litmus paper.
- **What would you do if the patient started to become cyanosed, grunting and wheezing?**
  - Remove the NG tube immediately, as these are signs that the tube is probably in the respiratory tree. Tube in bronchi.
- **Look at this CXR and comment on the position of the NG tube.**
  - NG tube in bronchial tree.

Demonstrates clear and logical diagnostic reasoning

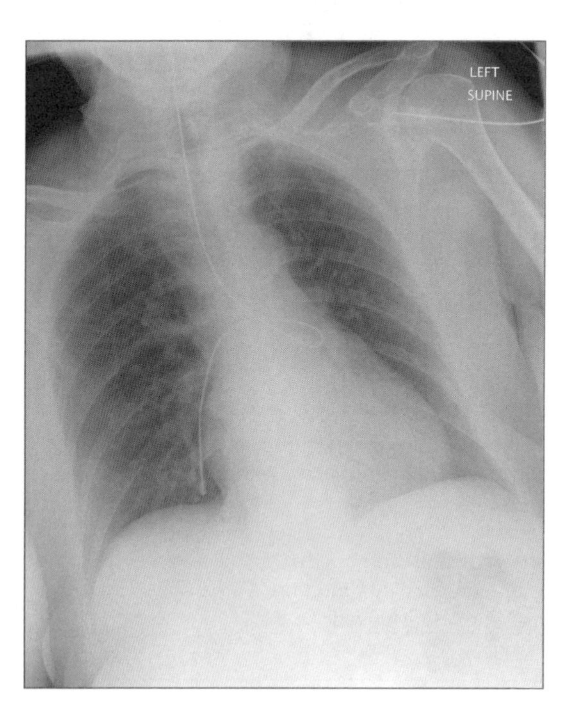

GLOBAL PROCEDURE MARK

A B C D E

Station 5 – Prescribing skills

Allergies, sensitivities and adverse drug reactions			Patient details/addressograph
No known allergies ☐		Initials RF	Gender (M)/ F
Not possible to ascertain ☐		Date 21.11.11	Weight (kg): 90 / Date:
Medicine/substance	Reaction & Severity	Initials & Date	Height: 184
PENICILLIN	SEVERE RASH	RF 044	Surface area (m²):
Alerts			

Patient details/addressograph	
NHS/ Hospital No:	236543
Surname:	DA COSTA
First name:	JACK
Date of birth:	15.01.88

IN-PATIENT MEDICATION PRESCRIPTION AND ADMINISTRATION RECORD

PasTest HOSPITAL

Consultant	Trainee Dr. Name and Bleep no.	Date of admission	Date chart reboarded	Estimated date of discharge
RICHARDS	FEATHER 044	21.11.11		
This chart is no. .... of	Transcribing Check by Pharmacy Sign .... Date	Ward 1. HDU .... 2.		

Supplementary Medication charts in use: Other (please specify): 1 .... 2 ....

Epidural/PCA ☐ Syringe driver ☐ TPN ☐ Chemotherapy ☐ Insulin sliding scale ☐

Once only medications – loading doses, pre-medication, PGDs or surgical antibiotic propylaxis

Date	Time to be given	Medicine (approved name)	Dose	Route	Signature and bleep no.	Pharmacy	Time given	Given by	Checked by
21.11	13.30	LEVOFLOXACIN	500mg	IV	RF 044				
21.11	13.30	CLARITHROMYCIN	500mg	IV	RF 044				

SCENARIO 11

Regular prescriptions						
Oral anticoagulation follow the anticoagulation guidelines available on the intranet						
Indication	Target INR	Baseline INR (if applicable)	Duration of therapy / Date therapy started	Date of anticoagulation follow-up appointment (clinic or other)*	Anticoagulant record book given or updated. Sign and date	Date patient counselled and sign

* A follow-up appointment must be booked with the anti-coagulant clinic or enhanced provider of primary care services. If not, the TTA will not be dispensed

Initiating warfarin	Perform baseline coagulation screen, LFTs, U&Es and FBC	Prescribe initiation dose as per guidelines	CHECK INR ON DAY 3	FOLLOW DOSING ALGORITHM IN GUIDELINE
Continuing warfarin	Maintenance therapy	FOLLOW MAINTENANCE DOSING ALGORITHM IN GUIDELINE		

Do not use the initiation protocol for patients already on warfarin. More frequent INR monitoring may be required for patients on interacting drug(s)

Medication				Date													
1				INR													
Route	Frequency OD	Time 18.00	Start	Dose													
			Stop	Dr sign													
Signature		Bleep no.	Pharmacy	Given													

Initiating warfarin – Reduced dosing regimen in red. Refer to anticoagulation policy

Day	One	Two	Three							Four and above								
INR	<1.4	No test	<2.0	2.0-2.1	2.2-2.5	2.6-2.9	3.0-3.3	3.4-4.0	>4.0	<1.4	1.4-1.5	1.6-1.7	1.8-1.9	2.0-2.3	2.4-3.0	3.1-4.0	4.1-4.5	>4.5
Dose mg	10 5	10 5	10	5	4	3	2	1	0	9	8	7	6	5	4	3	Miss 1 day	Miss 2 day

Thromboprophylaxis please prescribe treatment regimens in the regular medications section

Choice of mechanical prophylaxis and leg(s) to be applied to			Leg			Enter Time	Enter details below
Graduated elastic compression stockings	Intermittend pneumatic compression device (IPC)		Left	Right	Both		
☑ 21/11 Start Date:	☐ End Date:	Signature and Bleep No.	☐	☐	☑		
☐ Start Date:	☐ End Date:	Signature and Bleep No. AF	☐	☐	☐		

Medication		Dose	Dose Change	Enter Time	Enter details below
Please ensure you have completed the VTE risk assessment form	Date				
	Route				
	Signature			Instructions: NOT FOR HEPARIN - D.I.C	Pharmacy ☐
	Bleep no.				

Oxygen			
Target Saturation	88-92% ☐	94/98% ☑	If oxygen saturation falls below target range on prescribed oxygen, patient needs urgent clinical review. If oxygen saturation is above targent range on prescribed oxygen, ask for review.
Other specify)		*Device: N= nasal cannula, SM = simple face mask, V = venturi, H = humidified, RM = reservoir mask, OTHER = other eg. NCPAP/NIPPV	Pharmacy ☐
Target Saturation not applicable ☐			

	Date Changed	Date Changed	Enter Time	Enter details below
	21/11			
Device	NASAL CANNULAE			
% or L/min (specify a range eg 1-21 L/min)	21/ MIN			
Signature and Bleep no.	RF 044			

Regular prescriptions continued																	
Regular medications																	
For 7 Days	Dose			Date 21	22	23	24	25	26	27							
Date	21.11			Medication	LEVOFLOXACIN				Instructions	SEVERE C.A.P			Signature and bleep no.	RF 044		Pharmacy	☐
Route	IV																
Signature	RF																
06																	
(09)	500mg																
12																	
18																	
(22)	500mg																
24																	

Regular prescriptions continued																	
Regular medications																	
	Dose			Date 21	22	23	24	25	26	27							
Date	21.11			Medication	CLARITHROMYCIN				Instructions	SEVERE C.A.P			Signature and bleep no.	RF 044		Pharmacy	☐
Route	IV																
Signature	RF																
06																	
(09)	500mg																
12																	
18																	
(22)	500mg																
24																	

21/11 Infusion prescriptions continued										SC = subcutaneous		IVC = intravenous central IVP = intravenous peripheral		
Date & time	Route	Infusion Fluid		Medication		Duration	Rate	Prescriber's signature & bleep no.	Date given	Given by / Added by	Check by	Start time	Finish time	Pharmacy
		Name & strength	Volume	Approved name with expiry / unit number	Dose									
21/11	IV	0.9% SALINE Exp: Batch/unit no:	50ml	ACTRAPID INSULIN	50 units		0.1 units/kg/hr = 90 units/hr	RF 044						
21/11	IV	0.9% SALINE Exp: Batch/unit no:	1 LITRE	+20mmol KCl			1hr	RF 044						
21/11	IV	0.9% SALINE Exp: Batch/unit no:	1 LITRE	+20mmol KCl			2hr	RF 044						
21/11	IV	0.9% SALINE Exp: Batch/unit no:	1 LITRE	+20mmol KCl			2hr	RF 044						
21/11	IV	0.9% SALINE Exp: Batch/unit no:	1 LITRE	+20mmol KCl			4hr	RF 044						
21/11	IV	0.9% SALINE Exp: Batch/unit no:	1 LITRE	+20mmol KCl			4hr	RF 044						
21/11	IV	0.9% SALINE Exp: Batch/unit no:	1 LITRE	+20mmol KCl			4hr	RF 044						
21/11	IV	0.9% SALINE Exp: Batch/unit no:	1 LITRE	+20mmol KCl			6hr	RF 044						
21/11	IV	0.9% SALINE Exp: Batch/unit no:	1 LITRE	+20mmol KCl			8hr	RF 044						
		TITRATE FLUIDS TO MAINTAIN - BP > 100 SYSTOLIC; HR < 100 BPM; U.O > 0.5 ml/kg/HR > 45ML/HR												

SCENARIO 11

As required medications																								
Medication PARACETAMOL				Date																				
Indication				Time																				
Dose 1g	Route PR/ PO	Maximum frequency / dose 6 hour	Start date 21/11	Dose																				
			Stop date	Route																				
Signature RF			Bleep no. 044	Given																				
Additional instructions:											Pharmacy ☐													

As required medications																								
Medication CYCLIZINE				Date																				
Indication				Time																				
Dose 50 mg	Route IV/ IM	Maximum frequency / dose 8 hour	Start date 21/11	Dose																				
			Stop date	Route																				
Signature RF			Bleep no. 044	Given																				
Additional instructions:											Pharmacy ☐													

GLOBAL PRESCRIBING MARK

A B C D E

SCENARIO 11

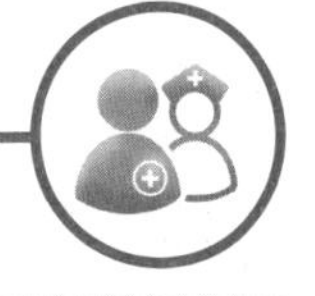

Station 6 – Clinical communication skills

Patient script

You are Mr Jack Da Costa, aged 24 years old (DOB 15 January 1988). You were admitted a few days ago and don't remember very much about the admission. Your girlfriend Dianne told you that you were admitted with a horrible chest infection. You have been told by the nursing staff on the other ward that you were very unwell due to a chest infection and sugar diabetes. You are in real shock about the new diagnosis. You realise now that this must be the reason why you have been feeling so unwell over the last few weeks and haven't been able to train.

You are a bright and intelligent man and are keen to learn as much as you can about your new illness. You are keen to hear what the doctors and nurses can do to make it better and how it may affect your life from now on (if at all). You are hopeful it may be cured with treatment.

Lifestyle: you're very fit as you are a competitive taekwando expert and train three to four times per week.

Diet – you're very strict about your diet – low fat with very few sweet things such as cakes, biscuits, sweets and chocolates.

You're a non-smoker and drink almost no alcohol.

FHx: as above

Ideas and concerns – you have some understanding about diabetes, as you have two older aunts who are diabetic but don't really know that much about it. You are worried as your grandfather became diabetic in later life and he went blind and died of a 'massive' stroke. Your aunts too have had lots of heart attacks and other problems.

Expectations – you haven't really given it much thought but hope you won't get the full-blown diabetes 'I'm young and very fit so should be OK, shouldn't I?'

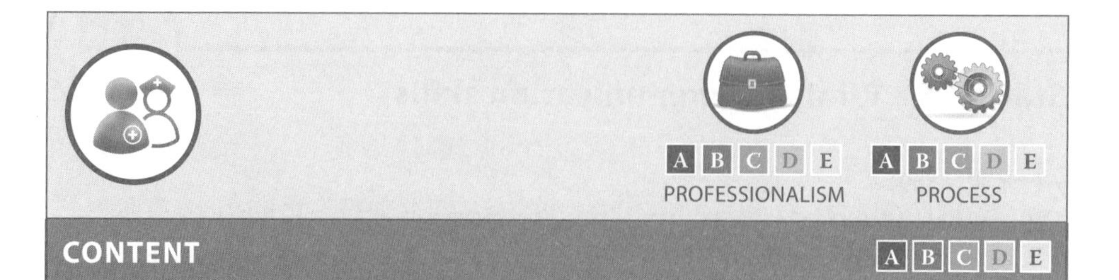

CONTENT

A B C D E

Investigates patient's present level of understanding of scenario

Summarises and confirms what has happened so far and reason for discussion today

- To discuss the new diagnosis, and the treatments and lifestyle changes the patient may have to make.

Asks what, and how much information the patient would like to be told

Establishes patient's ideas, concerns and expectations

Explains the key, important information

- **New diagnosis (in an appropriate/empathetic manner)**
- Normal physiology of the pancreas/insulin
- Why pancreas has failed (mechanism: autoimmune disease)
- Explains the term 'type 1 diabetes mellitus'; how it differs from type 2 diabetes
- Explains no cure.
- **Explains insulin therapy**
- Explains the role of injectable insulin; aim to maintain blood glucose as normal level as possible (normally 4–7 mmol/l)
- Different types of insulin – long-acting (once a day/evening) sets the basal level of control, and short-acting (with meals) covers the food intake with each meal.
- Given by self-administered injections under the skin of the thighs, buttocks and belly
- Administered by special devices, called pens, monitor control using blood taken by pinpricks from fingertips
- We will teach you how to administer the injections over the next few days, offers reassurance – very simple.
- **Goes through importance of lifestyle**
- Eating healthy foods – low fat and low carbohydrate, avoid short-acting sugars – don't need 'diabetic' foods, just sensible eating
- Weight – avoiding becoming fat/overweight
- Exercise – good cardiovascular fitness
- Reduce cardiovascular risk – no smoking, safe levels of alcohol, maintain good sugar and blood pressure control
- Sticking to medications, monitor treatment and attend regular 6-monthly review with HCPs.

Invites patient to ask questions as they proceed through the consultation and is able to deal with them appropriately

Summarises important areas of the consultation back to the patient

Formally ends the consultation and ensures appropriate follow-up has been discussed

CLINICAL DIAGNOSTIC REASONING

A B C D E

- **How will you monitor this patient's long-term control at the GP or outpatient review?**
  - Clinical assessment looking for macrovascular and microvascular complications; HBA1c or fructosamine.
- **Can you tell the patient any research evidence that backs up your claims about glycaemic control?**
  - T1DM – DCCT; T2DM – UKPDS

Demonstrates safe, sensible and appropriate management plan

Demonstrates clear and logical diagnostic reasoning

GLOBAL COMMUNICATION MARK

A B C D E

Scenario 11: Reflection and consolidation

History

Mr Jack Da Costa is a 23-year-old previously fit-and-well apprentice carpenter. He is a competitive taekwando expert and is normally very fit, training four times per week.
Since his last competition, 2 months ago, he has been telling Dianne that he hasn't felt well. Of note he has had marked polyuria and polydypsia, blurring of his vision, is losing weight and feels too tired to train. Over the last few days he has had a cough productive of greenish sputum and has had a high fever. Over the last 24 hours he has become increasingly confused and unwell, and today Dianne became so concerned that she phoned the GP, who immediately organised an ambulance to bring him to the Emergency Department.
He is otherwise well with no significant history of note.
He is a non-smoker and rarely drinks alcohol.
As far as Dianne knows his family history is unremarkable –grandad and two aunts diabetic.
He is an apprentice carpenter and doing well at work.

Examination

On examination of this young man, he was acutely unwell looking, confused and agitated; clinically very dehydrated and had marked oral candidasis.
His initial observations revealed a CBG >48 mmol/l, a temperature of 39.6 °C, HR 120 regular, low volume, BP = 82/54 mmHg; RR >30 bpm and his O_2 sats were 98% on room air.
He was cold and clammy to the touch and drenched in sweat.
On examination of his chest, the trachea was in the midline. Percussion was reduced in the right lower zone associated with coarse crackles. TVF was normal throughout.
Of note he had no signs of meningism, his abdomen was soft and non-tender and he had no signs of skin sepsis (the toe web spaces were normal).
In summary, this is a previously fit-and-well young man who now presents with signs consistent of hyperglycaemic pre-coma and a right lower zone chest infection. He is severely dehydrated and overtly septic.

Data interpretation

To confirm the clinical diagnoses, the essential investigations should include:

- FBC (infection), U&Es (dehydration), RBG (diabetes), blood ketones (if available), coagulation screen – DIC, blood cultures (bacteraemia)
- ABGs (acidosis/respiratory failure)
- CXR (chest infection)
- Sputum cultures
- Urinalysis (ketones).

Management

This patient is seriously unwell and requires care in a high-dependency environment.
He requires regular monitoring of:

- Vital observations – capillary blood glucose, BP, HR, fluid balance, temperature
- Blood tests – blood ketones (if available), blood pH/bicarbonate, serum K^+
- Intravenous fluids
- Intravenous insulin infusion – sliding scale or FRIVII
- Intravenous antibiotics
- Anti-pyretics.

Once he is better, he will need education and long-term follow-up for his new diagnosis of type 1 diabetes.

Further reading and web links

www.diabetes.org.uk/Documents/About%20Us/Our%20views/Care%20recs/Joint%20British%20Diabetes%20Societies%20Inpatient%20Care%20Group%20-%20The%20Management%20of%20Diabetic%20Ketoacidosis%20in%20Adults%20-%20Pathway%20Poster.pdf
http://emedicine.medscape.com/article/117739-overview

Scenario 12: 'Out of breath'

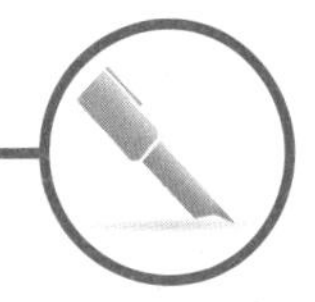

Station 1

History *10-minute station*

You are the FY1 doctor in the Emergency Department. Mr Brian Winter, a gentleman known to have COPD, has been brought in after his wife called the ambulance. He is in the resuscitation area of the Emergency Department. From the end of the bed he appears very short of breath and is unable to speak. Your Registrar has asked you to take a history from the patient's wife, while he completes an initial physical assessment.

- **Please take a comprehensive history from Mrs Winter to assess Mr Winter's pre-morbid status and the history of the presenting complaint. You will be asked to present your history to the examiner at the end of the station.**

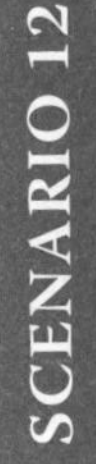

You will be assessed on the following areas, as well as the content and diagnostic reasoning of your history – take them into account in your presentation.

Professionalism

- Professional appearance (NHS dress code) – including general appearance, hair and jewellery
- Maintains patient and personal safety
- Polite introduction; identifies patient or interviewee correctly; confirms patient's date of birth from name band or other source
- Obtains informal consent; maintains patient's privacy
- Displays empathetic and caring attitudes and behaviours throughout.

Process

- Good organisation and structure; appropriate use of open and closed questions
- Appropriate fluency/rhythm/pace to the interview – this may change depending on environment and acute nature of problem
- Appropriate time for the patient to respond/reply to questions
- Appropriate acknowledgement of difficult or emotional areas of the patient's history.

Communication skills

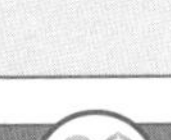

- Demonstrates caring and sympathetic attitude
- Asks open questions
- Invites patient to ask questions and answers them appropriately
- Addresses patient's ideas, concerns and expectations.

Station 2

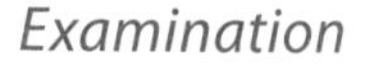

Examination *10-minute station*

Having completed your history taking from Mrs Winter, you join your Registrar in Resus and he asks you to complete an examination of Mr Winter while he takes a referral phone call from a GP.

- **Please perform the examination (from information within the station) and be ready to present your findings and a basic management plan when the Registrar returns in 10 minutes.**

You will be assessed on the following areas, as well as the content and skills of your examination – take them into account in your presentation.

Professionalism

- Professional appearance; maintains infection control standards, including hand cleaning and appropriate use of gloves and aprons
- Maintains patient and personal safety
- Polite introduction; identifies patient and confirms date of birth from name band or other source
- Obtains informal consent; maintains patient privacy and dignity
- Displays empathetic and caring attitudes and behaviours throughout.

Process

- Appropriate fluency/rhythm/pace to the examination – this may change depending on environment and acute nature of problem
- Good organisation and structure of examination; sensitive and empathetic approach
- Uses appropriate clinical techniques throughout
- Maintains privacy and dignity throughout.

Clinical communication

- Explains proposed examination/procedure: explains examination/procedure as it proceeds
- Offers information in a clear, structured and fluent manner, avoiding jargon
- Listens to patient and responds appropriately
- Demonstrates appropriate body language.

Please read the information below before presenting this case to the ST3 Medical Registrar as if you were on a busy medical take.
[NB If you have a model do not read this section]

Clinical findings

- o Patient thin and cachectic, appears dyspnoeic at rest, unable to complete sentences; plethoric, not cyanosed, no flap of CO_2 retention
- o Observations – HR 105 bpm, BP 165/85 mmHg, RR 34 bpm (using accessory muscles of respiration), O_2 sats 87% on air, temperature 36.7 °C
- o GCS – opens eyes spontaneously, speaking but confused at times, following commands (E4V4M6)
- o Respiratory examination – inspection, hyper-expanded 'barrel'-shaped chest; palpation, decreased chest expansion bilaterally; percussion, hyper-resonant percussion note throughout both lung fields; auscultation, widespread quiet vesicular breath sounds with expiratory wheeze
- o CV examination – peripheral capillary refill time 3 s; heart sounds easily heard, normal; JVP not elevated

Station 3

Procedural skills *10-minute station*

Procedure
Mr Winter has been in Resus and on oxygen for 10 minutes. He has been receiving high-flow O_2 via a reservoir mask.

- **Using the following equipment, please obtain an arterial blood gas sample in order to assess Mr Winter's oxygenation and ventilation.**

Equipment provided

- Manikin
- Identity bracelet
- Gloves
- Heparinised syringe
- 22 G needle
- Alcohol skin swab
- Gauze

- **Describe the abnormalities on the following arterial blood gas (ABG) results:**

ABG result on 85% O_2: pH 7.28, PO_2 11.4, PCO_2 10.8, HCO_3 27.4, BE 1.2

- **Please select and apply the most appropriate oxygen therapy for this patient.**

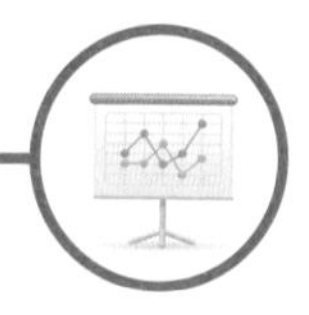

Station 4

Data interpretation *10-minute station*

Mr Winter's blood gas is given in the table below, as are four other samples from patients in the Medical Admissions Unit.

- **Match the patient histories with the most appropriate set of blood gas results (taken on air) and the therapy that should be initiated. You should write the inferred diagnoses for each set of blood gas results, eg type II respiratory failure with a metabolic acidosis.**

Patient	ABG	Treatment
1 A 24-year-old man with a recent respiratory tract infection now presenting with lower limb weakness and progressive dyspnoea	(A) pH 7.52 $PaCO_2$ 2.1 PaO_2 14.2 sats 100% HCO_3 22	(a) High-flow oxygen via a reservoir mask/heparin
2 A 47-year-old man admitted 4 hours ago after a large inferior myocardial infarction	(B) pH 7.20 $PaCO_2$ 8.4 PaO_2 4.7 sats 72% HCO_3 36	(b) Paper bag/ reassurance
3 A 69-year-old man who was a heavy smoker presenting with increased SOB and increased sputum	(C) pH 7.52 $PaCO_2$ 2.4 PaO_2 6.5 sats 86% HCO_3 24	(c) Intubation and ventilation (IPPV)/ plasmapheresis
4 A 24-year-old woman presenting with acute dyspnoea, haemoptysis and pleuritic chest pain	(D) pH 7.42 $PaCO_2$ 6.9 PaO_2 8.2 sats 89% HCO_3 24	(d) High-flow oxygen via a reservoir mask/diuretics
5 A 15-year-old girl who developed acute dyspnoea, dizziness and tetany while at a concert	(E) pH 7.20 $PaCO_2$ 4.5 PaO_2 7.5 sats 83% HCO_3 16	(e) 24% oxygen via venture mask and nebuliser

Station 5

Prescribing skills *10-minute station*

You have been asked to write up Mr Winter's drug and fluid charts (see page 368).

- **Using the BNF and charts provided, please write up the following interventions:**
  - **oxygen**
  - **nebulisers**
  - **steroids**
  - **antibiotics**
  - **fluids**

Details

Mr Brian Winter; DOB: 10/05/1944; No known allergies; Weight: 92 kg; Ward: MAU; Consultant: Dr Mackay

Blood results – FBC: Hb 15.4 g/dl, MCV 88 fl, WCC 18.9 × 10^9/l, neutrophils 16.4 × 10^9/l, platelets 134 × 10^9/l

U&Es: Na^+ 137 mmol/l, K^+ 4.2 mmol/l, urea 7.8 mmol/l, creatinine 98 μmol/l

RBG: 6.2 mmol/l

CCa^{2+} 2.43 mol/l, PO_4^- 0.98 mmol/l, Mg 0.9 mmol/l

Clotting screen: INR 0.9

CXR: hyper-expanded lung fields with flattening of the diaphragm, no focal consolidation

ECG: sinus tachycardia

Remember: DRUG DRs Don't Forget Signing Off (page 373)

Answers

Station 1 – History

Patient script

You are a 67-year-old lady who has been married to your husband, a 69-year-old retired lorry driver, for forty years.

He was diagnosed with COPD ten years ago.

He was a heavy smoker of forty cigarettes per day until that point but stopped 2 years ago.

He is currently using a number of inhalers and home nebulisers.

He has been admitted to hospital twice already this winter with infective exacerbations of his COPD and has once required the BiPAP mask on the high dependency unit. He has never been to the intensive care unit.

His COPD is looked after by the community Respiratory Nurse Specialist Team who visit every 1–2 weeks.

At best he is able to walk on the flat to the shops, 200 m away and finds a flight of stairs very difficult. He sleeps downstairs in your two floor home and there is a bathroom downstairs. He sleeps poorly and is often low in mood because of his breathlessness but is able to sleep on one pillow.

He has been unwell for three days, with increased sputum production, not green or offensive. He is now short of breath on minimal exertion and has not slept at night despite increased use of nebulisers. He has no fever or coryzal symptoms. He has not seen his GP as it was the weekend and is not on any antibiotics or steroids.

His only other medical problem is hypertension which is treated with ramipril. He has no allergies and does not drink alcohol.

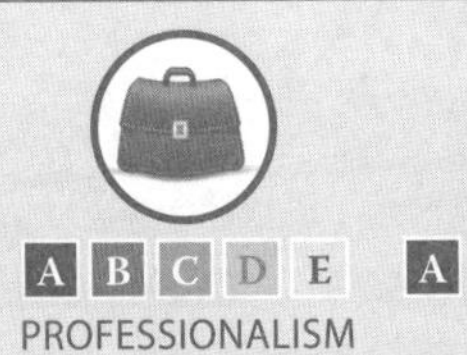
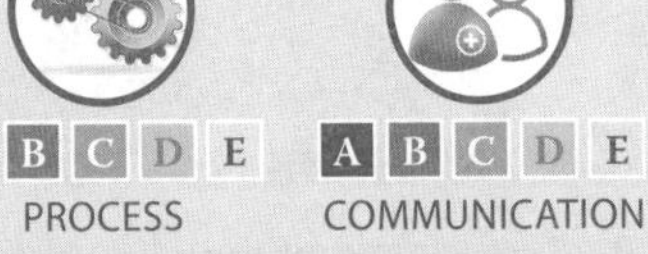

A B C D E PROFESSIONALISM | A B C D E PROCESS | A B C D E COMMUNICATION

CONTENT
A B C D E

Identifies key information

- Duration of illness
- Presence of increased shortness of breath and wheeze
- Presence of increased sputum production and characteristics
- No fever or coryzal symptoms.

History of COPD

- Exercise tolerance: 200 m on flat at best, less than one flight of stairs
- Current therapy: no long term oxygen therapy (LTOT) but on home nebulisers
- Previous admissions: no ICU but previous NIPPV (BiPAP)
- Ex-smoker
- Worsening clinical status on current treatment
- Mobilises to shops at best
- Poor sleep and mood.

Includes important negatives, including systemic enquiry

- No haemoptysis
- No weight loss
- No cardiac symptoms such as oedema, chest pain or orthopnoea.

Identifies key information from rest of history

- Under the care of Community Respiratory Nurse Specialist Team
- No current or recent courses of antibiotics or steroids.

Completing the patient history

- Drug and allergy history: on inhalers – tiotropium and Seretide® at home; nebulised salbutamol as required; ramipril 2.5 mg od
- Previous medical history: hypertension
- Social and occupational history: retired lorry driver; lives downstairs in two-floor house; no social care package; ex-smoker – 80 pack year history; no alcohol intake; no pets
- No relevant family history.

Summarises important areas of the history back to the patient

Invites Mrs Winter to ask questions and is able to deal with them appropriately

Establishes ideas, concerns and expectations

- Identifies that Mrs Winter is very concerned about Mr Winter and that he is 'the worst he has ever been'.

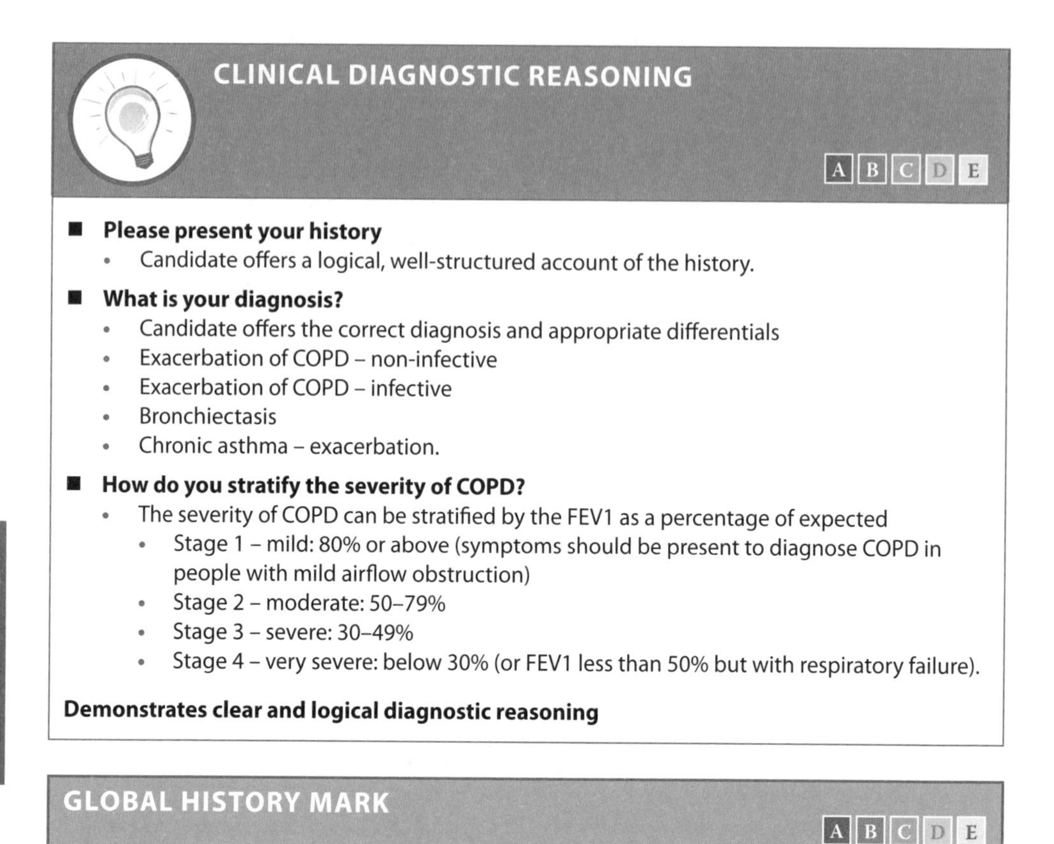

CLINICAL DIAGNOSTIC REASONING

A B C D E

- **Please present your history**
  - Candidate offers a logical, well-structured account of the history.
- **What is your diagnosis?**
  - Candidate offers the correct diagnosis and appropriate differentials
  - Exacerbation of COPD – non-infective
  - Exacerbation of COPD – infective
  - Bronchiectasis
  - Chronic asthma – exacerbation.
- **How do you stratify the severity of COPD?**
  - The severity of COPD can be stratified by the FEV1 as a percentage of expected
    - Stage 1 – mild: 80% or above (symptoms should be present to diagnose COPD in people with mild airflow obstruction)
    - Stage 2 – moderate: 50–79%
    - Stage 3 – severe: 30–49%
    - Stage 4 – very severe: below 30% (or FEV1 less than 50% but with respiratory failure).

Demonstrates clear and logical diagnostic reasoning

GLOBAL HISTORY MARK

A B C D E

Station 2 – Examination

Patient script

If you are an actor/patient, read the patient history and physical signs fully – when the candidate comes to an abnormal site in their examination, act-out tenderness and/or volunteer the relevant physical sign.

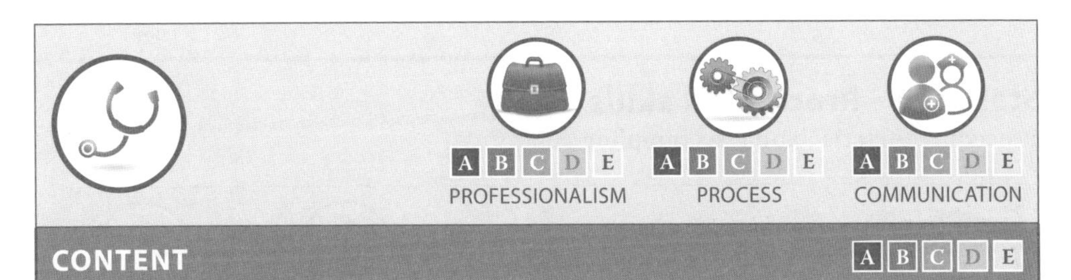

CONTENT

A B C D E

Exposes and positions patient correctly and maintains comfort

- Patient should be exposed to the waist and sitting at 45 degrees.

Comments on wellbeing of patient, ie well or unwell

'Feet to face'

- Observes and comments on patient and surroundings from foot of bed
- Short of breath at rest
- Not cyanotic but only able to complete short sentences.

Focused examination

- Inspection – inspects for scars on thorax
- Palpation – assesses trachea, assesses chest expansion anteriorly and posteriorly
- Auscultation – auscultates in all areas, anteriorly and posteriorly
- Assesses for either tactile vocal fremitus or vocal resonance.

Completes examination

- JVP not elevated, no peripheral oedema
- Assesses GCS.

Thanks patient, offers assistance, maintains patient's dignity and privacy until they are dressed

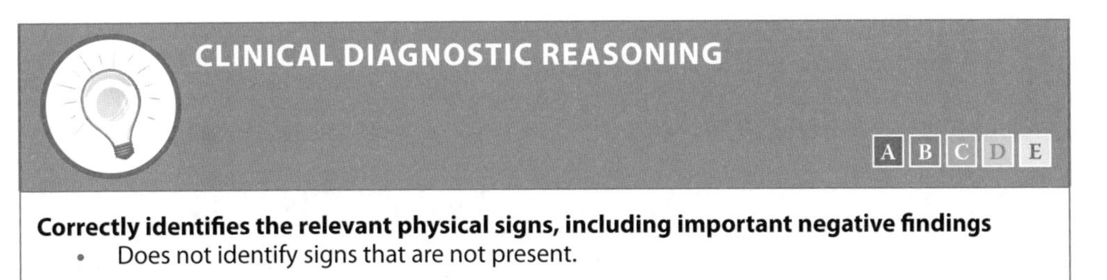

Correctly identifies the relevant physical signs, including important negative findings

- Does not identify signs that are not present.

Demonstrates a safe and sensible management plan

- Controlled oxygen therapy
- Treatment with steroids and nebulised B-agonists
- CXR, ABG, IV access
- Bloods
- FBC – looking for leucocytosis
- U&E – looking for renal impairment
- CRP – evidence of infection.

GLOBAL EXAMINATION MARK

A B C D E

Station 3 – Procedural skills

Procedure: Arterial blood gas sampling

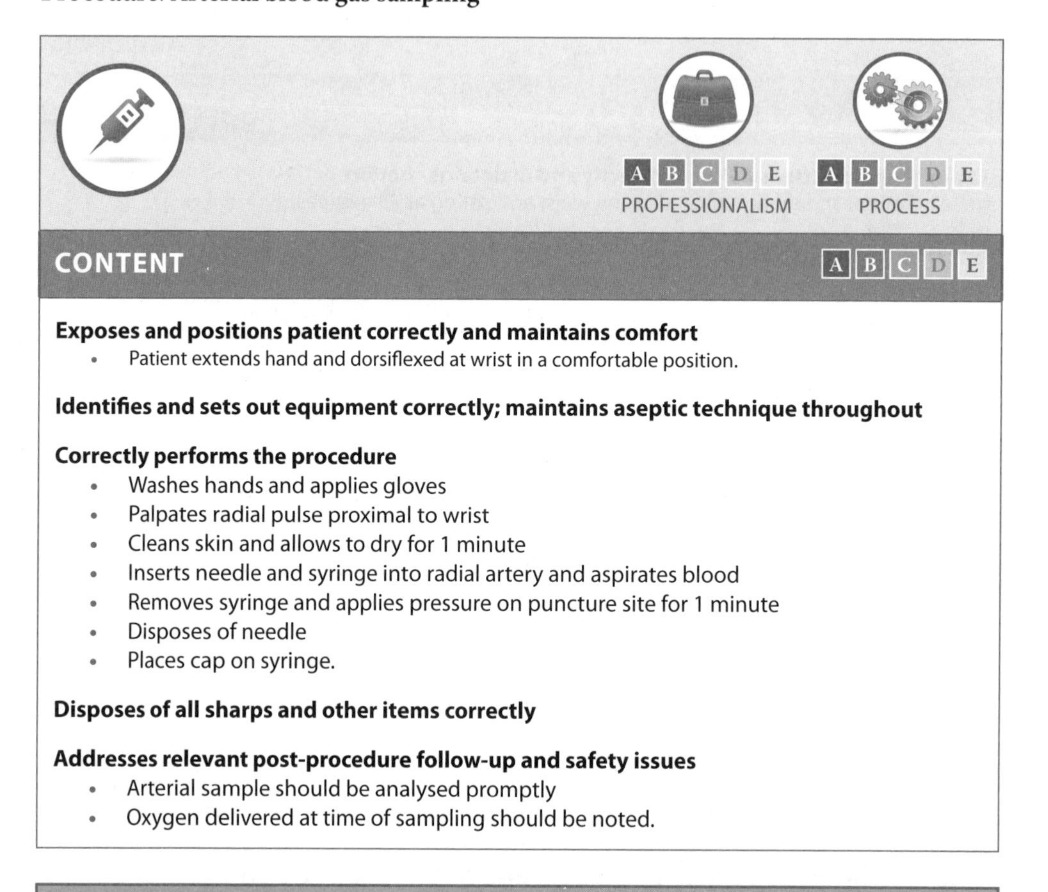

CONTENT A B C D E

Exposes and positions patient correctly and maintains comfort

- Patient extends hand and dorsiflexed at wrist in a comfortable position.

Identifies and sets out equipment correctly; maintains aseptic technique throughout

Correctly performs the procedure

- Washes hands and applies gloves
- Palpates radial pulse proximal to wrist
- Cleans skin and allows to dry for 1 minute
- Inserts needle and syringe into radial artery and aspirates blood
- Removes syringe and applies pressure on puncture site for 1 minute
- Disposes of needle
- Places cap on syringe.

Disposes of all sharps and other items correctly

Addresses relevant post-procedure follow-up and safety issues

- Arterial sample should be analysed promptly
- Oxygen delivered at time of sampling should be noted.

GLOBAL PROCEDURE MARK A B C D E

Station 4 – Data interpretation

1 (D) (c)

This patient has Guillain–Barré syndrome with both motor and sensory neuropathy; the blood gas results suggest type II respiratory failure, the pH is normal. The HCO_3 is normal, which shows this patient does not normally retain CO_2. The patient is young, and this set of blood gases imply he is tiring with poor respiratory effort; a similar picture may be found in severe asthma. The treatment of choice is ventilation and plasmapheresis.

2 (E) (d)

This man has acute pulmonary oedema, which causes a type I respiratory failure. He also has a metabolic acidosis, shown by the low pH and HCO_3 – this is probably due to a lactic acidosis caused by poor tissue oxygenation.

3 (B) (e) (Mr Winter)

These results are consistent with type II respiratory failure, a respiratory acidosis and compensatory metabolic alkalosis. This combination is seen in chronic CO_2 retainers, in which the respiratory acidosis is caused by the retention of CO_2 and the metabolic alkalosis by the retention of HCO_3. These patients should be given 24% (28% maximum) O_2 therapy.

4 (C) (a)

This patient has had a PE and demonstrates type I respiratory failure with a respiratory alkalosis. She is hypoxic, which is important to note, as occasionally such patients are diagnosed as 'hysterical' and are given a paper bag to rebreathe into! Type I failure in this age group is always pathological and should be taken seriously.

5 (A) (b)

This patient has a respiratory alkalosis but has no respiratory failure. She has been hyperventilating, and this is shown by the supersaturated high levels of oxygen with low CO_2. This patient should be treated with a rebreathing bag and reassurance.

GLOBAL DATA INTERPRETATION MARK

A B C D E

Station 5 – Prescribing skills

Check: DRUG DRs Don't Forget Signing Off (page 373)

Allergies, sensitivities and adverse drug reactions					Patient details/addressograph
No known allergies ✓		Initials GR	Gender (M) / F		NHS/ Hospital No: 1951958
Not possible to ascertain ☐		Date 13.01	Weight (kg)	Date	
Medicine/substance	Reaction & Severity	Initials & Date	92		Surname: WINTER
			Height		First name: BRIAN
			1.73m		
Alerts			Surface area (m²)		Date of birth: 10.05.42

IN-PATIENT MEDICATION PRESCRIPTION AND ADMINISTRATION RECORD

PasTest HOSPITAL

Consultant	Trainee Dr. Name and Bleep no.	Date of admission	Date chart reboarded	Estimated date of discharge
MACKAY	GREEN 604	13.01.12		
This chart is no. 1 of 1	Transcribing Check by Pharmacy Sign .... Date	Ward 1. MAU 2.		

Supplementary Medication charts in use: Other (please specify): 1 .... 2 ....

Epidural/PCA ☐ Syringe driver ☐ TPN ☐ Chemotherapy ☐ Insulin sliding scale ☐

Once only medications – loading doses, pre-medication, PGDs or surgical antibiotic propylaxis

Date	Time to be given	Medicine (approved name)	Dose	Route	Signature and bleep no.	Pharmacy	Time given	Given by	Checked by
13.01	16.00	PREDNISOLONE	40mg	PO	GR 604				
13.01	16.00	SALBUTAMOL	2.5mg	NEB	GR 604				
13.01	16.00	IPRATROPIUM	500mcg	NEB	GR 604				

Regular prescriptions continued

Regular medications

	Dose			Date 13	14	15											
Date	13.01			Medication: PREDNISOLONE					Instructions				Signature and bleep no.: GR 604			Pharmacy ☐	
Route	PO																
Signature	GR																
06																	
(09)	40mg			X													
12																	
18																	
22																	
24																	

SCENARIO 12

Regular prescriptions continued

Regular medications

		Dose			Date 13	14	15												
Date		13.01			Medication	SALBUTAMOL				Instructions				Signature and bleep no.	GR 604		Pharmacy		
Route		NEB																	
Signature		GR																	
06		2.4mg																	
10		2.4mg																	
14		2.4mg																	
18		2.4mg																	
22		2.4mg																	
02		2.4mg																	

Regular prescriptions continued

Regular medications

		Dose			Date 13	14	15												
Date		13.01			Medication	IPRATROPIUM				Instructions				Signature and bleep no.	GR 604		Pharmacy		
Route		NEB																	
Signature		GR																	
06																			
10		500mcg																	
14		500mcg																	
18		500mcg																	
22		500mcg																	
02																			

Regular prescriptions continued

Anti-infectives prescription *prescribe long term prophylaxis and anti-tuberculosis medications in regular medications section*

For 7 Days			Date 13	14	15	16	17	18								
Date		13/01	Medication	CO-AMOXICLAV				Indication	LRTI			Signature and bleep no.	GR 604		Pharmacy	
Route		IV														
Times		Dose														
06		1.2g														
09																
12		1.2g														
18																
22		1.2g														
24																

Regular prescriptions continued

Anti-infectives prescription *prescribe long term prophylaxis and anti-tuberculosis medications in regular medications section*

For 7 Days			Date 13	14	15	16	17	18								
Date		13/01	Medication	CLARITHROMYCIN				Indication	LRTI			Signature and bleep no.	GR 604		Pharmacy	
Route		PO														
Times		Dose														
06																
09		500mg														
12																
18																
22		500mg														
24																

Thromboprophylaxis please prescribe treatment regimens in the regular medications section								
Choice of mechanical prophylaxis and leg(s) to be applied to							Enter Time	Enter details below
Graduated elastic compression stockings		Intermittend pneumatic compression device (IPC)	Leg					
			Left	Right	(Both)			
13.01 Start Date:	End Date:	Signature and Bleep No.						
Start Date:	End Date:	Signature and Bleep No.						

Medication		Dose	Dose Change	Enter Time	Enter details below
CLEXANE		40mg			
Please ensure you have completed the VTE risk assessment form	Date	13.01.12			
	Route	SC			
	Signature	GR		Instructions	Pharmacy
	Bleep no.	604			

Oxygen					
Target Saturation	88-92% ☑	94/98% ☐		If oxygen saturation falls below target range on prescribed oxygen, patient needs urgent clinical review. If oxygen saturation is above targent range on prescribed oxygen, ask for review.	
Other specify)				*Device: N= nasal cannula, SM = simple face mask, V = venturi, H = humidified, RM = reservoir mask, OTHER = other eg. NCPAP/NIPPV	Pharmacy
Target Saturation not applicable ☐					
	Date Started	Date Changed	Date Changed	Enter Time	Enter details below
	13.01				
* Device	VENTURI				
% or L/min (Specify a range eg 1-12 L/min)	28%				
Signature and Bleep No.	GR 604				

As required prescriptions			Date	Time	Dose	Route	Date	Time	Dose	Route	Date	Time	Dose	Route	Date	Time	Dose	Route
Drug PARACETAMOL	Allergies Checked	Dose 1g																
Frequency 6 HOURLY	Max Dose/24 hrs 4g	Route PO																
Indication																		
Signature GR 604	Pharmacy	Start 13.01																

As required prescriptions			Date	Time	Dose	Route	Date	Time	Dose	Route	Date	Time	Dose	Route	Date	Time	Dose	Route
Drug METOCLOPRAMIDE	Allergies Checked	Dose 10mg																
Frequency 8 HOURLY	Max Dose/24 hrs	Route IM/IV																
Indication																		
Signature GR 604	Pharmacy	Start 13.01																

SCENARIO 12

As required prescriptions																		
			Date	Time	Dose	Route	Date	Time	Dose	Route	Date	Time	Dose	Route	Date	Time	Dose	Route
Drug SALBUTAMOL	Allergies Checked	Dose 2.5mg																
Frequency	Max Dose/24 hrs	Route NEB																
Indication																		
Signature GR 604	Pharmacy	Start 13.01																

GLOBAL PRECRIBING MARK A B C D E

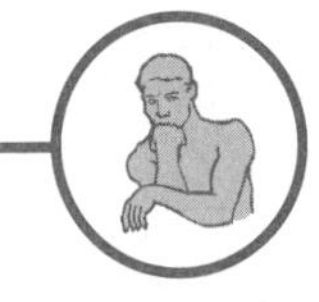

Scenario 12: Reflection and consolidation

History

Mr Winter is a 69-year-old man with severe COPD. He is on home nebulisers but not long-term oxygen therapy. He has been admitted to hospital twice already this year and has required non-invasive ventilation but has never been admitted to the Intensive Care Unit. He is reviewed in the community by the Respiratory Nurse Specialist Team. At best his exercise tolerance is less than 200 m on the flat and less than one flight of stairs.

Mr Winter has presented with a 3-day history of increased dyspnoea and wheeze, which has not improved with increased nebulised therapy. He is now breathless at rest. He describes an increase in sputum production but it is not green or offensive. This history suggests an acute exacerbation of severe COPD.

Examination

Mr Winter is a 69-year-old man who is obviously tachypnoeic at rest with increased work of breathing, a raised respiratory rate of 34 and increased use of his accessory muscles of respiration. He has decreased oxygen saturation on room air of 87% and is tachycardic at 105 bpm. He has widespread expiratory wheeze with a hyper-resonant percussion note throughout both lung fields.

He has signs in keeping with chronic obstructive pulmonary disease with a hyper-expanded chest and bilaterally symmetrically decreased chest expansion. He has a plethoric complexion and cachexia. He does not demonstrate signs of right heart failure.

Examination of the patient with chronic COPD can give useful information about the severity of the disease. The classical description of the 'pink puffer' and 'blue bloater' rarely exist in isolation, and most patients with COPD will have elements of both clinical pictures.

Emphysema – patients with predominant emphysema have destruction of the alveolar walls. This leads to a reduced surface area for gas exchange and to reduced ventilation and a raised PCO_2. Patients have to expend a great deal of energy to keep the airways open and have a chronically increased respiratory rate. This leads to chronic weight loss, increased respiratory effort and a plethoric appearance, the 'pink puffer'.

Chronic bronchitis – in COPD there is chronic inflammation and destruction of the tissues in the large airways leading to an increase in sputum production. This chronic bronchitis and eventually fibrosis leads to a limitation of airflow. This leads to chronic hypoxia, which in turn leads to pulmonary hypertension and right heart failure. This hypoxia and fluid retention leads to the clinical picture of a 'blue bloater'.

Investigation

The diagnosis of COPD should be considered in smokers or ex-smokers (over 35 years) with no clinical features of asthma and with any of the following symptoms:

- Exertional breathlessness,
- Chronic cough
- Regular sputum production (cough with sputum production on most days for 3 months of a year, for two consecutive years)
- Frequent winter 'bronchitis'
- Wheeze.

This diagnosis can be confirmed by spirometry, which will demonstrate an obstructive pattern. The diagnosis of COPD is made when the FEV1/FVC ratio is <70%.

Additional investigations that should be performed at the time of diagnosis:

- CXR to exclude other pathologies
- FBC to identify anaemia or polycythaemia.

In some circumstances, it may be appropriate to perform:

- Serial peak flow measurements – to exclude asthma
- Alpha-1-antitrypsin – if early onset, minimal smoking history or family history
- ECG and ECHO – to assess cardiac status if there are features of cor pulmonale
- Sputum culture – to identify organisms if sputum is persistently present and purulent.

Management

The care of patients with COPD requires a multidisciplinary approach and should include:

- Pharmacological treatments – starting with inhaled ß2-agonist therapy and escalating in a stepwise approach
- Smoking cessation
- Pulmonary rehabilitation
- Diet and nutrition
- Influenza and pneumococcal immunisation
- Management of cardiac complications (cor pulmonale)
- Domicillary oxygen in those patients who fulfil criteria
- Palliative care input
- Education of patients and advising patients on self-management strategies
- Evaluation for surgical intervention in selected patients.

Further reading and web links

Management of chronic obstructive pulmonary disease in adults in primary and secondary care. NICE guideline June 2010:
http://guidance.nice.org.uk/CG101
Patient information and support resources:
www.lunguk.org/you-and-your-lungs/conditions-and-diseases/copd

Scenario 13: 'Funny turns'

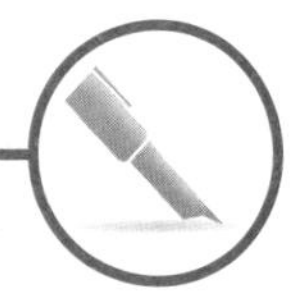

Station 1

History *10-minute station*

You are the FY1 on a Medicine for the Elderly firm. The Consultant has asked you to come down to Outpatients to clerk in a man who has been referred by his GP with 'funny turns'.

- **Please take a focused, diagnostic history from the patient, Mr Samuel Cohen, who is waiting in Room 3 of the Outpatient Clinic. The Consultant has asked you to present the history and differential diagnosis to her once you have finished.**

You will be assessed on the following areas, as well as the content and diagnostic reasoning of your history – take them into account in your presentation.

Professionalism

- Professional appearance (NHS dress code) – including general appearance, hair and jewellery
- Maintains patient and personal safety
- Polite introduction; identifies patient or interviewee correctly; confirms patient's date of birth from name band or other source
- Obtains informal consent; maintains patient's privacy
- Displays empathetic and caring attitudes and behaviours throughout.

Process

- Good organisation and structure; appropriate use of open and closed questions
- Appropriate fluency/rhythm/pace to the interview – this may change depending on environment and acute nature of the problem
- Appropriate time for the patient to respond/reply to questions
- Appropriate acknowledgement of difficult or emotional areas of the patient's history.

Communication skills

- Demonstrates caring and sympathetic attitude
- Asks open questions
- Invites patient to ask questions and answers them appropriately
- Addresses patient's ideas, concerns and expectations.

Station 2

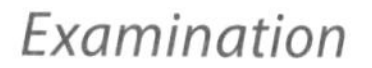

Examination *10-minute station*

The Consultant agrees that this is most likely to be a case of severe aortic stenosis. She asks you to perform a focused, diagnostic examination of Mr Cohen, with a view to proving this diagnosis and including or excluding its complications.

- **Please complete your assessment and then present the relevant findings (given within the station) to your Consultant.**

You will be assessed on the following areas, as well as the content and skills of your examination – take them into account in your presentation.

Professionalism

- Professional appearance; maintains infection control standards, including hand cleaning and appropriate use of gloves and aprons
- Maintains patient and personal safety
- Polite introduction; identifies patient and confirms date of birth from name band or other source
- Obtains informal consent; maintains patient privacy and dignity
- Displays empathetic and caring attitudes and behaviours throughout.

Process

- Appropriate fluency/rhythm/pace to the examination – this may change depending on environment and acute nature of problem
- Good organisation and structure of examination; sensitive and empathetic approach
- Uses appropriate clinical techniques throughout
- Maintains privacy and dignity throughout.

Clinical communication

- Explains proposed examination/procedure; explains examination/procedure as it proceeds
- Offers information in a clear, structured and fluent manner, avoiding jargon
- Listens to patient and responds appropriately
- Demonstrates appropriate body language.

Please read the information below before presenting this case to the Consultant as if you were in a busy outpatient clinic.
[NB If you have a model do not read this section]

Clinical findings

- o **Well-looking elderly man – short of breath at rest; AMTS = 10/10, no tar staining; face not cyanosed; no signs of anaemia; no stigmata of hyperlipidaemia**
- o **Observations – HR 86 bpm, BP 145/126 mmHg, irregular, low volume**
- o **CV examination – hands: cool peripheries; no clubbing, no stigmata of infective endocarditis; carotid pulse: sustained/slow rising in character; apex beat: undisplaced, hyperdynamic; no heaves or thrills; HS: S1 + soft S2 + soft ejection systolic murmur; ?S4; no radiation to carotids; no sacral or peripheral oedema; all peripheral pulses palpable; no bruits/no evidence of aneurysms**
- o **Respiratory examination – bibasal crackles**
- o **In summary, this is an elderly man with signs of significant aortic stenosis and pulmonary oedema.**

Station 3

Data interpretation *10-minute station*

Mr Cohen is admitted to CCU under the care of the cardiologists. On reviewing Mr Cohen the next day, you are approached by the Cardiology Registrar, who invites you to take part in the ECG teaching session she is just about to give. She has prepared questions on the ECG of several of the present inpatients on the CCU.

- **Please indicate whether the following statements are TRUE (T) or FALSE (F) regarding each of the ECGs shown below. You may assume all ECGs are running at 25 mm/s.**

1

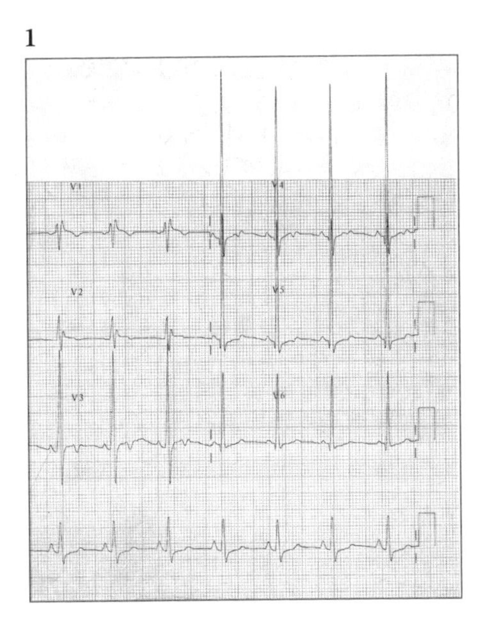

(A) **The rate is 85 bpm.**

(B) **The P-wave morphology is consistent with P mitrale.**

(C) **There is evidence of first-degree heart block.**

(D) **There are inverted T waves in the anterior leads.**

(E) **There are features to suggest left ventricular hypertrophy (LVH).**

2

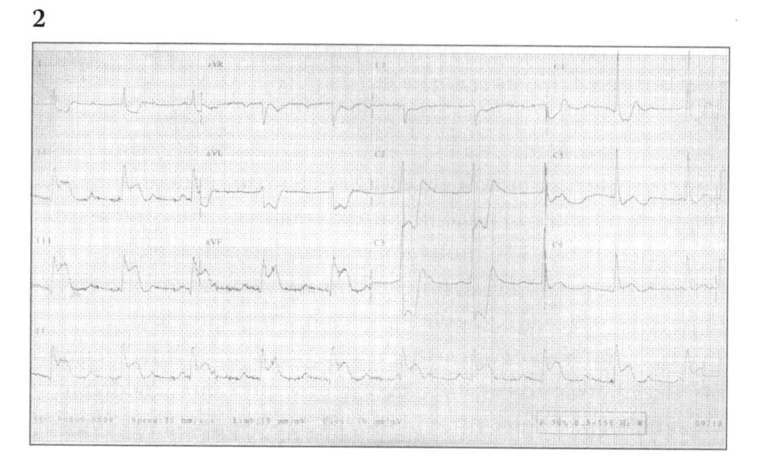

(A) The axis is deviated to the left.

(B) There is inferior ST segment elevation.

(C) There is ST elevation in the anterior leads.

(D) There is ST segment depression in the high lateral leads.

(E) There are features to suggest second-degree heart block.

3

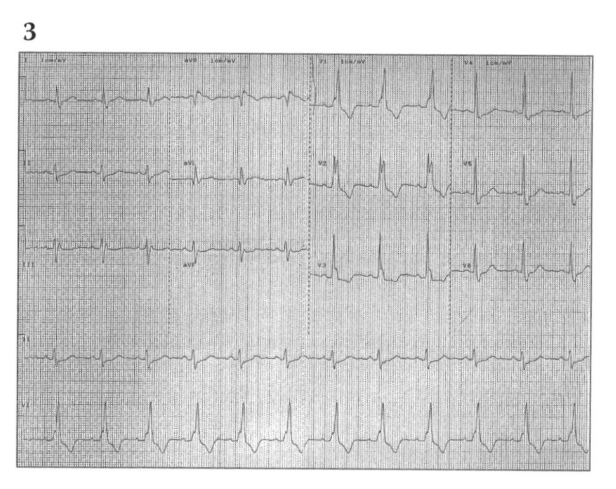

(A) The rate is over 100 bpm.

(B) The axis is deviated to the right.

(C) There is T-wave inversion in the infero-lateral leads.

(D) There are features of a right bundle branch block.

(E) There are features to suggest bifascicular block.

4

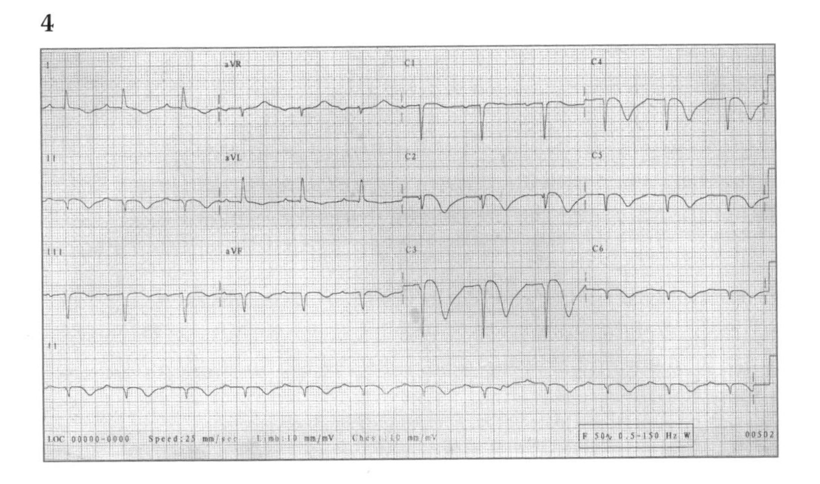

(A) The rate is approximately 70 bpm.

(B) The axis is deviated to the left.

(C) There is T-wave inversion in the infero-lateral leads.

(D) There are Q waves in the inferior leads.

(E) There is normal anterior R-wave progression.

5

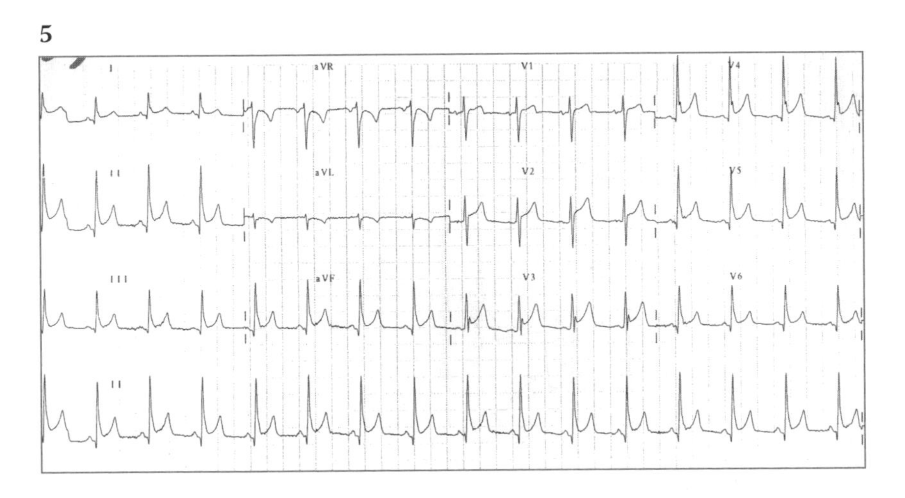

(A) The rate is approximately 75 bpm.

(B) The axis is normal.

(C) There is evidence of high take-off of the ST segment in the anterior leads.

(D) There is ST elevation in the infero-lateral leads.

(E) There is evidence to suggest an acute STEMI.

Station 4

Prescribing skills *10-minute station*

- **Using the BNF and the drug chart provided, write up Mr Cohen's regular medications (where appropriate) and the prescribed drugs listed below.**

Details

Mr Samuel Cohen; Hospital No. 109087; DOB: 06/05/1927; Drug allergies: penicillin – severe rash; Weight: about 82 kg; Ward: CCU; Consultant: Dr Syed

U&Es: Na^+ 139 mmol/l, K^+ 4.9 mmol/l, urea 9.9 mmol/l, creatinine 135 μmol/l

eGFR: 63 ml/min/1.73 m^2

Stat side: furosemide 40 mg od

Regular medications: bendroflumethiazide 2.5 mg od; ramipril 10 mg od

Added: furosemide 40 mg od; bisoprolol 1.25 mg od; aspirin 75 mg od; enoxaparin 40 mg od

PRN side: paracetamol 1 g max. qds (6 hourly); metoclopramide 10 mg max. tds (8 hourly)

> **Remember: DRUG DR**s **D**on't **F**orget **S**igning **O**ff (page 373)

Station 5

Clinical communication skills *10-minute station*

You are asked by the Senior Staff Nurse if you could give a teaching session to the student nurses on the ward regarding Mr Cohen's underlying condition, why he tends to collapse and why he suffers angina-like chest pain. They would also like to know why medications such as the ACEIs and his furosemide might make his condition worse.

- **Please give a talk, of up to 7 minutes, to the three student nurses regarding Mr Cohen's severe aortic stenosis. You should discuss physiological principles wherever you can, and address the students' questions at the end of the talk.**

Answers

Station 1 – History

Patient script

You are Mr Samuel Cohen (DOB 6 May 1927), an 84-year-old, retired furniture manufacturer. You have recently handed over your business to your two sons and were intending to finally start enjoying retirement, when 'all this started'. You have always been a keen golfer and had until your problems started been playing three to four times a week (handicap 12).

Over the last 2–3 months you have begun to feel increasingly unwell and have been unable to complete your round without a golf buggy. Initially you noticed you were getting increasingly short of breath, especially on the fairway of the third, which 'has quite a dramatic hill to it'. This has worsened and recently you have found it hard to walk on the flat for more than about 50–100 yards without feeling totally drained and breathless. You have also noticed that your ankles have been swelling and more recently you have developed a dry irritating cough. You sleep with three pillows (but this has not changed recently) and deny waking short of breath, wheeze, sputum or having any haemoptyis.

Since this started, you have had two or three funny turns, where you have suddenly felt faint and have blacked out, 'crashing' to the ground. These attacks come with no warning and your wife says you are out cold for about a minute or two, before coming round. She says you look 'deathly pale' and washed out. Once 'awake' you recover very quickly and are able to get up with little or no assistance. After a few minutes you feel totally well again.

You deny headache, loss of higher function, or focal neurological deficit. No features of seizures.

In the last few weeks the shortness of breath has now become associated with 'twinges' across the front of your chest. These come only on exertion, especially when you are carrying your golf bag. The 'twinges' last between 1 and 5 minutes, never longer, and are always relieved if you sit down and rest. They in turn are associated with feeling dizzy and unwell, 'like I'm going to pass out, but I don't'.

You are otherwise systemically well and have no other problems at the present time.

Previous medical history: known high blood pressure and diet-controlled type 2 diabetes mellitus; you were not allowed to do national service 'because I had a heart problem' but were never told what it was; you don't know if you have had rheumatic fever.

Vascular risk: no known IHD, stroke or PVD.
Cholesterol: normal (checked for life assurance).

You are a lifelong cigar smoker (no cigarettes), and you enjoy the occasional whiskey or brandy – never more than one or two per week.

Family history: two brothers died of strokes; father died of typhoid fever; mother died in childbirth.

Medications: allergy to penicillin (causes severe rash); ramipril 10 mg od; bendrofluomethiazide 5 mg od; paracetamol 1 g PRN

Social history: you live with your wife of 52 years – she is well; you have a detached house in the suburbs, with three flights of internal stairs; independent of ADLs – still driving; no formal or informal care; your two sons live nearby; one daughter lives in Cornwall; you have 11 grandchildren.

Ideas and concerns: you are very worried that you may have been having 'mini-strokes', as this is what your golf partner had last year. He had similar fainting attacks.

Expectations: you are hoping that you can be put on a bit of aspirin (like your golf partner was) and have the rest of your investigations as an outpatient.

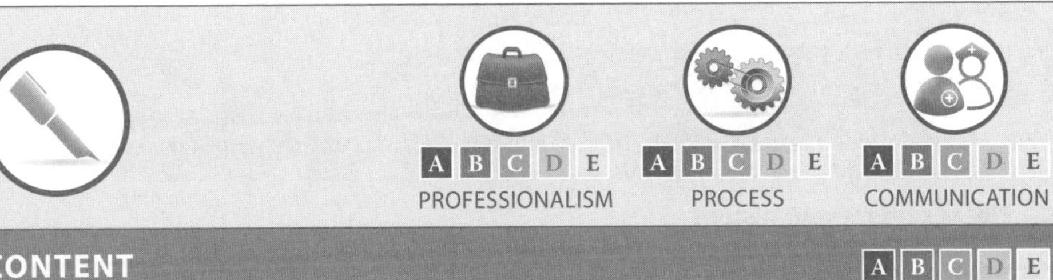

CONTENT

A B C D E

Identifies key information

- Very fit and well until recently
- Onset and progression
- Exertional dyspnoea – exercise tolerance pre-morbid and now; duration and progression, other symptoms of heart failure – SOA, PND, orthopnoea, cough, sputum, haemoptysis
- Chest pain/twinges – SOCRATES
- Episodes of loss of consciousness – frequency, pre – intra- and post-collapse symptoms and signs, cardiovascular and neurological symptoms
- Present state of health.

Identifies important negatives, including systemic enquiry

Completing the patient history

- Drug and allergy history: bendroflumethiazide, ramipril, paracetamol; penicillin allergy – severe skin rash
- Previous medical history: vascular risk
- Social and occupational history: married; children; grandchildren; recently retired furniture manufacturer; independent and well, no carers; wife well

Summarises important areas of the history back to the patient

Invites patient to ask questions and is able to deal with them appropriately

Establishes patient's ideas, concerns and expectations

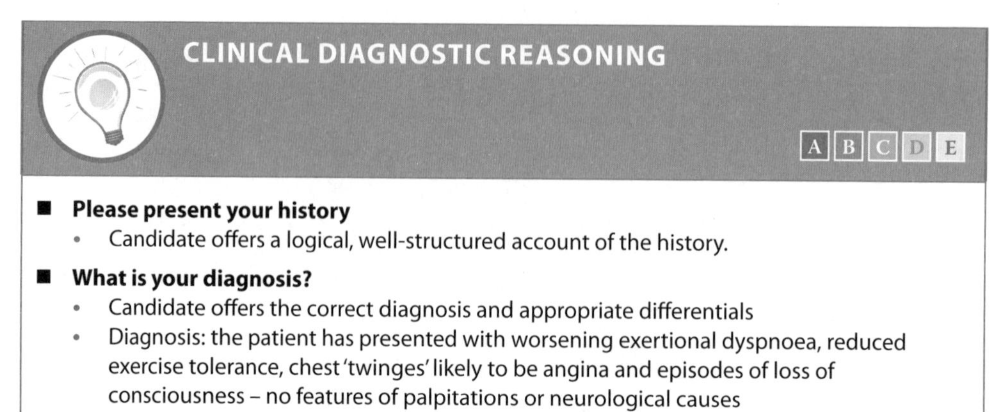

CLINICAL DIAGNOSTIC REASONING

A B C D E

- **Please present your history**
  - Candidate offers a logical, well-structured account of the history.
- **What is your diagnosis?**
  - Candidate offers the correct diagnosis and appropriate differentials
  - Diagnosis: the patient has presented with worsening exertional dyspnoea, reduced exercise tolerance, chest 'twinges' likely to be angina and episodes of loss of consciousness – no features of palpitations or neurological causes
  - The most likely unifying diagnosis is severe or significant aortic stenosis.
- **What are the common causes of this condition in the UK?**
  - Younger age group – congenital bicuspid valve
  - Older age group (and immigrant populations coming from endemic areas) – rheumatic fever.

Demonstrates clear and logical diagnostic reasoning

GLOBAL HISTORY MARK

A B C D E

Station 2 – Examination

Patient script

If you are an actor/patient, read the patient history and physical signs fully – when the candidate comes to an abnormal site in their examination, act-out tenderness and/or volunteer the relevant physical sign.

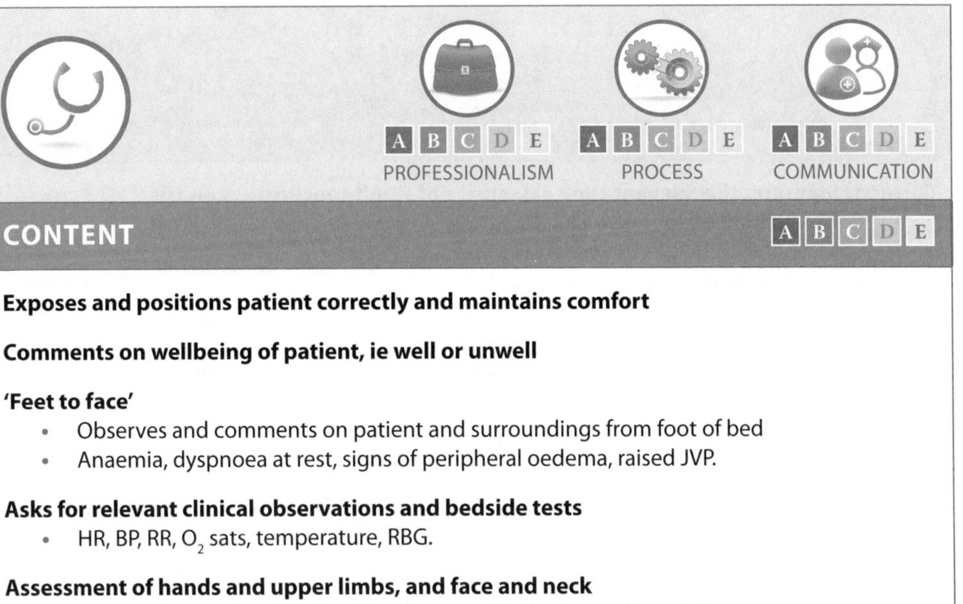

Exposes and positions patient correctly and maintains comfort

Comments on wellbeing of patient, ie well or unwell

'Feet to face'

- Observes and comments on patient and surroundings from foot of bed
- Anaemia, dyspnoea at rest, signs of peripheral oedema, raised JVP.

Asks for relevant clinical observations and bedside tests

- HR, BP, RR, O_2 sats, temperature, RBG.

Assessment of hands and upper limbs, and face and neck

- Tar staining, perfusion of hands, stigmata of infective endocarditis
- Takes patient's BP
- Face and neck including anaemia, central cyanosis, JVP.

Focused examination of the cardiovascular and respiratory systems, commenting on presence or absence on signs of significant aortic stenosis and its complications

- Hands – cool peripheries
- Radial pulse – low volume
- Blood pressure – narrow pulse pressure (systolic – diastolic <40 mmHg)
- Carotid character – slow rising or sustained
- Apex beat – undisplaced; sustained/hyperdynamic (heaving)
- Palpable systolic thrill (often lost in significant disease)
- Auscultation – ejection systolic murmur (very unlikely to have ejection click); S4, soft second heart sound
- Pulmonary oedema ± signs of right heart failure.

Completes examination

- Offers to examine for other signs of infective endocarditis.

Thanks patient, offers assistance, maintains patient's dignity and privacy until they are dressed

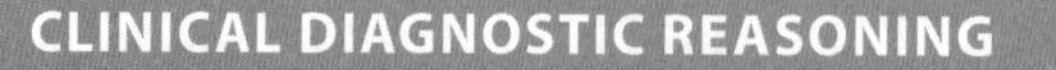

CLINICAL DIAGNOSTIC REASONING

A B C D E

Correctly identifies the relevant clinical features of significant aortic stenosis

- Cool peripheries
- Low volume pulse
- Narrow pulse pressure
- Sustained/slow rising carotid pulse
- Apex beat – hyperdynamic and undisplaced
- Ejection systolic murmur (intensity is independent of the degree of the stenosis)
- Soft S2
- S4
- Bibasal crackles suggestive of pulmonary oedema.

Is able to list three essential/diagnostic investigations that should be considered, with a reason for each

- ECG – features of IHD – old and new; features of left heart strain and hypertrophy – P mitrale, LAD, LBBB or voltage criteria of left ventricular hypertrophy
- CXR – signs of pulmonary oedema, calcified aortic valve
- Echo – confirm and define valvular heart disease, LVEF
- PCA/ventriculogram and pressure measurements – coronary arteries and defining the pressure gradient and degree of stenosis.

Is able to list three acute interventions that should be arranged for this patient once he is admitted to the wards

- Furosemide
- Stop ACEI until echo results
- Add aspirin and clopidogrel
- Consider GTN spray – PRN
- Consider addition of beta-blocker – hypertension and IHD.

Demonstrates safe, sensible and appropriate management plan

Demonstrates clear and logical diagnostic reasoning

GLOBAL EXAMINATION MARK

A B C D E

Station 3 – Data interpretation

1 (A) True, (B) False, (C) False, (D) True, (E) True

This ECG tracing shows only the chest leads V1–V6. The rhythm strip demonstrates a tall P wave, rather than a broad P wave of P mitrale. The PR interval is normal. There are inverted T waves in V1–V4 (the anteroseptal leads). There are very tall R waves in V4 and V5 (>25 mm) in keeping with the voltage criteria of LVH.

2 (A) False, (B) True, (C) False, (D) True, (E) False

This ECG shows a large infero-posterior STEMI with high lateral ST depression. The axis is normal as leads I, II and III are all positive. There is ST elevation in leads II, III and aVF (inferior) and deep ST depression in the anterior leads (consistent with posterior ischaemia). There is ST depression in leads I and aVL (high lateral leads). The rhythm is third degree or complete heart block.

3 (A) False, (B) False, (C) False, (D) True, (E) True

This ECG shows normal sinus rhythm at a rate of about 75 bpm. There is left axis deviation and right bundle branch block, consistent with bifascicular block.

4 (A) True, (B) True, (C) True, (D) True, (E) False

This ECG demonstrates widespread T-wave inversion in all territories of the ECG. There are very large, deep inverted T waves in the anterior leads that are consistent with 'hyperacute' T waves in acute ischaemia. The rate is 72 bpm and there is left axis deviation. There are no R waves in any of the anterolateral leads.

5 (A) True, (B) True, (C) True, (D) True, (E) False

This is an ECG demonstrating the changes of acute pericarditis. There is 'saddle-shaped' or concave ST elevation, particularly in leads II, III and aVF, V4, V5 and V6. There is evidence of high take-off of the ST segment in the anterior leads – this means the ST segment takes off from above the baseline.

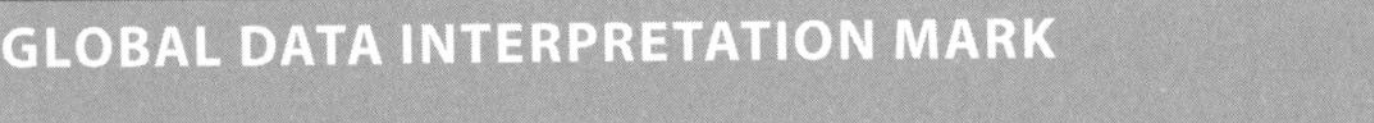

A B C D E

SCENARIO 13

Station 4 – Prescribing skills

Check: DRUG DRs Don't Forget Signing Off (page 373)

Allergies, sensitivities and adverse drug reactions					Patient details/addressograph
No known allergies ✓		Initials AF	Gender (M)/ F		NHS/ Hospital No: 109087
Not possible to ascertain ☐		Date 21.11.11	Weight (kg)	Date	
Medicine/substance	Reaction & Severity	Initials & Date	63kg		Surname: COHEN
PENICILIN	SEVERE RASH	AF 21.11			
			Height		First name: SAMUEL
			1.70m		
Alerts			Surface area (m²)		Date of birth: 06.05.27

IN-PATIENT MEDICATION PRESCRIPTION AND ADMINISTRATION RECORD

PasTest HOSPITAL

Consultant	Trainee Dr. Name and Bleep no.	Date of admission	Date chart reboarded	Estimated date of discharge
SYED	FEATHER 311	21.11.11		

This chart is no.	Transcribing Check by Pharmacy	Ward
.... of	Sign .... Date	1. CCU .... 2. ....

Supplementary Medication charts in use: Other (please specify): 1 .... 2 ....

Epidural/PCA ☐ Syringe driver ☐ TPN ☐ Chemotherapy ☐ Insulin sliding scale ☐

Once only medications – loading doses, pre-medication, PGDs or surgical antibiotic propylaxis

Date	Time to be given	Medicine (approved name)	Dose	Route	Signature and bleep no.	Pharmacy	Time given	Given by	Checked by
21.11	14.00	FUROSEMIDE	40mg	IV	AF 311				

Regular prescriptions						
Oral anticoagulation follow the anticoagulation guidelines available on the intranet						
Indication	Target INR	Baseline INR (if applicable)	Duration of therapy / Date therapy started	Date of anticoagulation follow-up appointment (clinic or other)*	Anticoagulant record book given or updated. Sign and date	Date patient counselled and sign
* A follow-up appointment must be booked with the anti-coagulant clinic or enhanced provider of primary care services. If not, the TTA will not be dispensed						

Initiating warfarin	Perform baseline coagulation screen, LFTs, U&Es and FBC	Prescribe initiation dose as per guidelines	CHECK INR ON DAY 3	FOLLOW DOSING ALGORITHM IN GUIDELINE
Continuing warfarin	Maintenance therapy	FOLLOW MAINTENANCE DOSING ALGORITHM IN GUIDELINE		

Do not use the initiation protocol for patients already on warfarin. More frequent INR monitoring may be required for patients on interacting drug(s)

Medication				Date													
1				INR													
Route	Frequency OD	Time 18.00	Start	Dose													
			Stop	Dr sign													
Signature		Bleep no.	Pharmacy	Given													

Initiating warfarin – Reduced dosing regimen in red. Refer to anticoagulation policy

Day	One	Two	Three							Four and above									
INR	<1.4	No test	<2.0	2.0-2.1	2.2-2.5	2.6-2.9	3.0-3.3	3.4-4.0	>4.0	<1.4	1.4-1.5	1.6-1.7	1.8-1.9	2.0-2.3	2.4-3.0	3.1-4.0	4.1-4.5	>4.5
Dose mg	10 5	10 5	10	5	4	3	2	1	0	9	8	7	6	5	4	3	Miss 1 day	Miss 2 day

Thromboprophylaxis please prescribe treatment regimens in the regular medications section

Choice of mechanical prophylaxis and leg(s) to be applied to						Enter Time	Enter details below
Graduated elastic compression stockings	Intermittend pneumatic compression device (IPC)		Leg				
			Left	Right	Both		
21/11 Start Date: ☑	End Date: ☐	Signature and Bleep No.	☐	☐	☑		
Start Date: ☐	End Date: ☐	Signature and Bleep No. AF	☐	☐	☐		

Medication		Dose	Dose Change	Enter Time	Enter details below
CLEXANE		40mg			
Please ensure you have completed the VTE risk assessment form	Date	21/11			
	Route	SC			
	Signature	AF		Instructions	Pharmacy ☐
	Bleep no.	311			

Oxygen			
Target Saturation	88-92% ☐	94/98% ☐	If oxygen saturation falls below target range on prescribed oxygen, patient needs urgent clinical review. If oxygen saturation is above targent range on prescribed oxygen, ask for review.
Other specify)		*Device: N= nasal cannula, SM = simple face mask, V = venturi, H = humidified, RM = reservoir mask, OTHER = other eg. NCPAP/NIPPV	Pharmacy ☐
Target Saturation not applicable ☐			

	Date Changed	Date Changed	Enter Time	Enter details below
Device				
% or L/min (specify a range eg 1-21 L/min)				
Signature and Bleep no.				

SCENARIO 13

Regular prescriptions continued									
Regular medications									
Date	21/11	Medication	BENDROFLUMETHIAZIDE	Instructions		Signature and bleep no.	AF 311	Pharmacy	
Route	PO								
Times	Dose								
Date			21	22	23	24	25	26	
06									
(09)		2.5g							
12									
18									
22									
24									

Regular prescriptions continued									
Regular medications									
Date	21/11	Medication	FUROSEMIDE	Instructions		Signature and bleep no.	AF 311	Pharmacy	
Route	IV								
Times	Dose								
Date			21	22	23	24	25	26	27
06									
(09)		40mg							
12									
18									
22									
24									

Regular prescriptions continued									
Regular medications									
Date	21/11	Medication	BISOPROLOL	Instructions		Signature and bleep no.	AF 311	Pharmacy	
Route	PO								
Times	Dose								
Date			21	22	23	24	25	26	27
06									
(09)		1.25mg							
12									
18									
22									
24									

Regular prescriptions continued									
Regular medications									
Date	21/11	Medication	RAMIPRIL	Instructions	NOT BEFORE ECHO	Signature and bleep no.	AF 311	Pharmacy	
Route	PO								
Times	Dose								
Date			21	22	23	24	25	26	27
06									
(09)		10mg							
12									
18									
22									
24									

Regular prescriptions continued								
Regular medications								
Date	21/11	Medication ASPRIN		Instructions		Signature and bleep no. AF 311	Pharmacy ☐	
Route	PO							
Times	Dose							
Date		21	22	23	24	25	26	27
06								
09	75mg							
12								
18								
22								
24								

As required medications					
Medication PARACETAMOL				Date	
Indication				Time	
Dose 0.5-1 mg	Route PO	Maximum frequency / dose 6 hourly	Start date 21/11	Dose	
			Stop date	Route	
Signature AF			Bleep no. 311	Given	
Additional instructions:				Pharmacy ☐	

As required medications					
Medication METOCLOPRAMIDE				Date	
Indication				Time	
Dose 10 mg	Route IV/IM	Maximum frequency / dose 8 hourly	Start date 21/11	Dose	
			Stop date	Route	
Signature AF			Bleep no. 311	Given	
Additional instructions:				Pharmacy ☐	

GLOBAL PRESCRIBING MARK

A B C D E

SCENARIO 13

Station 5 – Clinical communication skills

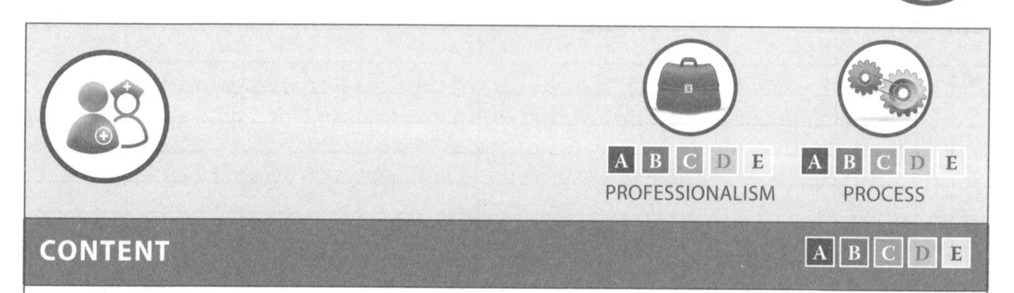

CONTENT A B C D E

Doctor introduces him/herself and the topic

Confirms only has limited time (6–7 minutes); recommends any questions be reserved for end of talk

Confirms the discussion topics

- Severe aortic stenosis and its complications
- Effects of treatments such as ACEI and diuretics
- Will be attempting to utilise first principles wherever possible.

Ascertains present understanding of the students

- Normal anatomy of the left ventricle, including relation to the coronary sinuses
- Pathology of aortic stenosis
- Concepts of PRE and AFTER LOAD.

Explains effects of severe aortic stenosis

- Obstruction of coronary sinuses by stenosed valve leads to cardiac ischaemia
- Collapse of patient is due to severely reduced cardiac output – this leads to reduced blood pressure, cerebral perfusion and thus collapse
- From first principles cardiac output = Stroke volume (SV) × Heart rate
- Stroke volume is determined by the Frank Starling law (degree of stretch of the cardiac muscle fibres determines the force of contractility; in turn determines the stroke volume)
- The degree of stretch is in turn determined by:
  (a) The health of the muscle fibres – in severe aortic stenosis, LV hypertrophy leading reduced ability to stretch
  (b) Volume of blood in the left ventricle just before contraction (systole) = End diastolic volume (EDV)
- EDV is determined by pre-load (venous return), filling time (ventricular diastole) and the 'atrial kick'
  - SV (and thus CO) is significantly reduced if one of these factors is significantly impaired
  - Thus if we give such patients large doses of diuretics or ACEI, which both reduces venous return, they will cause a reduction in EDV and so a reduction in stretch of the LV
  - A simple rule 'It's a mechanical/physical blockage – it needs physical removal (ie stretching of blockage or surgical excision/replacement)

Summarises important areas of the talk back to the nurses

Invites questions, attempts clarification of areas of concern

Suggests reading materials that may clarify issues

Formally ends the discussion

CLINICAL DIAGNOSTIC REASONING

A B C D E

- **I read that the addition of an ACEI make the effects of renal artery stenosis (RAS) worse. Is this similar to the mechanism involved with aortic stenosis or is it different?**
  - For the mechanism of how ACEIs make renal artery stenosis we have to go back to the concepts of preload and afterload; if aortic stenosis is primarily about PRE-load, in renal artery stenosis, the main focus is AFTER-load.
  - In renal artery stenosis: the kidney has reduced preload because of the arterial stenosis, ie less blood is able to enter the kidney and thus the filtration system; the normal glomerular filtration is maintained by producing a 'clamp' (through increased sympathetic vasoconstriction) on the efferent (outgoing) blood vessels, ie increasing the afterload
  - Thus the blood flow is slowed through the kidney and thus filtration is maintained.
  - If you give such patients with RAS an ACEI or indeed an A2RB, the efferent 'clamp' is removed (ACEI reduce sympathetic vasoconstriction).
  - So although the blood travels quicker through the filtration system, paradoxically less is actually filtered – thus making the renal impairment worse.
- **So can you give these patients A2 receptor blockers instead?**
  - No A2RB produces the same effects as the ACEI.

Demonstrates safe, sensible and appropriate management plan

Demonstrates clear and logical diagnostic reasoning

GLOBAL COMMUNICATION MARK

A B C D E

Scenario 13: Reflection and consolidation

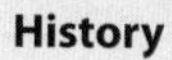

History

Mr Samuel Cohen is an 84-year-old recently retired furniture manufacturer. He has known hypertension and diet-controlled type 2 diabetes mellitus but is normally very fit and well and is a keen golfer.
He now presents with a 2- to 3-month history of exertional dyspnoea, ankle oedema and a dry cough. His exercise tolerance has always been very good, but is now reduced to about 100 m on the flat. He is unable to climb inclines and is now using a golf buggy to complete his rounds of golf. In the last few weeks the shortness of breath has become associated with 'twinges' across the chest. These come only on exertion, and last between 1 and 5 minutes. They are always relieved by rest but are associated with feeling dizzy and unwell.
Of note he has also suffered two or three 'funny turns' where without warning he feels faint and then has lost consciousness. His wife witnessed these episodes and says he goes cold, grey and clammy.
He was unable to serve in the army 'because of a heart problem but was never told what it was. He doesn't know if he ever had rheumatic fever when younger.
He is otherwise systemically well.

Examination

On examination, this is a well-looking elderly man who is short of breath at rest (his AMTS = 10/10).
He has several features of significant aortic stenosis, including: cool peripheries, low volume pulse (irregular and rate of 88 bpm), narrow pulse pressure with a BP of 145/126 mmHg, carotid pulse that is sustained/slow rising in character, apex beat undisplaced but hyperdynamic in nature, and no heaves or thrills.
On auscultation he had a soft second heart sound and grade 2/6 ejection systolic murmur that did not radiate. There was possibly a fourth heart sound as well.
He had signs of pulmonary oedema with bibasal crackles heard on auscultation of his lung fields.
Of note there was no tar staining of his fingers or stigmata of hyperlipidaemia and no peripheral stigmata of infective endocarditis.
In summary, this is a previously fit and well elderly man now presenting with signs of significant aortic stenosis and pulmonary oedema.

Data interpretation

If he agrees, this gentleman should be 'worked up' for an aortic valve replacement and possible CABG

- Bloods: FBC, U&Es, RBG, HBA1c, LFTs, clotting
- CXR
- ECG
- Echocardiogram
- Cardiac catheterisation – coronary angiography and pressure measurements across aortic valve
- Newer modalities such as cardiac MRI may become increasingly utilised over the next few years.

Management

In view of the likely severity of the aortic stenosis, aortic valve replacement is the treatment of choice (valvuloplasty may be used in some cases but does not offer a long-term 'cure'). Medical management of both his heart failure and angina should be initiated but without surgical intervention. Mr Cohen will become increasingly symptomatic and will not survive.

Further reading and web links

Explanation of CO, SV and HR from first principles:
http://skillstat.com/PDF/mceCO.pdf
www.med-ed.virginia.edu/courses/rad/cardiacmr/Pathology/Valvular/Valvular.html
Video images of cardiac MRI scans:
http://emedicine.medscape.com/article/780702-overview

Scenario 14: 'Fallen community leader'

Station 1

History *10-minute station*

You are the FY1 in a busy GP practice. The next patient, Mr Baljit Singh, has agreed to talk to you before seeing the GP.

- **Please take a focused, diagnostic history from the patient, with a view to presenting the history to the GP once you have finished.**

You will be assessed on the following areas, as well as the content and diagnostic reasoning of your history – take them into account in your presentation.

Professionalism

- Professional appearance (NHS dress code) – including general appearance, hair and jewellery
- Maintains patient and personal safety
- Polite introduction; identifies patient or interviewee correctly; confirms patient's date of birth from name band or other source
- Obtains informal consent; maintains patient's privacy
- Displays empathetic and caring attitudes and behaviours throughout.

Process

- Good organisation and structure; appropriate use of open and closed questions
- Appropriate fluency/rhythm/pace to the interview – this may change depending on environment and acute nature of the problem
- Appropriate time for the patient to respond/reply to questions
- Appropriate acknowledgement of difficult or emotional areas of the patient's history.

Communication skills

- Demonstrates caring and sympathetic attitude
- Asks open questions
- Invites patient to ask questions and answers them appropriately
- Addresses patient's ideas, concerns and expectations.

Station 2

Examination *10-minute station*

The GP agrees that this man has a history of long-term alcohol excess. He asks you to perform an appropriate assessment of the patient and then present the relevant findings (given within the station) to him.

- **Please include the following in your assessment:**
  - **A formal abdominal examination**
  - **Assessment for signs of chronic liver disease**
  - **Signs of acute hepatic decompensation and delirium tremens.**

You will be assessed on the following areas, as well as the content and skills of your examination – take them into account in your presentation.

Professionalism

- Professional appearance; maintains infection control standards, including hand cleaning and appropriate use of gloves and aprons
- Maintains patient and personal safety
- Polite introduction; identifies patient and confirms date of birth from name band or other source
- Obtains informal consent; maintains patient privacy and dignity
- Displays empathetic and caring attitudes and behaviours throughout.

Process

- Appropriate fluency/rhythm/pace to the examination – this may change depending on environment and acute nature of problem
- Good organisation and structure of examination; sensitive and empathetic approach
- Uses appropriate clinical techniques throughout
- Maintains privacy and dignity throughout.

Clinical communication

- Explains proposed examination/procedure; explains examination/procedure as it proceeds
- Offers information in a clear, structured and fluent manner, avoiding jargon
- Listens to patient and responds appropriately
- Demonstrates appropriate body language.

Please read the information below before presenting this case to the GP as if you were in a busy GP surgery.
[NB If you have a model do not read this section]

Clinical findings

- o **Patient is unkempt, dishevelled and looks chronically unwell; feet to face – patient is slightly agitated but no signs of delirium tremens (DTs), apyrexial**
- o **Observations – HR 86 bpm, BP 130/73 mmHg; regular and normal; CBG 3.7 mmol/l**
- o **No signs of acute liver decompensation – no jaundice, or signs of hepatic encephalopathy – no asterixis, no confusion, drowsiness or hepatic fetor; of note he has several signs of chronic liver disease, including Dupuytren's contracture, leuconychia, palmar erythema, bruising over his arms and truncal areas, gynaecomastia and several spider naevi; he also has marked tar staining of the fingers of his right hand**
- o **Abdominal examination: abdomen distended but soft and non-tender, no palpable masses, hepatomegaly 5 cm below right costal margin associated with 3–4 cm splenomegaly below left costal margin, no evidence of renal masses, demonstrable ascites with shifting dullness; no DRE or examination of external genitalia.**

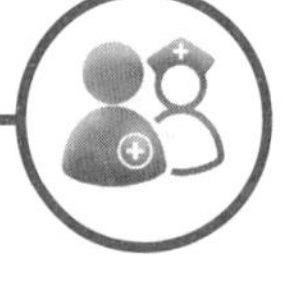

Station 3

Clinical communication skills *10-minute station*

- **The GP asks you to counsel Mr Singh regarding his alcohol intake and discuss with him:**
  The possible underlying causes for his drinking
  The likely effects of his drinking if he continues
  Agencies that may help him stop drinking.

Station 4

Data interpretation *10-minute station*

Despite going to a few Alcoholics Anonymous group meetings and promising his wife and family he would give up, Mr Singh continues to drink heavily. Three months later he is admitted to his local hospital with a large, fresh haematemesis.

Part 1:

You are the FY1 on call for Medicine and are asked to chase up Mr Singh's investigation results.

- **Please fill in the table below with the abnormal results. You should state the likely cause in Mr Singh's case, and a secondary differential cause of each abnormality.**

FBC: Hb 8.9 g/dl, MCV 104 fl, WCC 3.6 × 10^9/l, neutrophils 1.9, platelets 67 × 10^9/l
U&Es: Na^+ 123 mmol/l, K^+ 3.9 mmol/l, urea 22.6 mmol/l, creatinine 94 μmol/l
RBG: 3.1 mmol/l
Coagulation: INR 1.7, APTT 54 s
LFTs: TBil 66.5,ALT 432 IU/l, AST 523 IU/l, Alk Phos 1812 IU/l, γGT 432 IU/l, ALB 18 g/l

Abnormality	Likely cause	Differential cause
1.		
2.		
3.		
4.		
5.		
6.		
7.		
8.		
9.		

Part 2:
While awaiting the results, the Gastroenterology ST5 hands you a set of results from another jaundiced man who has recently been admitted under her care.

- Please read the scenario she gives you and then answer the questions on the data below.

Mr JA is a 25-year-old trainee engineer who has recently returned from Thailand. He was admitted 2 days ago with jaundice, nausea and vomiting and several episodes of loose stool. On further questioning he admits to having had unprotected sex with several 'bar hostesses' at a party. His LFTs showed a hepatitic derangement; his viral hepatitis screen is shown below:

HAV – aHAV IgM negative; aHAV IgG negative
HCV – aHCV antibody 'weakly positive'; HCV RIBA negative
HBs antigen positive
aHBs antibody negative
HBc antigen negative
aHBc IgG negative
aHBc IgM positive
HBe antigen positive
aHBe antibody negative
HBV DNA (copies/ml) 5 × 106

SCENARIO 14

1 The HAV results indicate he had previously been immunised against HAV infection.
2 The HCV results indicate he is likely to have a low-grade HCV infection.
3 The HBs antigen positivity indicates previous HBV immunisation.
4 The HBs antibody negativity indicates no HBV immunity.
5 The aHBc IgM positivity indicates acute viral replication.
6 The HBe antigen positivity indicates the patient is at high risk of infecting others.
7 This patient has an acute on chronic HBV infection.
8 The HBV DNA (copies/ml) is a marker of viral load, and thus infectivity.
9 This patient can donate blood after receiving treatment.
10 Untreated, this condition predisposes to hepatocellular carcinoma.

Station 5

Procedural skills *10-minute station*

A technician in the Haematology Laboratory bleeps you to say that the sample taken for Mr Singh's crossmatch was accidentally broken in transit to the lab. She apologises (it was not her fault) but asks if you could send a second sample as soon as possible.

Procedure A

- Using the following equipment, please take an appropriate sample of blood from the manikin arm provided and complete the details required on the crossmatch bottle and the form. You should crossmatch Mr Singh for six units of blood. You should talk to the examiner as if they were the patient.

Equipment provided

- Phlebotomy manikin arm with hospital identity bracelet containing patient's correct details
- Box of vacutainers and appropriate needles
- Different blood bottles
- Tourniquet
- Alcohol wipes
- Gauze or similar to press on puncture wound
- Gloves
- Crossmatch form

Details

Mr Baljit Singh; Hospital No. 4545422; DOB: 16/09/1973; Weight: approx. 70 kg; Height: 1.78 m; Allergies: NKDA; Blood group: not known; Hb: 8.9 g/dl, but has bled since then; No previous operations/blood transfusions; Hospital: The Central Hospital; Ward: Emergency Department; Consultant: Dr Odoje.

Procedure B

- Using the following equipment, please demonstrate how you would put up an emergency unit of O negative blood, while awaiting the first unit of crossmatched blood. You may assume the prescription for the O negative unit has been written up by another doctor.

Equipment provided

- Phlebotomy manikin arm with cannula inserted and hospital identity bracelet containing patient's correct details
- One blood unit – labelled as O negative/for emergency use
- Blood-giving set and ordinary fluid-giving set
- Gloves

In addition to the patient details already given, the following observations were taken 5 minutes ago:

BP 93/65 mmHg
HR 124 bpm
RR 22 bpm
CBG 4.1 mmol/l
O_2 sats 96% on 2 l/min
Temperature 36.7 °C

Station 6

Prescribing skills *10-minute station*

Mr Singh is admitted for an emergency endoscopy and treatment. The ST5 asks you to complete the drug chart on page 368.

- Using the BNF and chart provided, please complete Mr Singh's drug chart and prescribe:

  A six-unit blood transfusion
  An anti-encephalopathy regime
  An alcohol-withdrawal regime, including sedatives and appropriate vitamin therapy.

Remember: DRUG DRs Don't Forget Signing Off (page 373)

Answers

Station 1 – History

Patient script

You are sad, desperate and slightly agitated.

You are Mr Baljit Singh, DOB 16 September 1973, a 38-year-old Sikh man. If/when asked, you came to see the doctor today because you are 'at the end of your tether'. If pushed further 'it's because I'm drinking myself to death doctor'.

You were previously working as a foreman in a car factory but were made redundant when the car industry started to slow down about 3 years ago. Prior to this you were a proud family man, who was a leader in the local Sikh community and was thinking of running for the council, and possibly later, for parliament. In your adult life you have 'always enjoyed a drink' but 'never let it rule or ruin you'. You would describe yourself as a 'social drinker' who drank a few 'large' (if pushed about two 'quadruple') whiskies most weeknights, and a few more with friends at the weekend. If asked, a litre bottle of Johnny Walker Red Label (your favourite) would last about 10 days or so. You don't drink any other alcohol, ie no wine or beer, no other spirits.

Since being made redundant you have been unable to find a new job (despite applying for almost 100) and became increasingly frustrated, angry and then depressed. You began to drink very heavily (two to three bottles of whisky per day), which meant you missed job interviews and important appointments. This made you feel 'disgusted with yourself' and caused you to be more depressed, and so you drank more.

You became increasingly reclusive, and only went out to buy whisky. Over the last 18 months you became 'impossible to live with' and your wife and three daughters have gone to live with your mother-in-law, as you were becoming increasingly aggressive and unpleasant. You were never physically abusive but constantly shouted and screamed at the family, especially when challenged about your drinking. You have not stopped drinking for any appreciable time over the last 3 years and most recently have been drinking heavily (when able). You have never thought about Alcoholics Anonymous or similar groups. At present you're drinking 'anything I can get my hands on'. You still drink whisky but now drink the cheap own brand of the local supermarket. You eat very little and are feeling increasingly weak and unable to go on.

No previous, or family, history of mental health problems, alcohol or drug addiction.

No suicidal ideation; no self-harm.

'Just feel very low and need help'.

Ideas and concerns – you realise that if you carry on like this you will lose everything precious, including your family, your house and maybe even your life.

Expectations – you know it won't be easy but know you need to stop drinking or you may die. You really want the help of anyone who will listen.

If the candidate attempts the CAGE questionnaire:

C – 'I know I need to cut down but I just can't stop myself'

A – 'Yes, I often get very angry when challenged about my drinking' (see above)

G – 'I'm not sure if guilty is the right word, but I know I am going to lose everything precious to me soon and am desperate to stop'

E – 'I drink all hours I am awake – the first thing I often do before getting out of bed is to take a swig from the bottle on my bedside table. Recently it has often been empty'

You have no jaundice or other hepatobiliary symptoms. There are no other systemic symptoms of note, but you are feeling increasingly weak and tired and are sleeping for long periods.

You have never taken any regular medications and have no allergies as far as you know.

You have no significant medical or surgical history and no mental health problems.

You live in a four-bedroom house; your mortgage was paid off after a rich uncle died in India and left you some money.

You have three daughters – aged 9, 10 and 12 years.

Cigarette smoker – since 16-yo; smoke 15–20 per day; no illicit drug taking

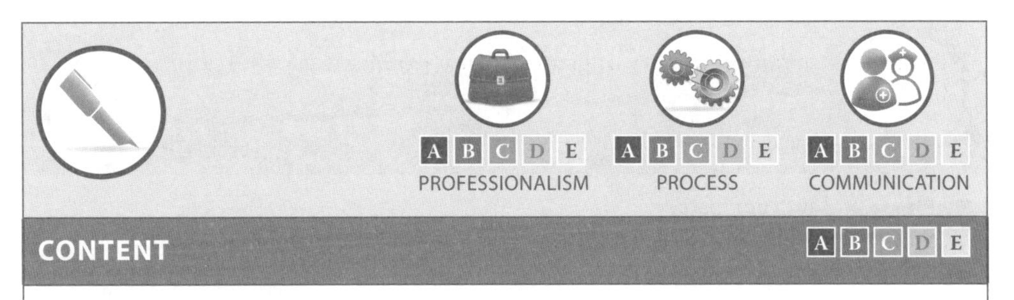

Identifies key information

- Fit and well until redundancy and inability to secure new job
- 'Social drinker' – defines social drinking (actually drinking over 30 units per week)
- Progression of drinking after becoming redundant – previous alcohol consumption compared to present
- Defines: what, when, where, quantity of alcohol he is drinking; excludes consumption of other alcohol – other spirits, wines and beer
- How drinking is impacting on his life – family, friends, work, social
- Mood; asks directly about suicidal ideation; self-harm
- CAGE questionnaire or similar
- Periods of abstinence; attendance at AA or similar groups
- Hepatobiliary and systemic symptoms.

Completing the history

- Drug and allergy history: nil medication, allergies NKDA
- Previous medical history
- Social history: cigarette smoking, illicit drug taking, prior to redundancy and now; married, children, housing, financial circumstances.

Summarises important areas of the history back to the patient

Invites patient to ask questions and is able to deal with them appropriately

Establishes patient's ideas, concerns and expectations

CLINICAL DIAGNOSTIC REASONING

A B C D E

- **Please present your history**
  - Candidate offers a logical, well-structured account of the history.
- **What conclusions would you draw from this history?**
  - This is a man who has always 'enjoyed' alcohol in large amounts
  - Became a real problem when he lost his job and then couldn't find another
  - Now drinking in real excess (two to three bottles of whisky per day)
  - Increasingly aware that his life is falling apart – family now living with other family members; not able to do anything else apart from drinking – increasingly weak/not eating
  - Seems genuine about trying to give up – although no period of abstinence in over 3 years.
- **What advice would you give this patient today?**
  - Acknowledges that giving up is not going to be easy for Mr Singh but if he doesn't his life may well be in danger
  - Patient has taken a major first step by coming to talk to the GP BUT has not shown any evidence of actually trying to stop drinking
  - He must be encouraged to go to community agencies that will help with both physical and mental withdrawal; you can supply details if he is interested
  - He needs to seek support through family and agencies such as Alcoholics Anonymous.

Demonstrates safe, sensible and appropriate management plan

Demonstrates clear and logical diagnostic reasoning

GLOBAL HISTORY MARK

A B C D E

Station 2 – Examination

Patient script

If you are an actor/patient, read the patient history and physical signs fully – when the candidate comes to an abnormal site in their examination, act-out tenderness and/or volunteer the relevant physical sign.

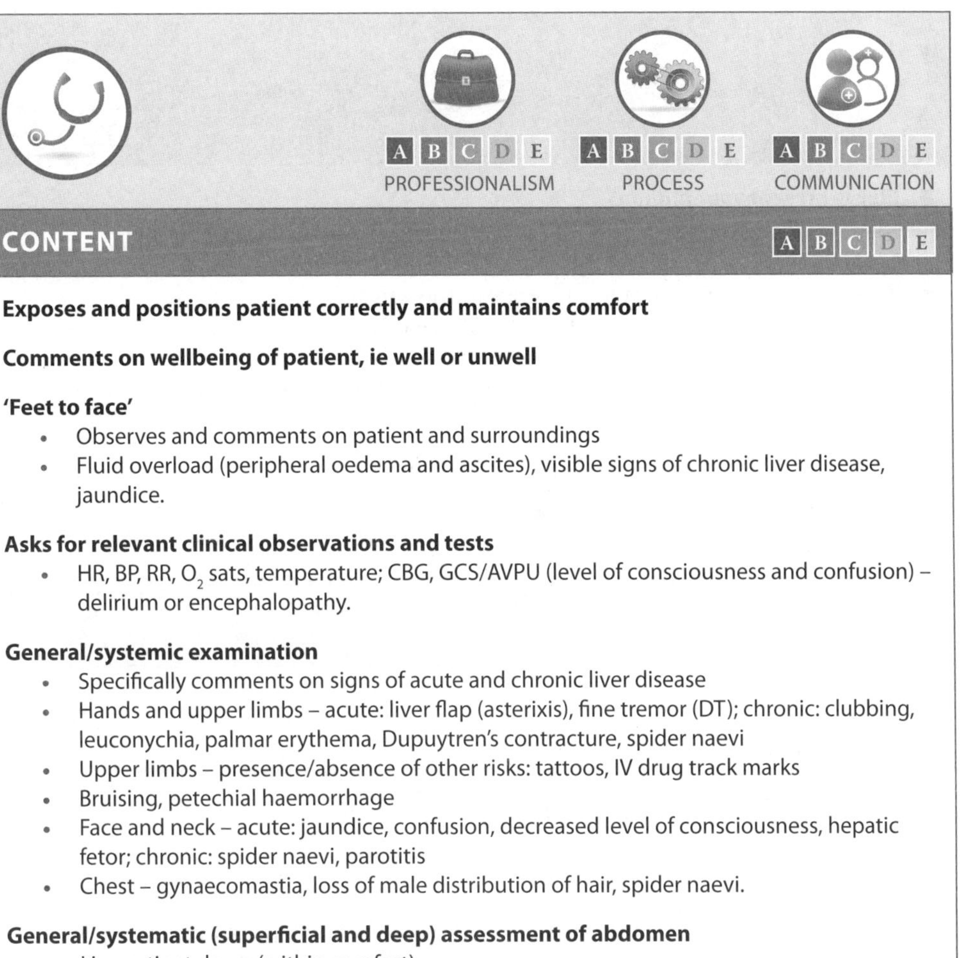

CONTENT

A B C D E

Exposes and positions patient correctly and maintains comfort

Comments on wellbeing of patient, ie well or unwell

'Feet to face'

- Observes and comments on patient and surroundings
- Fluid overload (peripheral oedema and ascites), visible signs of chronic liver disease, jaundice.

Asks for relevant clinical observations and tests

- HR, BP, RR, O_2 sats, temperature; CBG, GCS/AVPU (level of consciousness and confusion) – delirium or encephalopathy.

General/systemic examination

- Specifically comments on signs of acute and chronic liver disease
- Hands and upper limbs – acute: liver flap (asterixis), fine tremor (DT); chronic: clubbing, leuconychia, palmar erythema, Dupuytren's contracture, spider naevi
- Upper limbs – presence/absence of other risks: tattoos, IV drug track marks
- Bruising, petechial haemorrhage
- Face and neck – acute: jaundice, confusion, decreased level of consciousness, hepatic fetor; chronic: spider naevi, parotitis
- Chest – gynaecomastia, loss of male distribution of hair, spider naevi.

General/systematic (superficial and deep) assessment of abdomen

- Lies patient down (within comfort)
- Assesses for: masses, hepatomegaly, splenomegaly, renal enlargement, ascites, bowel sounds.

Completes examination by offering to perform DRE and assessment of external genitalia:

■ **Why would you do these assessments?**

- DRE: stool assessment, eg constipation, melaena, diarrhoea
- External genitalia – atrophy in chronic liver disease.

Thanks patient, offers assistance, maintains patient's dignity and privacy until they are dressed

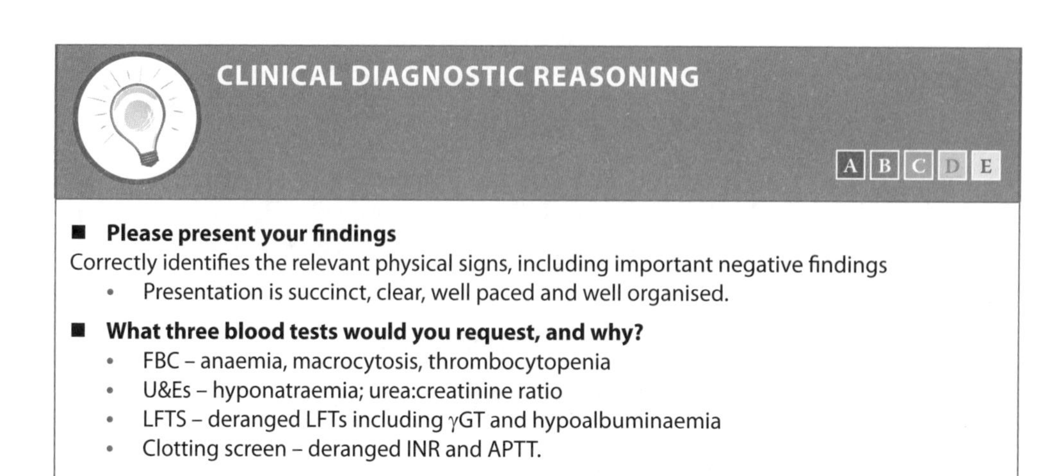

CLINICAL DIAGNOSTIC REASONING

A B C D E

- **Please present your findings**

Correctly identifies the relevant physical signs, including important negative findings

- Presentation is succinct, clear, well paced and well organised.

- **What three blood tests would you request, and why?**
  - FBC – anaemia, macrocytosis, thrombocytopenia
  - U&Es – hyponatraemia; urea:creatinine ratio
  - LFTS – deranged LFTs including γGT and hypoalbuminaemia
  - Clotting screen – deranged INR and APTT.

Demonstrates a safe, sensible and appropriate management plan

Demonstrates clear and logical diagnostic reasoning

GLOBAL EXAMINATION MARK

A B C D E

Station 3 – Clinical communication skills

Patient script

You are sad, desperate and slightly agitated. You are Mr Baljit Singh – see script for the History station to recap alcohol and pre-morbid history.

You should be open to suggestions about any agencies that may help you stop drinking. **You realise that if you carry on like this you will lose everything precious including your family, your house and maybe even your life.**

You have heard that you can be given an injection to make you sleep for a day or so (rapid detoxification) and when you wake up you don't feel like drinking. You would really like to try this, as you are desperate.

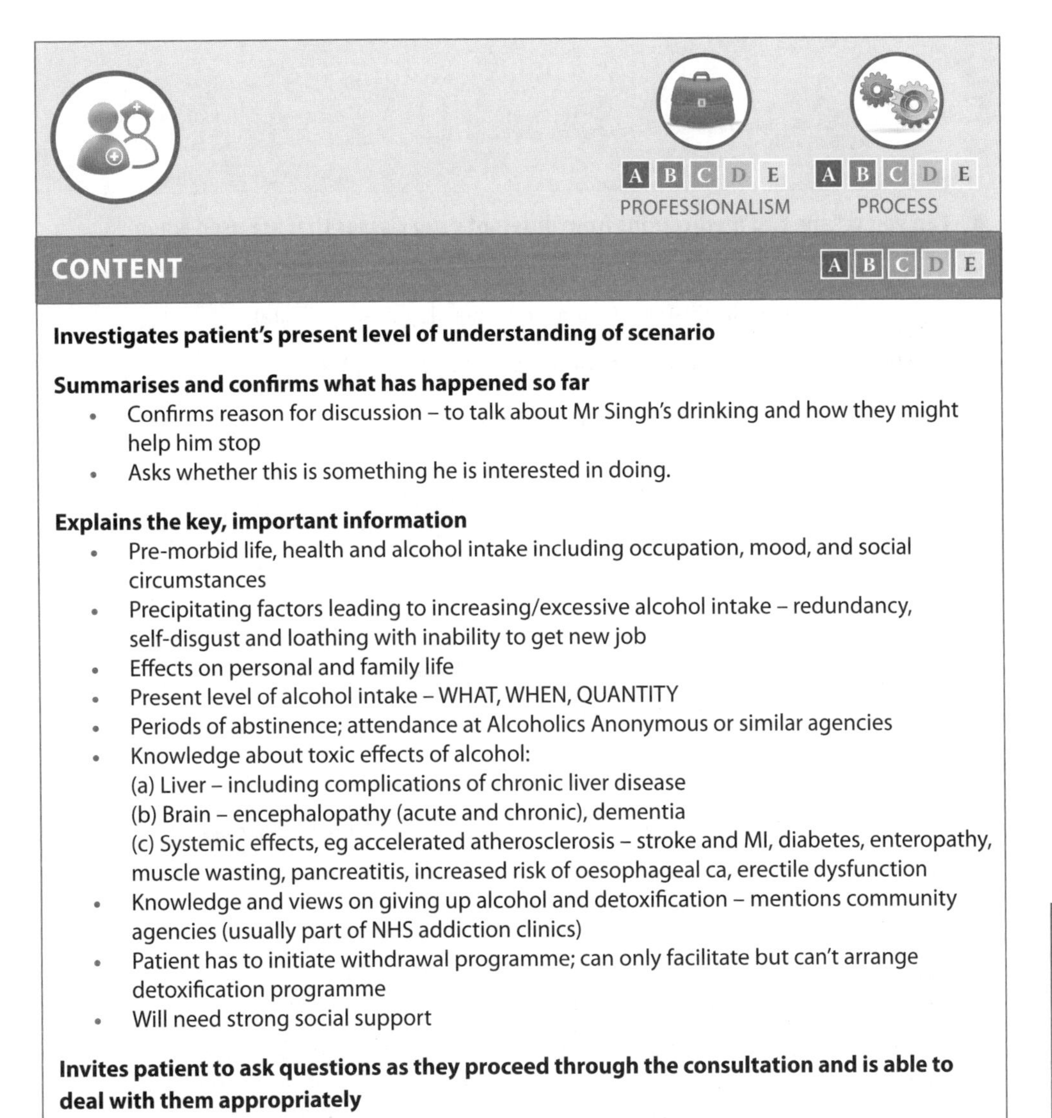

A B C D E
PROFESSIONALISM

A B C D E
PROCESS

CONTENT

A B C D E

Investigates patient's present level of understanding of scenario

Summarises and confirms what has happened so far

- Confirms reason for discussion – to talk about Mr Singh's drinking and how they might help him stop
- Asks whether this is something he is interested in doing.

Explains the key, important information

- Pre-morbid life, health and alcohol intake including occupation, mood, and social circumstances
- Precipitating factors leading to increasing/excessive alcohol intake – redundancy, self-disgust and loathing with inability to get new job
- Effects on personal and family life
- Present level of alcohol intake – WHAT, WHEN, QUANTITY
- Periods of abstinence; attendance at Alcoholics Anonymous or similar agencies
- Knowledge about toxic effects of alcohol:
  (a) Liver – including complications of chronic liver disease
  (b) Brain – encephalopathy (acute and chronic), dementia
  (c) Systemic effects, eg accelerated atherosclerosis – stroke and MI, diabetes, enteropathy, muscle wasting, pancreatitis, increased risk of oesophageal ca, erectile dysfunction
- Knowledge and views on giving up alcohol and detoxification – mentions community agencies (usually part of NHS addiction clinics)
- Patient has to initiate withdrawal programme; can only facilitate but can't arrange detoxification programme
- Will need strong social support

Invites patient to ask questions as they proceed through the consultation and is able to deal with them appropriately

Summarises important areas of the consultation back to the patient

Formally ends the consultation and ensures appropriate follow-up has been discussed

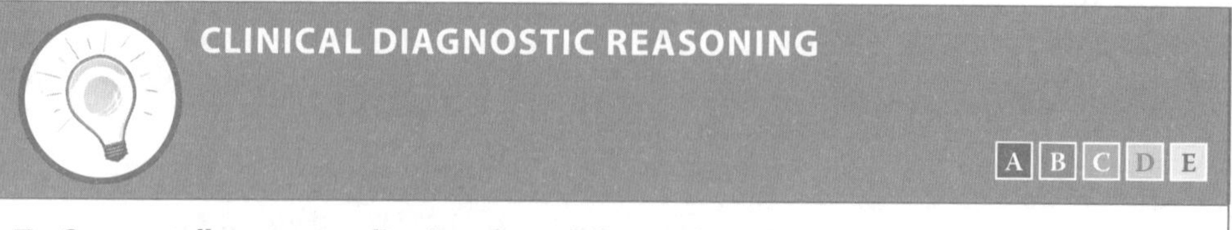

CLINICAL DIAGNOSTIC REASONING

A B C D E

- **Can you tell me two medications from different drug classes that are used when patients are placed on a withdrawal programme?**
  - Benzodiazepenes – chlordiazepoxide, diazepam, lorazepam
  - Vitamins – especially thiamine (vitamin B_1), multivitamins (B_{12}, folate).

Demonstrates a safe, sensible and appropriate management plan

Demonstrates clear and logical diagnostic reasoning

GLOBAL COMMUNICATION MARK

A B C D E

Station 4 – Data interpretation

Part 1:

Abnormality	Likely cause	Differential cause
Hb 8.9 g/dl, MCV 104 fl	Alcohol toxicity	B_{12}/folate deficiency
WCC 3.6 × 10^9/l	Alcohol toxicity on the bone marrow	Immunosuppression
Platelets 67 × 10^9/l	Alcohol toxicity on the bone marrow; splenic sequestration (splenomegaly)	DIC; drugs
Patient has a mild pancytopenia most likely as a direct toxic effect of alcohol on the bone marrow. Other causes, eg marrow failure (myelodysplasia), haematological malignancies (eg myeloma), or toxicity (eg drugs causing aplastic anaemia) should be excluded and a blood film should be requested.		
Na^+ 123 mmol/l	Fluid overload and secondary hyperaldosteronism	SIADH – need to ensure no signs of raised intracranial pressure and a normal, clear CXR
Urea 22.6 mmol/l, creatinine 94 μmol/l	Acute GI bleed; note the grossly elevated urea compared to the creatinine. This is due to the protein load of the blood in the upper GI tract. This is then absorbed and broken down to urea.	Any cause of pre-renal impairment, eg dehydration – but the degree of raised urea:creatinine is classical of an upper GI bleed

Abnormality	Likely cause	Differential cause
RBG: 3.1 mmol/l	Chronic liver disease plus poor nutrition leads to loss of glycogen stores and hypoglycaemia	Insulin or sulphonylurea therapy
INR 1.7, APTT 54 s	Coagulopathy secondary to chronic liver dysfunction and resultant poor protein synthesis	Anti-coagulation; any cause of chronic liver disease
TBil 66.5, ALT 432 IU/l, AST 523 IU/l, Alk Phos 1812 IU/l, γGT 432 IU/l	Grossly deranged mixed liver profile consistent with chronic alcoholic liver disease	Any cause of cirrhosis will produce this picture
ALB 18 g/l	Chronic liver disease due to alcohol excess (or indeed any other cause)	Poor nutrition, malabsorption and chronic loss, eg nephrotic syndrome or enteropathy

Part 2:

1. False – the results suggest no previous exposure to HAV.

2. False – HCV is an RNA virus; in the acute infection anti-HCV antibodies are measured. A positive anti-HCV antibody result indicates acute viral infection; occasionally a false positive result, often weakly positive, is obtained. In this case an HCV recombinant immunoblast assay (RIBA) is performed. If this is negative it excludes infection.

3. False – the combination of HBs antigen positivity (confirming viral exposure) with aHBc IgM positivity indicates acute viral infection and replication.

4. True – aHBs antibody positivity indicates previous viral exposure with subsequent development of immunity, commonly seen with immunisation, or after acute infection.

5. True – see answer to question 3.

6. True – HBe antigen is a marker of acute infectivity.

7. False – this patient has all the markers of acute viral infection; carriers' status is defined by the ongoing positivity of the HBs antigen, with negative expression of aHBs antibody. Their status as high and low risk is defined by expression of the aHBc and aHBe antibodies. High-risk carriers will be positive for HBs antigen, aHBc IgG and HBe antigen. Low-risk carriers will be positive for HBs antigen, aHBc IgG and aHBe antibody.

8. True – this newer test is used as a marker of viral replication infectivity. Acute infection may be represented by millions (or even billions) of copies/ml, where fewer than 2000 copies per ml indicates an 'inactive infection'.

9. False – anyone who has ever had HBV infection cannot presently donate blood or organs.

10. True – chronic HBV infection predisposes to HCC.

GLOBAL DATA INTERPRETATION MARK

A B C D E

Station 5 – Procedural skills

Procedure A: Taking blood sample for crossmatch

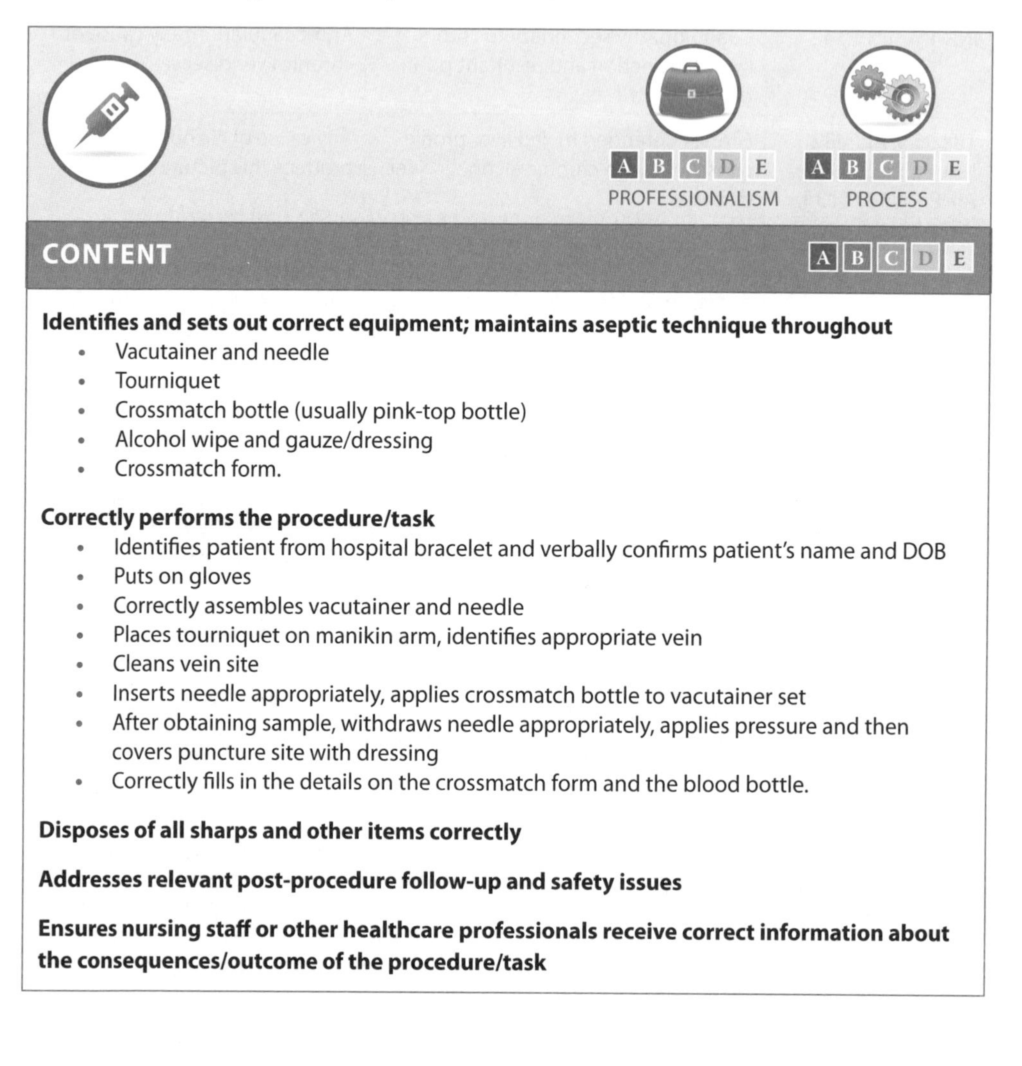

CONTENT A B C D E

Identifies and sets out correct equipment; maintains aseptic technique throughout

- Vacutainer and needle
- Tourniquet
- Crossmatch bottle (usually pink-top bottle)
- Alcohol wipe and gauze/dressing
- Crossmatch form.

Correctly performs the procedure/task

- Identifies patient from hospital bracelet and verbally confirms patient's name and DOB
- Puts on gloves
- Correctly assembles vacutainer and needle
- Places tourniquet on manikin arm, identifies appropriate vein
- Cleans vein site
- Inserts needle appropriately, applies crossmatch bottle to vacutainer set
- After obtaining sample, withdraws needle appropriately, applies pressure and then covers puncture site with dressing
- Correctly fills in the details on the crossmatch form and the blood bottle.

Disposes of all sharps and other items correctly

Addresses relevant post-procedure follow-up and safety issues

Ensures nursing staff or other healthcare professionals receive correct information about the consequences/outcome of the procedure/task

Procedure B: Setting up and connecting emergency unit of O negative blood

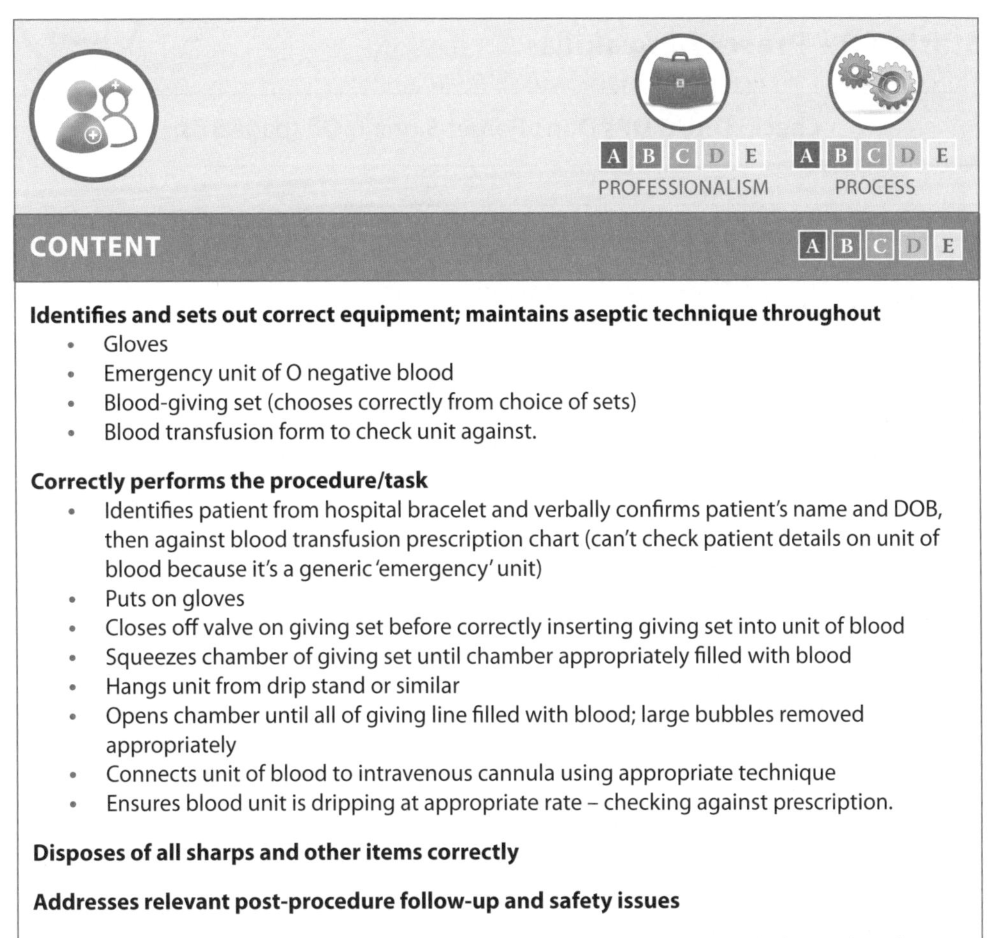

A B C D E PROFESSIONALISM

A B C D E PROCESS

CONTENT A B C D E

Identifies and sets out correct equipment; maintains aseptic technique throughout

- Gloves
- Emergency unit of O negative blood
- Blood-giving set (chooses correctly from choice of sets)
- Blood transfusion form to check unit against.

Correctly performs the procedure/task

- Identifies patient from hospital bracelet and verbally confirms patient's name and DOB, then against blood transfusion prescription chart (can't check patient details on unit of blood because it's a generic 'emergency' unit)
- Puts on gloves
- Closes off valve on giving set before correctly inserting giving set into unit of blood
- Squeezes chamber of giving set until chamber appropriately filled with blood
- Hangs unit from drip stand or similar
- Opens chamber until all of giving line filled with blood; large bubbles removed appropriately
- Connects unit of blood to intravenous cannula using appropriate technique
- Ensures blood unit is dripping at appropriate rate – checking against prescription.

Disposes of all sharps and other items correctly

Addresses relevant post-procedure follow-up and safety issues

Ensures nursing staff or other healthcare professionals receive correct information about the consequences/outcome of the procedure/task

GLOBAL PROCEDURE MARK

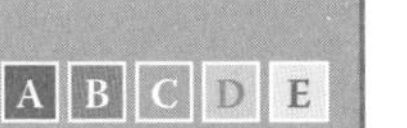

Station 6 – Prescribing skills

Check: DRUG DRs Don't Forget Signing Off (page 373)

Allergies, sensitivities and adverse drug reactions					Patient details/addressograph
No known allergies ✓	Initials AF		Gender (M) F		NHS/ Hospital No: 4545422
Not possible to ascertain ☐	Date 21.11.11		Weight (kg)	Date	
Medicine/substance	Reaction & Severity	Initials & Date	70		Surname: SINGH
			Height		First name: BALJIT
			1.78m		
Alerts			Surface area (m²)		Date of birth: 16.09.73

IN-PATIENT MEDICATION PRESCRIPTION AND ADMINISTRATION RECORD

PasTest HOSPITAL

Consultant	Trainee Dr. Name and Bleep no.	Date of admission	Date chart reboarded	Estimated date of discharge
This chart is no. .... of	Transcribing Check by Pharmacy Sign .... Date	Ward 1. .... 2.		

Supplementary Medication charts in use: Other (please specify): 1 .... 2 ....

Epidural/PCA ☐ Syringe driver ☐ TPN ☐ Chemotherapy ☐ Insulin sliding scale ☐

Once only medications – loading doses, pre-medication, PGDs or surgical antibiotic propylaxis

Date	Time to be given	Medicine (approved name)	Dose	Route	Signature and bleep no.	Pharmacy	Time given	Given by	Checked by
21.11	STAT	CHLORDIAZEPOXIDE	30mg	PO	AF 231				

SCENARIO 14

Regular prescriptions continued							
Regular medications							
For 7 Days	Dose	Date 21	22	23	24	25	26
Date	21.11	Medication	CHLORDIAZEPOXIDE	Instructions		Signature and bleep no. AF 231	Pharmacy ☐
Route	PO						
Signature	AF						
06							
(09)	30mg						
(12)	30mg						
(18)	30mg						
(22)	30mg						
24							

Regular prescriptions continued							
Regular medications							
	Dose	Date 21	22	23	24	25	26
Date	21.11	Medication	PABRINEX I+II	Instructions	Give 3 x doses	Signature and bleep no. AF 231	Pharmacy ☐
Route	IV						
Signature	AF						
06							
(09)	I+II						
12							
(18)	I+II						
22							
24							

Regular prescriptions continued							
Regular medications							
	Dose	Date 21	22	23	24	25	26
Date	21.11	Medication	THIAMINE	Instructions		Signature and bleep no. AF 231	Pharmacy ☐
Route	PO						
Signature	AF						
06							
(09)	100mg						
12							
(18)	100mg						
22							
24							

Regular prescriptions continued							
Regular medications							
	Dose	Date 21	22	23	24	25	26
Date	21.11	Medication	MULTIVITAMINS	Instructions		Signature and bleep no. AF 231	Pharmacy ☐
Route	PO						
Signature	AF						
06							
(09)	ii						
12							
18							
22							
24							

SCENARIO 14

Regular prescriptions						
Oral anticoagulation follow the anticoagulation guidelines available on the intranet						
Indication	Target INR	Baseline INR (if applicable)	Duration of therapy Date therapy started	Date of anticoagulation follow-up appointment (clinic or other)*	Anticoagulant record book given or updated. Sign and date	Date patient counselled and sign

* A follow-up appointment must be booked with the anti-coagulant clinic or enhanced provider of primary care services. If not, the TTA will not be dispensed

Initiating warfarin	Perform baseline coagulation screen, LFTs, U&Es and FBC	Prescribe initiation dose as per guidelines	CHECK INR ON DAY 3	FOLLOW DOSING ALGORITHM IN GUIDELINE
Continuing warfarin	Maintenance therapy	FOLLOW MAINTENANCE DOSING ALGORITHM IN GUIDELINE		

Do not use the initiation protocol for patients already on warfarin. More frequent INR monitoring may be required for patients on interacting drug(s)

Medication																		
Medication				Date														
1				INR														
Route	Frequency OD	Time 18.00	Start	Dose														
			Stop	Dr sign														
Signature		Bleep no.	Pharmacy	Given														

Initiating warfarin – Reduced dosing regimen in red. Refer to anticoagulation policy

Day	One	Two	Three							Four and above								
INR	<1.4	No test	<2.0	2.0-2.1	2.2-2.5	2.6-2.9	3.0-3.3	3.4-4.0	>4.0	<1.4	1.4-1.5	1.6-1.7	1.8-1.9	2.0-2.3	2.4-3.0	3.1-4.0	4.1-4.5	>4.5
Dose mg	10 5	10 5	10	5	4	3	2	1	0	9	8	7	6	5	4	3	Miss 1 day	Miss 2 day

Thromboprophylaxis please prescribe treatment regimens in the regular medications section

Choice of mechanical prophylaxis and leg(s) to be applied to						Enter Time	Enter details below
Graduated elastic compression stockings	Intermittend pneumatic compression device (IPC)		Leg: Left	Right	Both		
21/11 Start Date:	End Date:	Signature and Bleep No.	☐	☐	☑		
Start Date:	End Date:	Signature and Bleep No.	☐	☐	☐		

Medication		Dose	Dose Change	Enter Time	Enter details below
Please ensure you have completed the VTE risk assessment form	Date				
	Route				
	Signature			Instructions NOT FOR HEPARIN - ↑/NR/↓PLATELETS	Pharmacy
	Bleep no.				

Oxygen					
Target Saturation	88-92% ☐	94/98% ☐	If oxygen saturation falls below target range on prescribed oxygen, patient needs urgent clinical review. If oxygen saturation is above targent range on prescribed oxygen, ask for review.		
Other specify)			*Device: N= nasal cannula, SM = simple face mask, V = venturi, H = humidified, RM = reservoir mask, OTHER = other eg. NCPAP/NIPPV	Pharmacy ☐	
Target Saturation not applicable ☐					

	Date Changed	Date Changed	Enter Time	Enter details below
Device				
% or L/min (specify a range eg 1-21 L/min)				
Signature and Bleep no.				

SCENARIO 14

As required medications																							
Medication CHLORDIAZEPOZIDE				Date																			
Indication				Time																			
Dose 10-20 mg	Route PO	Maximum frequency / dose	Start date 21/11	Dose																			
			Stop date	Route																			
Signature AF			Bleep no. 231	Given																			
Additional instructions:														Pharmacy									

21/11 Infusion prescriptions continued										SC = subcutaneous		IVC = intravenous central IVP = intravenous peripheral		
Date & time	Route	Infusion Fluid		Medication		Duration	Rate	Prescriber's signature & bleep no.	Date given	Given / Added by	Check by	Start time	Finish time	Pharmacy
		Name & strength	Volume	Approved name with expiry / unit number	Dose									
21/11	IVP	BLOOD Exp: Batch/unit no:	1 UNIT				1hr	AF 231						
21/11	IVP	BLOOD Exp: Batch/unit no:	1 UNIT				1hr	AF 231						
21/11	IVP	BLOOD Exp: Batch/unit no:	1 UNIT				1hr	AF 231						
21/11	IVP	BLOOD Exp: Batch/unit no:	1 UNIT				1hr	AF 231						
21/11	IVP	BLOOD Exp: Batch/unit no:	1 UNIT				1hr	AF 231						
21/11	IVP	0.9% SALINE Exp: Batch/unit no:	1 LITRE				6hr	AF 231						

Check: DRUG DRs Don't Forget Signing Off (page 373)

GLOBAL PRESCRIBING MARK

A B C D E

Scenario 14: Reflection and consolidation

History

Mr Baljit Singh is a 38-year-old British-born Asian man, who presented today with a 3-year history of alcohol excess. He was previously fit and well with no medical history of note until losing his job as a foreman in the local car factory some 3 years ago. (The car factory closed due to the economic downturn).
In terms of his alcohol consumption, he says that before losing his job he always enjoyed a drink, describing himself as a 'social drinker'. He in fact drank over 30 units of whisky per week, drinking a litre bottle of Johnny Walker Red Label to himself over 10 days or so.
After being made redundant he became increasingly frustrated, angry and depressed.. His community work and aspirations stopped. He began to drink very heavily (two to three bottles of whisky per day) which meant he missed several job interviews and important appointments. This made him feel 'disgusted with himself' and caused him to be more depressed and so drink more.
He became increasingly reclusive, and only went out to buy whisky. Over the last 18 months he has become aggressive and unpleasant to his wife and daughters, and they have now gone to live with his mother-in-law. Of note he was never physically abusive but constantly shouted and screamed at the family, especially when challenged around his drinking.
He is still drinking heavily 'anything he can get his hands on'. He has not had any sustained periods of abstinence and has not tried to cut down or stop. He has never tried to attend Alcoholics Anonymous or similar groups. He has good insight into his drinking and realises that if he doesn't stop he may well die. Of note there is no previous personal or family history of mental health problems, alcohol or drug addiction. He has not suffered any suicidal ideation or self-harm.
He has been otherwise systemically well but has eaten very little recently and is feeling increasingly tired and 'can't go on'.
He doesn't take any regular medications and has no known drug allergies.
Mr Singh lives in a four-bedroom house, presently alone. He is an unemployed car factory worker. He has three daughters, aged 12, 10 and 9 years. He is a cigarette smoker – since 16 years old and smokes 15–20 per day; he does not take illicit drugs.

Examination

On examination, Mr Singh was unkempt and dishevelled and looked chronically unwell. He was slightly agitated, but there were no signs of delirium tremens (DTs). He was fully conversant and showed no signs of acute liver decompensation or encephalopathy. (Of note there was no jaundice, asterixis, confusion, drowsiness or hepatic fetor.)
He did, however, have several signs of chronic liver disease, including Dupuytren's contracture, leuconychia, palmar erythema, bruising over his arms and truncal areas, gynaecomastia and several spider naevi. He also has marked tar staining of the fingers of his right hand. He was apyrexial and haemodynamically stable; his CBG was 3.7 mmol/l.
Examination of his abdomen revealed a distended, soft and non-tender abdomen with no palpable masses. There was 5 cm hepatomegaly below the right costal margin associated with 3–4 cm splenomegaly below the left costal margin. There was no evidence of renal masses.
There was demonstrable ascites with shifting dullness.
I did not perform a DRE or assessment of the external genitalia.

Management

Initially Mr Singh should be sent for counselling and to a community detoxification programme using diazepam or chlordiazepoxide. He needs to volunteer for these programmes and cannot be 'forced to go'. If he doesn't attend (as in this case) he will invariably suffer fulminant liver failure over the next few years.

Further reading and web links
www.transfusionguidelines.org.uk/docs/pdfs/htm_edition-4_all-pages.pdf
www.patient.co.uk/doctor/Acute-Alcohol-Withdrawal-and-Delirium-Tremens.htm
http://ccn.aacnjournals.org/content/25/3/40.full.pdf
www.sign.ac.uk/pdf/sign74.pdf

Scenario 15: 'Off legs'

Station 1

History *10-minute station*

You are the FY1 on call with the Acute Medical Team. The Medical Registrar has asked you to take a focused, diagnostic history from a patient who has been referred by her GP after a home visit. She doesn't give you any further details other than the patient's name, Mrs Jean Simmons.

- **Please take a diagnostic, focused history from the patient with a view to presenting it to the Registrar as if you were in a busy Emergency Department.**

You will be assessed on the following areas, as well as the content and diagnostic reasoning of your history – take them into account in your presentation.

Professionalism

- Professional appearance (NHS dress code) – including general appearance, hair and jewellery
- Maintains patient and personal safety
- Polite introduction; identifies patient or interviewee correctly; confirms patient's date of birth from name band or other source
- Obtains informal consent; maintains patient's privacy
- Displays empathetic and caring attitudes and behaviours throughout.

Process

- Good organisation and structure; appropriate use of open and closed questions
- Appropriate fluency/rhythm/pace to the interview – this may change depending on environment and acute nature of the problem
- Appropriate time for the patient to respond/reply to questions
- Appropriate acknowledgement of difficult or emotional areas of the patient's history.

Communication skills

- Demonstrates caring and sympathetic attitude
- Asks open questions
- Invites patient to ask questions and answers them appropriately
- Addresses patient's ideas, concerns and expectations.

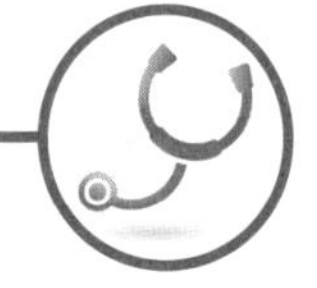

Station 2

Examination *10-minute station*

After completing and presenting the history, the Medical Registrar asks you to perform a focused examination of the patient. Mrs Simmons has already been seen by one of the Emergency Department nurses, who has recorded her observations on the chart. You may ask for these during your assessment.

- **Please perform the examination and present the relevant findings (given within the station) to the Medical Registrar in an appropriate manner for a busy medical doctor on call.**

You will be assessed on the following areas, as well as the content and skills of your examination – take them into account in your presentation.

Professionalism

- Professional appearance; maintains infection control standards, including hand cleaning and appropriate use of gloves and aprons
- Maintains patient and personal safety
- Polite introduction; identifies patient and confirms date of birth from name band or other source
- Obtains informal consent; maintains patient privacy and dignity
- Displays empathetic and caring attitudes and behaviours throughout.

Process

- Appropriate fluency/rhythm/pace to the examination – this may change depending on environment and acute nature of problem
- Good organisation and structure of examination; sensitive and empathetic approach
- Uses appropriate clinical techniques throughout
- Maintains privacy and dignity throughout.

Clinical communication

- Explains proposed examination/procedure; explains examination/procedure as it proceeds
- Offers information in a clear, structured and fluent manner, avoiding jargon
- Listens to patient and responds appropriately
- Demonstrates appropriate body language.

Please read the information below before presenting this case to the Medical Registrar as if you were a busy medical doctor on call. ***[NB If you have a model do not read this section]***

Clinical findings

- **Patient is a thin-looking middle-aged woman, looking chronically unwell**
- **Feet to face – patient is alert and orientated, and co-operative throughout**
- **Observations – HR 108 bpm, BP 112/78 mmHg, RR 18 bpm, O_2 sats 95% on air, temperature 36.8 °C, CBG 4.4 mmol/l, Urinalysis – NAD**
- **General examination – patient is clinically dehydrated; tenderness over anterior ribs, right shoulder and left mid thigh**
- **Focused examination of breasts – reconstructed left breast, scars clean, no masses; nil of note for right breast; no cervical or axillary lymphadenopathy**
- **RS and CV examinations – tender over several anterior ribs; otherwise unremarkable – no evidence effusions**
- **Focused examination of abdomen – 4 cm hepatomegaly, no ascites, bladder not palpable; DRE – loaded rectum, anal tone normal**
- **Neurological assessment of the upper limbs – motor and sensory assessment NAD**
- **Neurological assessment of the lower limbs, left and right – bulk, thin legs, no fasciculation; tone flaccid; power 1/5 left and 1–2/5 right; reflexes difficult to elicit; co-ordination and gait, not assessed (because of reduced power); plantars, bilateral extensor response; sensation – left and right, reduced LT and pinprick from feet to level of umbilicus (T10)**
- **In summary, this is a 52-year-old woman with known cancer of the left breast who now presents with signs consistent with lower thoracic spinal cord compression, hepatomegaly and bony tenderness over the mid-left thigh, right shoulder and several anterior ribs.**

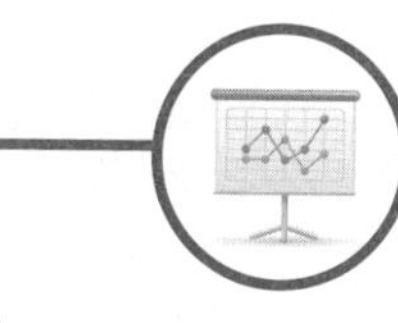

Station 3

Data interpretation *10-minute station*

Part 1:

- **You have been asked to review Mrs Simmons' investigation results, shown below. For each of the statements given below the results, please indicate whether it is TRUE (T) or FALSE (F).**

FBC: Hb 6.8 g/dl, MCV 89 fl, WCC 14.6 × 109/l, neutrophils 12 × 109/l, platelets 405 × 109/l

U&Es: Na+ 149 mmol/l, K+ 4.9 mmol/l, urea 15.9 mmol/l, creatinine 145 mmol/l

RBG: 4.8 mmol/l

LFTs: TBil 23.9 mmol/l, ALB 34 g/l, ALT 123 IU/l, AST 112 IU/l, alkaline phosphatase 676 IU/l

Corrected calcium 3.76 mmol/l, phosphate 0.98 mmol/l, alkaline phosphatase 676 IU/l

1 The Hb/MCV is consistent with an anaemia of chronic disease.
2 The likeliest explanation for her WCC and differential is a bacterial infection.
3 The Ur:Cr ratio suggests there is obstructive nephropathy.
4 The most likely cause of the abnormal calcium is secondary hyperparathyroidism.
5 The deranged LFTs are consistent with a hepatitic jaundice.
6 The hypoalbuminaemia is probably secondary to a malignancy-induced nephrotic syndrome.

Part 2:

- The Medical Registrar shows you Mrs Simmons' MRI scan and a normal scan for comparison. Please decide which is which, identify bony and nervous structures, and note any abnormalities.

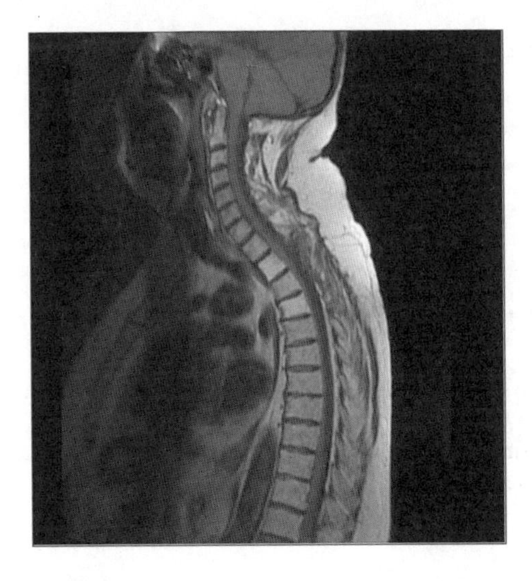

Figure 15.1

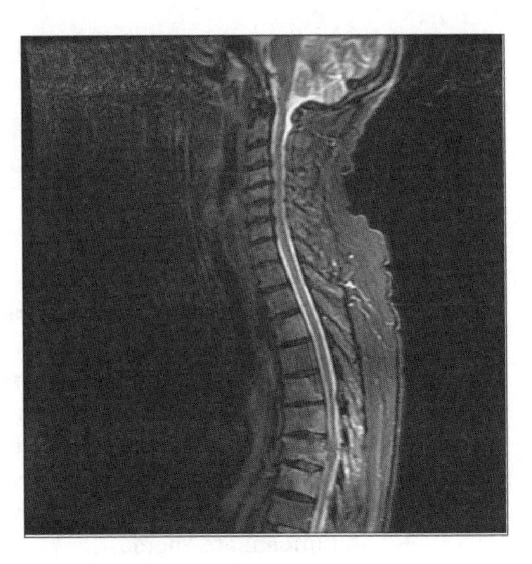

Figure 15.2

Station 4

Procedural skills *10-minute station*

Procedure

The Medical Registrar asks you to insert an indwelling urinary catheter for Mrs Simmons.

- Please insert a urinary catheter into the manikin provided, talking to the examiner as if they were the patient.
- Once inserted, please write up the procedure and discuss with the nurse the observations you require for Mrs Simmons.

Equipment provided

- Female catheterisation manikin
- Catheter pack – urinary catheter, gauze, container and cotton-wool balls
- Catheter bag
- Drapes
- Saline or antiseptic solution
- Water for injection (10 ml)
- Appropriate needles and syringes to draw up water
- Instillagel or similar
- Two sets of sterile gloves

Details

Mrs Jean Simmons; DOB: 13/09/1959; Unit No. 673121; Ward: MAU; Consultant: Dr Jones

Station 5

Prescribing skills *10-minute station*

The Medical Registrar has asked you to write up the drug and fluid charts for Mrs Simmons.

- Using a BNF and the charts provided, please write up:
  (a) An appropriate infusion of intravenous pamidronate
  (b) A fluid regime for the next 24 hours
  (c) VTE prophylaxis, including TEDs and LMWH
  (d) Regular codeine and paracetamol; dexamethasone
  (e) Stat phosphate enema
  (f) PRN cyclizine.

Details

Mrs Jean Simmons; DOB: 13/09/1959; Unit No. 673121; Ward: MAU; Consultant: Dr Jones

U&Es: Na^+ 145 mmol/l, K^+ 4.9 mmol/l, urea 15.9 mmol/l, creatinine 145 µmol/l

Corrected calcium 3.76 mmol/l, phosphate 0.98 mmol/l, alkaline phosphatase 676 IU/l

Height: 1.6 m

Weight: approx. 45 kg

Allergies: nil known

Remember: DRUG DRs Don't Forget Signing Off (page 373)

Station 6

Clinical communication skills *10-minute station*

Several days later you ask your Consultant if you can present Mrs Simmons' case in a case-based discussion (CbD). He thinks it would be a better learning experience if you were to role play a discussion about the investigation results and possible therapeutic intervention with him as if he were the patient. Mrs Simmons' MRI confirmed a compression of her spinal cord at T10/T11 and she was sent for emergency radiotherapy at St Richards, the local teaching hospital.

- **Please discuss the investigation results and the subsequent therapeutic intervention as if the Consultant was Mrs Simmons.**

Answers

Station 1 – History

Patient script

You are Mrs Jean Simmons, DOB 13 September 1959, a 52-year-old woman who was brought into the Emergency Department by ambulance this afternoon at about 2 pm after having been seen by your GP at home this lunchtime.

You were diagnosed as having cancer of the left breast 2 years ago at the local teaching hospital. After having several months of chemo- and radiotherapy, you then underwent breast reconstruction with excision of the lump and some of the glands in your left armpit.

Oncology history: all your care has been with the team at St Richards, the local teaching hospital. You are under the care of Dr Martin, Oncologist for DXT and CXT, and Ms Harris, Breast Surgeon. You have been having 6-monthly reviews with Dr Martin and were discharged from the care of Ms Harris last year. 'As far as I know I was doing well – no recurrence on last scan 4-months ago.'

You had been followed up and were really very well until a few weeks ago, when you started to get a 'gnawing' pain in your lower back. Initially the pain was 'held at bay' by regular co-dydramol that you had left over from your operation. You thought the pain might be due to some heavy gardening you had been doing. Over the last week, however, the pain has becoming increasingly severe, and is now almost unbearable. You now rate it as 8/10.

You called the GP out this morning because of sudden weakness in your legs. Despite your best efforts you were simply unable to get out of bed, and your husband had to carry you to the toilet, where you found it almost impossible to pass urine. (If asked) you have not had your bowels open for nearly 2 days (you had put this down to the co-dydramol). As well as feeling weak, your legs don't feel 'right', they are 'heavy' and 'woody', but if asked you don't have any pins and needles or but some loss of feeling in legs and up to your belly button.

Your arms feel normal, and you have not had any headaches, visual, speech or comprehension problems. You have not had any nausea and vomiting, blurred vision, seizures or loss of consciousness.

Apart from the pain in your back, you have also had pain in the middle of your left thigh, your right shoulder and in some of your ribs.

You have not had any respiratory or other abdominal symptoms.

Medications: co-dydramol, 2 tablets 6 hourly; naproxen 2 tablets once or twice a day (for the last week). No known allergies.

You live with your husband and youngest daughter (18 years old), who is studying medicine at Oxford. You are a chartered accountant – part time over the last 6 months.

Your three other children – Adam 27 years, Jack 25 years, and Lucy 21 years – all live within 50 miles of home. Adam is married with two young children.

In your house there are two flights of internal stairs; you were independent of all ADLs prior to admission.

You are a non-smoker; you have two to three glasses of wine at the weekends but very little alcohol over the last 8–12 months.

Previous medical history: nil of note prior to your breast cancer diagnosis.

Ideas and concerns: you think you may have damaged your back and this has caused the problem in your legs. However, if pushed, you admit that in the back of your mind you think that it may be the cancer causing this.

Expectations: you are hoping that the doctors can do some tests (like a scan or something) and have an answer for you today. You hope they can make it better.

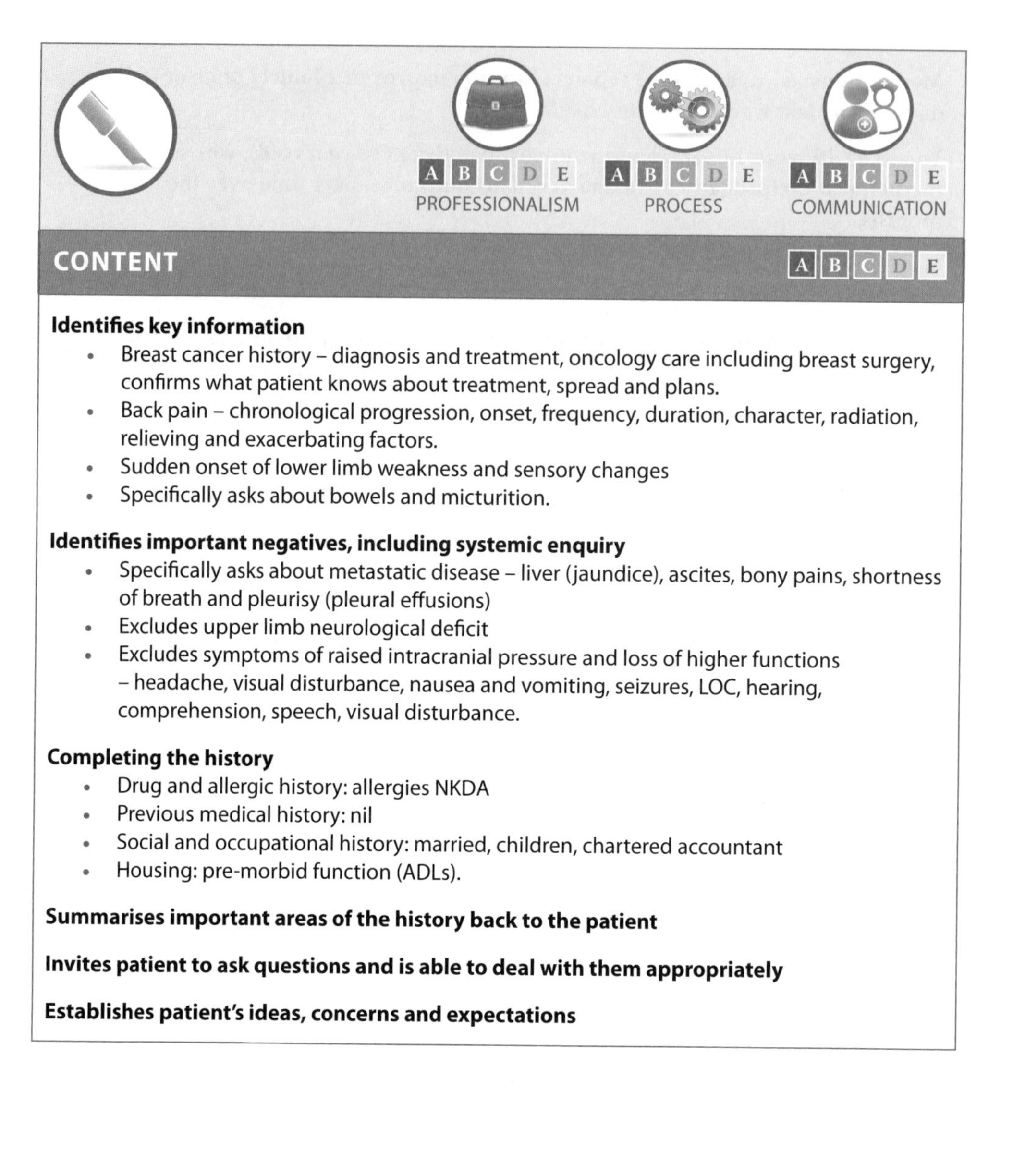

CONTENT

A B C D E

Identifies key information

- Breast cancer history – diagnosis and treatment, oncology care including breast surgery, confirms what patient knows about treatment, spread and plans.
- Back pain – chronological progression, onset, frequency, duration, character, radiation, relieving and exacerbating factors.
- Sudden onset of lower limb weakness and sensory changes
- Specifically asks about bowels and micturition.

Identifies important negatives, including systemic enquiry

- Specifically asks about metastatic disease – liver (jaundice), ascites, bony pains, shortness of breath and pleurisy (pleural effusions)
- Excludes upper limb neurological deficit
- Excludes symptoms of raised intracranial pressure and loss of higher functions – headache, visual disturbance, nausea and vomiting, seizures, LOC, hearing, comprehension, speech, visual disturbance.

Completing the history

- Drug and allergic history: allergies NKDA
- Previous medical history: nil
- Social and occupational history: married, children, chartered accountant
- Housing: pre-morbid function (ADLs).

Summarises important areas of the history back to the patient

Invites patient to ask questions and is able to deal with them appropriately

Establishes patient's ideas, concerns and expectations

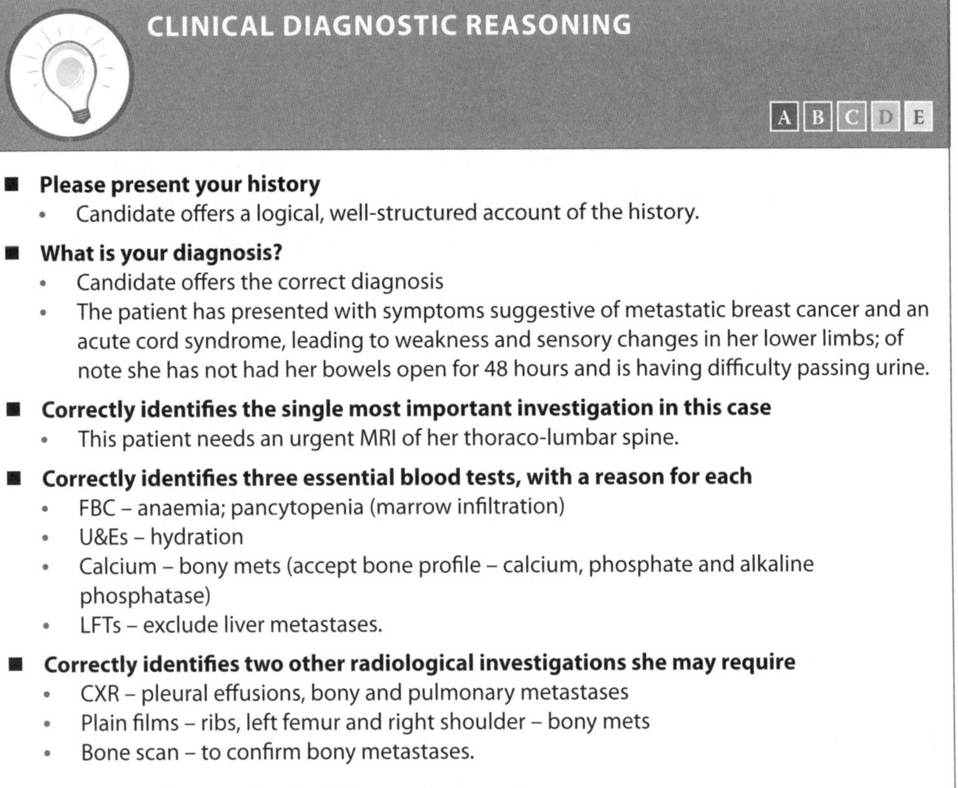

CLINICAL DIAGNOSTIC REASONING

A B C D E

- **Please present your history**
  - Candidate offers a logical, well-structured account of the history.
- **What is your diagnosis?**
  - Candidate offers the correct diagnosis
  - The patient has presented with symptoms suggestive of metastatic breast cancer and an acute cord syndrome, leading to weakness and sensory changes in her lower limbs; of note she has not had her bowels open for 48 hours and is having difficulty passing urine.
- **Correctly identifies the single most important investigation in this case**
  - This patient needs an urgent MRI of her thoraco-lumbar spine.
- **Correctly identifies three essential blood tests, with a reason for each**
  - FBC – anaemia; pancytopenia (marrow infiltration)
  - U&Es – hydration
  - Calcium – bony mets (accept bone profile – calcium, phosphate and alkaline phosphatase)
  - LFTs – exclude liver metastases.
- **Correctly identifies two other radiological investigations she may require**
  - CXR – pleural effusions, bony and pulmonary metastases
  - Plain films – ribs, left femur and right shoulder – bony mets
  - Bone scan – to confirm bony metastases.

Demonstrates clear and logical diagnostic reasoning

GLOBAL HISTORY MARK

A B C D E

Station 2 – Examination

Patient script

If you are an actor/patient, read the patient history and physical signs fully – when the candidate comes to an abnormal site in their examination, act-out tenderness and/or volunteer the relevant physical sign.

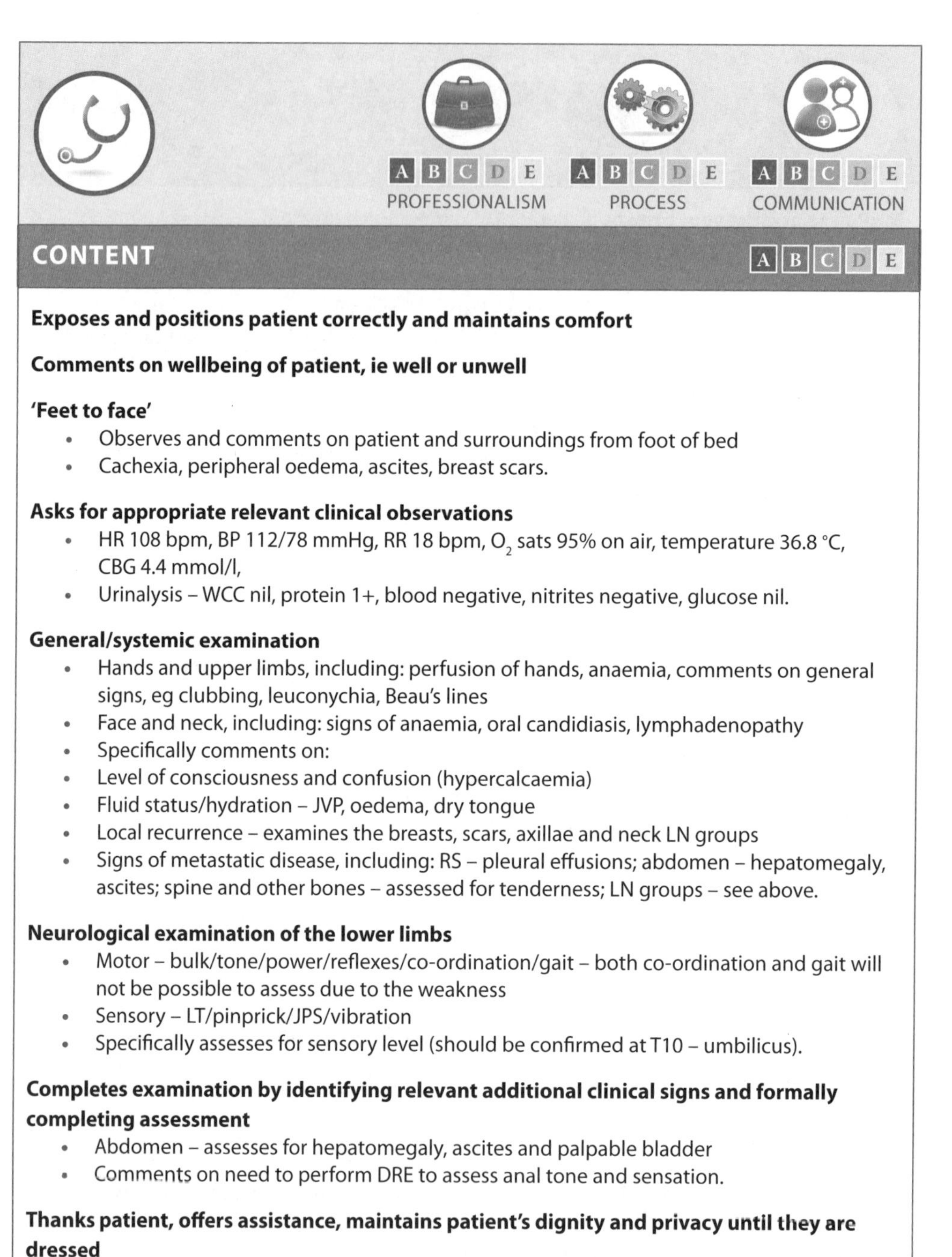

A B C D E
PROFESSIONALISM

A B C D E
PROCESS

A B C D E
COMMUNICATION

CONTENT

A B C D E

Exposes and positions patient correctly and maintains comfort

Comments on wellbeing of patient, ie well or unwell

'Feet to face'

- Observes and comments on patient and surroundings from foot of bed
- Cachexia, peripheral oedema, ascites, breast scars.

Asks for appropriate relevant clinical observations

- HR 108 bpm, BP 112/78 mmHg, RR 18 bpm, O_2 sats 95% on air, temperature 36.8 °C, CBG 4.4 mmol/l,
- Urinalysis – WCC nil, protein 1+, blood negative, nitrites negative, glucose nil.

General/systemic examination

- Hands and upper limbs, including: perfusion of hands, anaemia, comments on general signs, eg clubbing, leuconychia, Beau's lines
- Face and neck, including: signs of anaemia, oral candidiasis, lymphadenopathy
- Specifically comments on:
- Level of consciousness and confusion (hypercalcaemia)
- Fluid status/hydration – JVP, oedema, dry tongue
- Local recurrence – examines the breasts, scars, axillae and neck LN groups
- Signs of metastatic disease, including: RS – pleural effusions; abdomen – hepatomegaly, ascites; spine and other bones – assessed for tenderness; LN groups – see above.

Neurological examination of the lower limbs

- Motor – bulk/tone/power/reflexes/co-ordination/gait – both co-ordination and gait will not be possible to assess due to the weakness
- Sensory – LT/pinprick/JPS/vibration
- Specifically assesses for sensory level (should be confirmed at T10 – umbilicus).

Completes examination by identifying relevant additional clinical signs and formally completing assessment

- Abdomen – assesses for hepatomegaly, ascites and palpable bladder
- Comments on need to perform DRE to assess anal tone and sensation.

Thanks patient, offers assistance, maintains patient's dignity and privacy until they are dressed

CLINICAL DIAGNOSTIC REASONING

A B C D E

Correctly identifies the relevant physical signs, including important negative findings

- Normal level of consciousness/absence of confusion
- Hydration
- Breast examination and excludes evidence of local recurrence
- Evidence of metastases – hepatomegaly and bony tenderness
- Neurological assessment of lower limbs – confirming spinal cord compression with sensory level at approximately T10
- Comments if bladder is palpable and if anal tone is normal.

Correctly identifies three clinical interventions that should be arranged for this patient

- Insertion of an indwelling urinary catheter
- Phosphate enema
- Intravenous fluids
- Analgesia – may require opiates, NSAIDs, subsequent radiotherapy may be indicated to the bony metastases
- Place patient on pressure-relieving mattress – skin care.

Correctly identifies the single most important emergency intervention that should be arranged for this patient

- This is an oncological/medical emergency and the patient requires urgent referral for radiotherapy.

Correctly identifies the single oral or intravenous agent that might be prescribed in an attempt to improve the patient's neurological symptoms

- Dexamethasone may be beneficial here, reducing inflammation.

Demonstrates safe, sensible and appropriate management plan

Demonstrates clear and logical diagnostic reasoning

GLOBAL EXAMINATION MARK

A B C D E

Station 3 – Data interpretation

Part 1:

1. True – Hb 6.8 g/dl, MCV 89 fl is consistent with a normocytic anaemia. This is most likely because of her chronic illness and therapies over the last few months but could also be a marker of bone marrow involvement. Anaemia of chronic disease may also present with a microcytosis. There are two simple rules for diagnosing an anaemia of chronic disease: (1) there must be an anaemia; and (2) the patient must have a chronic disease! If they do not have a chronic disease, you need to find another cause for their normocytic anaemia.

2. False – WCC 14.6 × 10^9/l, neutrophils 12 × 10^9/l – although a neutrophilic leucocytosis is commonly associated with a bacterial infection, it may also be commonly caused by any acute inflammatory process, eg trauma, or in this case spinal cord compression.

3. False – urea 15.9 mmol/l, creatinine 145 μmol/l – the urea:creatinine ratio is 15.9:145 (normal is approximately urea = 4, creatinine = 70), thus the urea has risen approximately fourfold (15.9/4.0), while the creatinine has risen twofold (145/70). Thus urea has proportionally risen higher than the creatinine, indicating likely pre-renal failure. Obstructive nephropathy is indistinguishable from renal impairment on Ur:Cr ratio, and may only be confirmed or excluded by radiological imaging, usually ultrasound scanning.

4. False – the likeliest cause of the hypercalcaemia and elevated alkaline phosphatase is bony metastases. Secondary hyperparathyroidisim occurs in response to prolonged hypocalcaemia, most commonly seen in chronic renal failure.

5. False – the rise in transaminases and alkaline phosphatase indicates a 'mixed picture' probably because of liver metastases.

6. True – hypoalbminaemia reflects either severe acute illness or chronic illness. In this case it is most likely the result of her malignancy and treatment. A nephrotic syndrome may occur more commonly with lung cancer and multiple myeloma.

Part 2:

Figure 15.1 is a normal MRI scan; Figure 15.2 shows signal changes of multiple spinal secondary deposits, mainly involving the T6 – T9 vertebral bodies.

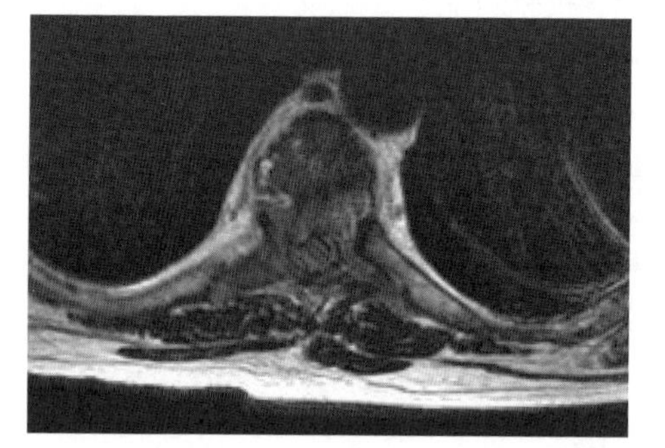

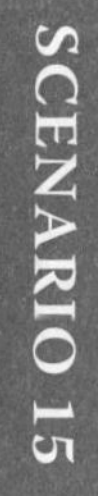

Figure 15.3 The T2 Axial view at the level of T8 shows destruction of vertebral body and effacement of the CSF and minor compression of the spinal cord.'

GLOBAL DATA INTERPRETATION MARK

A B C D E

Station 4 – Procedural skills

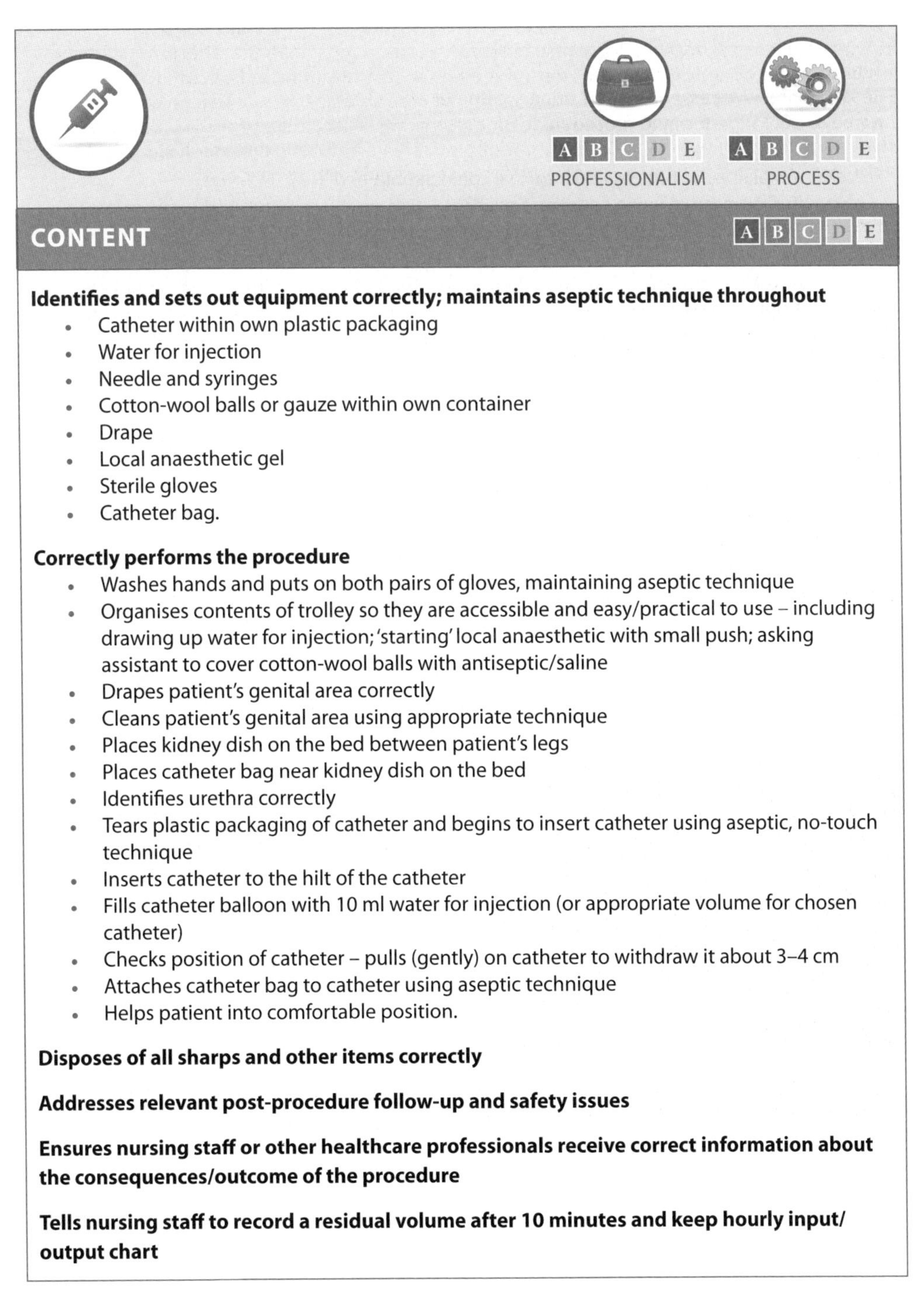

A B C D E
PROFESSIONALISM

A B C D E
PROCESS

CONTENT

A B C D E

Identifies and sets out equipment correctly; maintains aseptic technique throughout

- Catheter within own plastic packaging
- Water for injection
- Needle and syringes
- Cotton-wool balls or gauze within own container
- Drape
- Local anaesthetic gel
- Sterile gloves
- Catheter bag.

Correctly performs the procedure

- Washes hands and puts on both pairs of gloves, maintaining aseptic technique
- Organises contents of trolley so they are accessible and easy/practical to use – including drawing up water for injection; 'starting' local anaesthetic with small push; asking assistant to cover cotton-wool balls with antiseptic/saline
- Drapes patient's genital area correctly
- Cleans patient's genital area using appropriate technique
- Places kidney dish on the bed between patient's legs
- Places catheter bag near kidney dish on the bed
- Identifies urethra correctly
- Tears plastic packaging of catheter and begins to insert catheter using aseptic, no-touch technique
- Inserts catheter to the hilt of the catheter
- Fills catheter balloon with 10 ml water for injection (or appropriate volume for chosen catheter)
- Checks position of catheter – pulls (gently) on catheter to withdraw it about 3–4 cm
- Attaches catheter bag to catheter using aseptic technique
- Helps patient into comfortable position.

Disposes of all sharps and other items correctly

Addresses relevant post-procedure follow-up and safety issues

Ensures nursing staff or other healthcare professionals receive correct information about the consequences/outcome of the procedure

Tells nursing staff to record a residual volume after 10 minutes and keep hourly input/output chart

Name Mrs Jean Simmons	DOB 13.09.59
Unit Number 673121	Consultant Team Dr Jones
Date ** /**/ **	Ward MAU

Time
Reason for review – asked to insert urinary catheter
Name of Doctor performing procedure

Procedure explained to patient and informal consent obtained
Trolley cleaned using antiseptic swabs
Equipment placed on trolley using aseptic technique
14G catheter

Patient cleaned and area draped
Urethra identified; catheter inserted using aseptic technique
Balloon inflated using 10 ml water for injection
Catheter withdrawn 3–4 cm
Catheter bag attached – draining clear urine
5 ml urine sent for MC+S

Patient assisted to sit upright and helped to dress into hospital gown
Drapes and other equipment disposed of appropriately.

Nurses asked to record residual volume at 10 minutes.
Fluid balance to continue over next 24 hours.

Signature and printing of name
Bleep number

If you hold an on-call bleep or will not be the doctor caring for this patient after the on-call period finishes it is worth telling the nursing staff or writing your everyday bleep number in the notes so they can contact you, or find out who is caring for the patient.

CLINICAL DIAGNOSTIC REASONING

A B C D E

- **Could you tell me two common complications of inserting an indwelling urinary catheter?**
  - Urinary infection
  - Haematuria (traumatic insertion)
  - Blockage and obstruction of the catheter.

Demonstrates safe, sensible and appropriate management plan

Demonstrates clear and logical diagnostic reasoning

GLOBAL PROCEDURE MARK

A B C D E

Station 5 – Prescribing skills

Check: DRUG DRs Don't Forget Signing Off (page 373)

Allergies, sensitivities and adverse drug reactions					Patient details/addressograph
No known allergies ✓		Initials AF	Gender M (F)		NHS/ Hospital No: 673121
Not possible to ascertain ☐		Date 21.11.11	Weight (kg)	Date	
Medicine/substance	Reaction & Severity	Initials & Date	~45		Surname: SIMMONS
			Height		First name: JEAN
			160		
Alerts			Surface area (m²)		Date of birth: 13.09.59

IN-PATIENT MEDICATION PRESCRIPTION AND ADMINISTRATION RECORD

PasTest HOSPITAL

Consultant	Trainee Dr. Name and Bleep no.	Date of admission	Date chart reboarded	Estimated date of discharge
JONES	FEATHER 622	21.11.11		
This chart is no. .... of	Transcribing Check by Pharmacy Sign .... Date	Ward 1. .... 2.		

Supplementary Medication charts in use: Other (please specify): 1 .... 2 ....

Epidural/PCA ☐ Syringe driver ☐ TPN ☐ Chemotherapy ☐ Insulin sliding scale ☐

Once only medications – loading doses, pre-medication, PGDs or surgical antibiotic propylaxis

Date	Time to be given	Medicine (approved name)	Dose	Route	Signature and bleep no.	Pharmacy	Time given	Given by	Checked by
21.11	STAT	PHOSPHATE ENEMA	X1	PR	AF 622				

SCENARIO 15

Regular prescriptions continued									
Regular medications									
Date		21/11	Medication: CODEINE PHOSPHATE			Instructions		Signature and bleep no.: AF 622	Pharmacy
Route		PO							
Times		Dose							
Date			21	22	23	24	25	26	
06									
(09)		60mg							
(12)		60mg							
(18)		60mg							
(22)		60mg							
24									

Regular prescriptions continued									
Regular medications									
Date		21/11	Medication: PARACETAMOL			Instructions		Signature and bleep no.: AF 622	Pharmacy
Route		PO							
Times		Dose							
Date			21	22	23	24	25	26	27
06									
(09)		1g							
(12)		1g							
(18)		1g							
(22)		1g							
24									

Regular prescriptions continued									
Regular medications									
Date		21/11	Medication: LACTULOSE			Instructions		Signature and bleep no.: AF 622	Pharmacy
Route		PO							
Times		Dose							
Date			21	22	23	24	25	26	27
06									
(09)		10ml							
12									
(18)		10ml							
22									
24									

Regular prescriptions continued									
Regular medications									
Date		21/11	Medication: SENNA			Instructions		Signature and bleep no.: AF 622	Pharmacy
Route		PO							
Times		Dose							
Date			21	22	23	24	25	26	27
06									
(09)		ii							
12									
18									
22									
24									

SCENARIO 15

Regular prescriptions						
Oral anticoagulation follow the anticoagulation guidelines available on the intranet						
Indication	Target INR	Baseline INR (if applicable)	Duration of therapy Date therapy started	Date of anticoagulation follow-up appointment (clinic or other)*	Anticoagulant record book given or updated. Sign and date	Date patient counselled and sign
* A follow-up appointment must be booked with the anti-coagulant clinic or enhanced provider of primary care services. If not, the TTA will not be dispensed						

Initiating warfarin	Perform baseline coagulation screen, LFTs, U&Es and FBC	Prescribe initiation dose as per guidelines	CHECK INR ON DAY 3	FOLLOW DOSING ALGORITHM IN GUIDELINE
Continuing warfarin	Maintenance therapy	FOLLOW MAINTENANCE DOSING ALGORITHM IN GUIDELINE		
Do not use the initiation protocol for patients already on warfarin. More frequent INR monitoring may be required for patients on interacting drug(s)				

Medication				Date													
1				INR													
Route	Frequency OD	Time 18.00	Start	Dose													
			Stop	Dr sign													
Signature		Bleep no.	Pharmacy	Given													

Initiating warfarin – Reduced dosing regimen in red. Refer to anticoagulation policy																	
Day	One	Two	Three							Four and above							
INR	<1.4	No test	<2.0	2.0-2.1	2.2-2.5	2.6-2.9	3.0-3.3	3.4-4.0	>4.0	<1.4	1.4-1.5	1.6-1.7	1.8-1.9	2.0-2.3	2.4-3.0	3.1-4.0	4.1-4.5	>4.5
Dose mg	10 5	10 5	10	5	4	3	2	1	0	9	8	7	6	5	4	3	Miss 1 day	Miss 2 day

Thromboprophylaxis please prescribe treatment regimens in the regular medications section

Choice of mechanical prophylaxis and leg(s) to be applied to						Enter Time	Enter details below
Graduated elastic compression stockings	Intermittend pneumatic compression device (IPC)		Leg: Left	Right	Both		
☑ 21/11 Start Date:	☐ End Date:	Signature and Bleep No.	☐	☐	☑		
☐ Start Date:	☐ End Date:	Signature and Bleep No.	☐	☐	☐		

Medication		Dose	Dose Change	Enter Time	Enter details below
CLEXANE		40 mg			
Please ensure you have completed the VTE risk assessment form	Date	21/11			
	Route	SC			
	Signature	AF		Instructions HIGH RISK - METASTIC Ca.	Pharmacy ☐
	Bleep no.	622			

Oxygen			
Target Saturation	88-92% ☐	94/98% ☐	If oxygen saturation falls below target range on prescribed oxygen, patient needs urgent clinical review. If oxygen saturation is above targent range on prescribed oxygen, ask for review.
Other specify)		*Device: N= nasal cannula, SM = simple face mask, V = venturi, H = humidified, RM = reservoir mask, OTHER = other eg. NCPAP/NIPPV	Pharmacy ☐
Target Saturation not applicable ☐			

	Date Changed	Date Changed	Enter Time	Enter details below
Device				
% or L/min (specify a range eg 1-21 L/min)				
Signature and Bleep no.				

21/11 Infusion prescriptions continued										SC = subcutaneous		IVC = intravenous central IVP = intravenous peripheral		
Date & time	Route	Infusion Fluid		Medication		Duration	Rate	Prescriber's signature & bleep no.	Date given	Given by / Added by	Check by	Start time	Finish time	Pharmacy
		Name & strength	Volume	Approved name with expiry / unit number	Dose									
21/11	IVP	0.9% SALINE Exp: Batch/unit no:	250ml	DISODIUM PAMIDRONATE	60 mg	3 hrs @ 20mg/hr		AF 622						
21/11	IVP	0.9% SALINE Exp: Batch/unit no:	1 LITRE	+20mmol KCl		2 hours		AF 622						
21/11	IVP	0.9% SALINE Exp: Batch/unit no:	1 LITRE			4 hours		AF 622						
21/11	IVP	0.9% SALINE Exp: Batch/unit no:	1 LITRE	+20mmol KCl		4 hours		AF 622						
21/11	IVP	0.9% SALINE Exp: Batch/unit no:	1 LITRE			8 hours		AF 622						
21/11	IVP	0.9% SALINE Exp: Batch/unit no:	1 LITRE	+20mmol KCl		8 hours		AF 622						
		TO MAINTAIN - BP > 100 SYSTOLIC; HR < 100 BPM; U.O > 0.5 ml/kg/HR > 30ML/HR												

As required medications					
Medication: OROMORPH				Date	
Indication: Breakthrough Pain				Time	
Dose: 2.5 - 5 ml	Route: PO	Maximum frequency / dose: 6 hour	Start date: 21/11	Dose	
			Stop date:	Route	
Signature: AF			Bleep no. 622	Given	
Additional instructions:				Pharmacy	☐

As required medications					
Medication: CYCLIZINE				Date	
Indication:				Time	
Dose: 50 mg	Route: IV/ IM	Maximum frequency / dose: 8 hour	Start date: 21/11	Dose	
			Stop date:	Route	
Signature: AF			Bleep no. 622	Given	
Additional instructions:				Pharmacy	☐

SCENARIO 15

As required medications																									
Medication PHOSPHATE ENEMA				Date																					
Indication				Time																					
Dose X1	Route PR	Maximum frequency / dose	Start date 21/11	Dose																					
			Stop date	Route																					
Signature AF			Bleep no. 622	Given																					
Additional instructions:															Pharmacy										

GLOBAL PRESCRIBING MARK

A B C D E

Station 5 – Clinical communication skills

Patient script

You are very anxious when the doctor comes to see you as you have heard the doctors and nurses talking, and it seems your cancer has spread. You are happy to talk to the doctor – you have met already.

Ideas and concerns – you suspected that this may be caused by the spread of the cancer several days ago but just didn't want to believe it. You are very concerned that you may be 'paralysed' forever.

Expectations – you would like to be 'totally informed' of what is going on and what, if anything, can be done. You have been very positive throughout your treatment and want to try everything available.

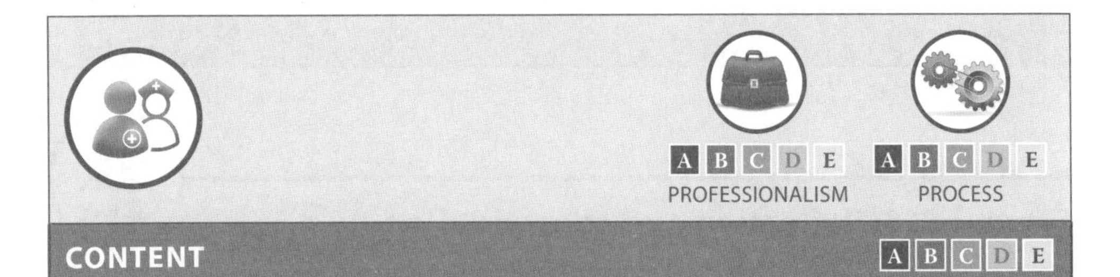

CONTENT A B C D E

Investigates patient's present level of understanding of scenario

Summarises and confirms what has happened so far and reason for discussion today

- Presentation with lower limb weakness, sensory changes, constipation and urinary retention
- Examination suggested signs of spinal cord compression, which was confirmed by the MRI scan.

Asks what, and how much information the patient would like to be told

Establishes patient's ideas, concerns and expectations

Explains the key, important information

- Confirms cord compression is secondary to spread of cancer (metastases); also found to have possible spread to liver, and other bones (where she is experiencing pain)
- The cord compression needs urgent treatment to stop permanent damage; if this (damage) were to occur she would be unable to walk again
- The way to treat it is by radiotherapy at St Richards under the care of the oncology (cancer) doctors – this is required as soon as possible
- This will reduced to pressure on the spine and will hopefully allow recovery.

Invites patient to ask questions as they proceed through the consultation and is able to deal with them appropriately

Summarises important areas of the consultation back to the patient

Formally ends the consultation and ensures appropriate follow-up has been discussed

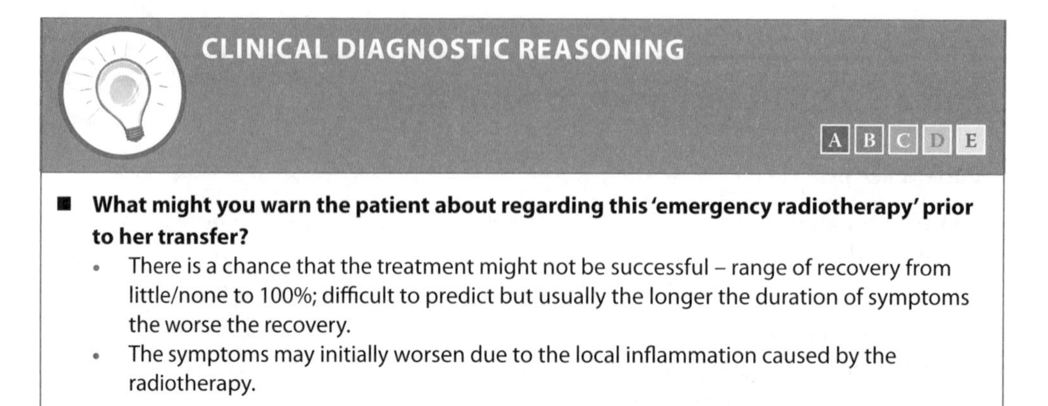

CLINICAL DIAGNOSTIC REASONING

A B C D E

- **What might you warn the patient about regarding this 'emergency radiotherapy' prior to her transfer?**
  - There is a chance that the treatment might not be successful – range of recovery from little/none to 100%; difficult to predict but usually the longer the duration of symptoms the worse the recovery.
  - The symptoms may initially worsen due to the local inflammation caused by the radiotherapy.

Demonstrates safe, sensible and appropriate management plan

Demonstrates clear and logical diagnostic reasoning

GLOBAL COMMUNICATION MARK

A B C D E

Scenario 15: Reflection and consolidation

History

Mrs Jean Simmons is a 53-year-old chartered accountant who was brought into the ED by ambulance at about 14:30 after a home visit by her GP.
Of note she was diagnosed as having cancer of the left breast two years ago at St Richards under the care of Dr Martin (oncology) and Ms Harris (Breast Surgeon). She had courses of pre-operative chemotherapy and radiotherapy, breast reconstruction with axillary clearance. She is presently having 6-monthly reviews with Dr Martin and was discharged from Ms Harris' care last year. Her last scan 4 months ago was apparently 'clear'.
She was very well until a few weeks ago when she started to get a 'gnawing' pain in her lumbar spine. Initially the pain was 'held at bay' by regular co-dydramol, but over the last week the pain has becoming increasingly severe, and is now rated 8/10.
This morning she had sudden weakness of her lower limbs and was unable to get out of bed. Her husband carried her to the toilet, where she found it very difficult to pass urine. She has been constipated for over 48 hours. As well as feeling weak, she describes her legs as feeling 'heavy' and 'woody'. Numb below umbilicus. She has no neurological symptoms in the upper limbs and no symptoms suggestive of raised intracranial pressure.
On direct questioning she also admits to pain in the middle of her left thigh, right shoulder and some of her ribs. She denies any other systemic symptoms of note.
Meds: co-dydramol two tablets 6 hourly; naproxen two tablets once or twice a day (for the last week).
Allergies: nil known
Mrs Simmons lives with husband and youngest daughter (18 years old) and has three other children who live relatively closely. She is a chartered accountant – over last 6-months part time. She is a non-smoker and drinks a few glasses of wine at weekends.
Previous medical history: nil of note prior to her breast cancer.

Examination

On examination, this was a chronically unwell-looking, thin, middle-aged woman.
Alert and orientated; co-operative throughout
Clinically dehydrated

Breast examination

Left: reconstructed left breast, scars clean; no masses
Right – nil of note
No cervical or axillary lymphadenopathy
Tenderness over anterior ribs, right shoulder and left mid thigh

Vital observations

HR 108 bpm, BP = 112/78 mmHg, RR 18 bpm, O_2 sats 95% on air, temperature 36.8 °C, CBG 4.4 mmol/l,
Urinalysis – NAD

RS, CV and abdominal examination

- Tender over several anterior ribs; otherwise unremarkable – no evidence effusions
- Abdomen – 4 cm hepatomegaly; no ascites; bladder – not palpable
- DRE: Loaded rectum – anal tone? Normal

Neurological assessment of the limbs
Lower limbs – left and right
Motor
Bulk – thin legs; no fasciculation
Tone – flaccid
Power – 1/5 left and 1 – 2/5 right
Reflexes – difficult to elicit
Co-ordination and gait – not assessed (because of reduced power)
Plantars – bilateral extensor response
Sensation – left and right
Reduced LT and pinprick from feet to level of umbilicus (T10).
In summary, this is a 52-year-old woman with known treated cancer of the left breast who now presents with signs consistent with lower thoracic spinal cord compression, hepatomegaly and bony tenderness over the mid left thigh, right shoulder and ribs.

Data interpretation

The history and examination are highly suggestive of an acute cord syndrome, with a cord level of about T10/T11, bony and possible liver and bony metastases.
The patient requires a routine set of blood tests including FBC, U&Es, RBG, LFTs, calcium and phosphate. She needs a plain CXR, and X-rays of her thoraco-lumbar spine. However, most urgently she needs an immediate MRI of her thoraco-lumbar spine.

Management

This is a medical emergency: *'Time equals neurones'*. Acute cord compression requires emergency decompression, either by neurosurgical intervention or, as in this case, radiotherapy. The patient, if willing, needs transfer to a tertiary referral centre where she can undergo the appropriate emergency therapy.
Her hypercalcaemia requires treatment with intravenous fluids and an intravenous bisphosphonate. She will require an indwelling urinary catheter and a phosphate enema.
Subsequently she may need further radiotherapy to her other bony metastases and possibly further chemotherapy.

Further reading and web links

www.nice.org.uk/nicemedia/pdf/CG80NICEGuideline.pdf

Scenario 16: 'All of a sudden'

Station 1

History *10-minute station*

You are the FY1 doctor on call for general medicine. A 62-year-old woman, Mrs Eleanor Reilly, has been referred to the hospital by her GP with a 1-day history of sudden-onset shortness of breath.

- **Please take a history from Mrs Reilly and present it along with your differential diagnosis to your Registrar.**

You will be assessed on the following areas, as well as the content and diagnostic reasoning of your history – take them into account in your presentation.

Professionalism

- Professional appearance (NHS dress code) – including general appearance, hair and jewellery
- Maintains patient and personal safety
- Polite introduction; identifies patient or interviewee correctly; confirms patient's date of birth from name band or other source
- Obtains informal consent; maintains patient's privacy
- Displays empathetic and caring attitudes and behaviours throughout.

Process

- Good organisation and structure; appropriate use of open and closed questions
- Appropriate fluency/rhythm/pace to the interview – this may change depending on environment and acute nature of problem
- Appropriate time for the patient to respond/reply to questions
- Appropriate acknowledgement of difficult or emotional areas of the patient's history.

Communication skills

- Demonstrates caring and sympathetic attitude
- Asks open questions
- Invites patient to ask questions and answers them appropriately
- Addresses patient's ideas, concerns and expectations.

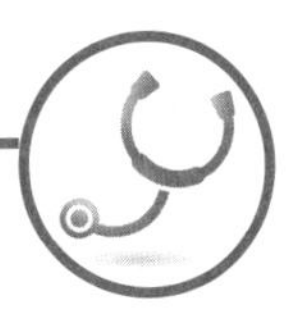

Station 2

Examination *10-minute station*

Your Registrar has asked you to examine Mrs Reilly.

- **Please examine Mrs Reilly's respiratory system and any other areas you feel are relevant (using information from within the station). Present your findings to your Registrar.**

You will be assessed on the following areas, as well as the content and skills of your examination – take them into account in your presentation.

Professionalism

- Professional appearance; maintains infection control standards, including hand cleaning and appropriate use of gloves and aprons
- Maintains patient and personal safety
- Polite introduction; identifies patient and confirms date of birth from name band or other source
- Obtains informal consent; maintains patient privacy and dignity
- Displays empathetic and caring attitudes and behaviours throughout.

Process

- Appropriate fluency/rhythm/pace to the examination – this may change depending on environment and acute nature of problem
- Good organisation and structure of examination; sensitive and empathetic approach
- Uses appropriate clinical techniques throughout
- Maintains privacy and dignity throughout.

Clinical communication

- Explains proposed examination/procedure: explains examination/procedure as it proceeds
- Offers information in a clear, structured and fluent manner, avoiding jargon
- Listens to patient and responds appropriately
- Demonstrates appropriate body language.

Please read the information below before presenting this case to the ST4 Medical Registrar as if you were on a busy medical take.
[NB If you have a model do not read this section]

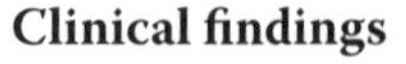

Clinical findings

- o **Patient appears dyspnoeic at rest**
- o **Able to speak in sentences**
- o **Observations – HR 110 bpm, BP 125/75 mmHg, RR 24 bpm, sats 90% on air, temperature 36.9 °C**
- o **CV examination – heart sounds easily heard, no rubs, no third heart sound, pulse regular in rhythm volume and JVP not elevated, apex beat not displaced peripheral capillary refill time <2 s**
- o **RS examination – trachea central, chest expansion normal bilaterally, percussion note normal throughout, breath sounds vesicular throughout both lung fields**
- o **Focused examination of right leg – swollen calf with erythema and dilated superficial veins and pitting oedema; Homans' sign positive (pain in calf on dorsiflexion of affected foot).**

Station 3

Data interpretation

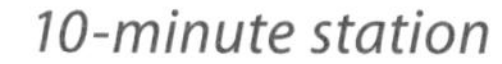

10-minute station

After presenting the history and examination for your Registrar, you have been asked to assess Mrs Reilly's risk of having a pulmonary embolism (PE) in order to guide further investigation.

- **Using the data provided in the following table, please calculate the Wells' score for PE for Mrs Reilly.**

Variable	Points
Clinical signs and symptoms of deep vein thrombosis (minimum of leg swelling and pain with palpation of the deep veins)	3.0
Alternative diagnosis less likely than pulmonary embolism	3.0
Heart rate >100/min	1.5
Immobilization (>3 days) or surgery in previous 4 weeks	1.5
Previous pulmonary embolism or deep vein thrombosis	1.5
Hemoptysis	1.0
Malignancy (receiving treatment, treated in the last 6 months, or palliative)	1.0

SCENARIO 16

Data interpretation and management

CXR normal

ABG on room air – pH 7.48, PO_2 7.9, PCO_2 3.5, HCO_3 23

FBC – HB 11.4, Plts 165, WCC 6.5

U&E – Na 129, K 3.5, urea 4.5 creatinine 89

Clotting screen – normal, D-dimer 1450

Decision made to perform CT pulmonary angiography.

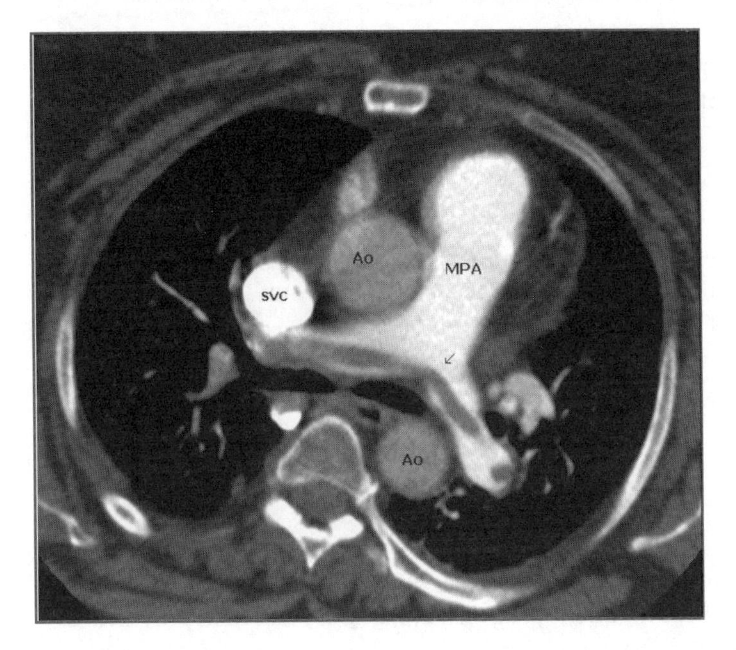

Figure 16.1 Mrs Reilly's CTPA shows a large pulmonary embolus in the pulmonary arterial trunk. This is termed a 'saddle embolus'. Ao = aorta; MPA = main pulmonary artery; SVC = superior vena cava

- Your Registrar asks you to take blood samples for a coagulopathy screen. He asks you to match some other patients who have been admitted with thromboembolic events to their investigations (given in the table overleaf).

Patient history	Haematology result	Diagnosis
1 A 69-year-old man with severe chronic airways disease	(A) INR 2.8 Plats 22	(a) Drug-induced coagulopathy
2 A 37-year-old woman with spontaneous bruising, recurrent infection and intracerebral haemorrhage	(B) INR 9.4	(b) Autocoagulation, and thrombocytopenia
3 A 51-year-old woman with recent DVT and thrombosis of the right upper limb	(C) Hb 19.2 Hct 0.59	(c) Pancytopenia secondary to aplastic anaemia
4 A 41-year-old alcohol abuser	(D) Hb 11.4 WCC 5.9 Plats 2076	(d) Secondary polycythaemia
5 A 39-year-old woman with a prosthetic mitral valve, on erythromycin for chest infection now presenting in coma	(E) Hb 6.2 WCC 2.1 Plats 6	(e) Primary thrombocythaemia

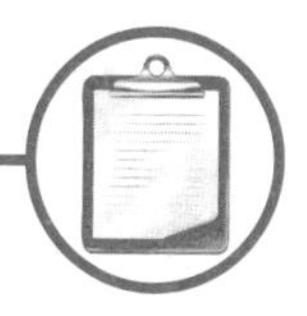

Station 4

Prescribing skills *10-minute station*

- **Using the BNF and information provided, please prescribe the required medications on Mrs Reilly's inpatient drug chart (page 368) and BNF provided, to include:**
  - **Anticoagulation**
  - **Analgesia**
  - **Oxygen.**

Details

Mrs Eleanor Reilly; Hospital No. 5672341; DOB: 1/12/1949; Drug allergies: nil; Weight: approx. 70 kg; Ward: MAU; Consultant: Dr Appleby

Remember: DRUG DRs Don't Forget Signing Off (page 373)

Station 5

Procedural skills *10-minute station*

Procedure

As a training exercise you have asked the Charge Nurse in the Emergency Department to supervise you drawing up and administering the subcutaneous injection of enoxaparin (low molecular weight heparin).

- **Using the following equipment, please perform the procedure.**

Equipment provided

- Alcohol swab
- Orange 24 G needle
- Syringe 1 ml or 2 ml
- Latex skin (or an orange if needed)
- Vial of low molecular weight heparin
- Drug chart for Mrs Reilly

Station 6

Clinical communication skills *10-minute station*

- **While on the Medical Admissions Unit Mrs Reilly undergoes further investigation for the possible underlying reason for DVT and PE. On close questioning she admits she has been suffering from abdominal bloating for the last 6 months. An abdominal ultrasound reveals a large ovarian mass lesion and associated metastases in her liver. You and your Registrar are going to break the news to Mrs Reilly and her husband. You have discussed the news you must break, and your Registrar is happy for you to explain this news as you have met them over the last few days. He will supervise your consultation.**

Answers

Station 1 – History

Patient script

You are a 62-year-old woman (DOB 1 December 1949) who attended your GP after developing shortness of breath yesterday evening at home. It happened suddenly and is associated with a sharp left-sided chest pain that is worse when you breathe in. You have not had a fever or productive cough, but you did notice a small amount of blood when you coughed this morning. You have not felt light-headed. You are currently short of breath at rest. You have been feeling quite run down and lethargic over recent months but have no specific symptoms.

You have no medical history. You are a current smoker of 20 per day. You drink no alcohol. You live with your husband and are still working part-time in a local shop. You take no regular medication and have no allergies.

On direct questioning: you noticed that your right leg was swollen about a week ago. It is sore and painful to walk on. It has increased in size since you first noticed it. You have never had a clot in the leg or lung, although your sister did have a DVT and an operation some years ago. You are not on HRT. You have been on no recent journeys and have had no recent operations. You have had three uncomplicated pregnancies (fit children 30, 28, 24) with no leg problems.

Ideas: you believe that you have a chest infection and are keen to get some antibiotics and go home.

Concerns: you are very worried about staying in the hospital, as you have an old pet cat at home.

Expectations: you reluctantly agreed to attend hospital for a CXR and expect to get home later today.

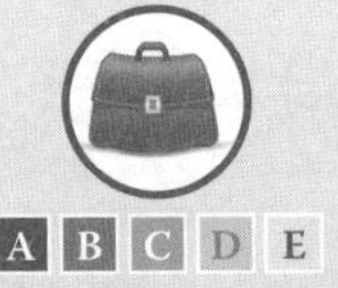

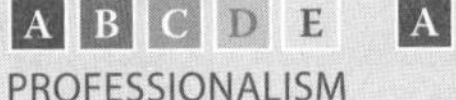

A B C D E PROFESSIONALISM | A B C D E PROCESS | A B C D E COMMUNICATION

CONTENT

A B C D E

Identifies key information

- Duration of illness – sudden-onset shortness of breath
- Presence of pleuritic chest pain
- Presence of haemoptysis – volume and colour
- Presence of clinical picture of right leg DVT.

Includes important negatives, including systemic enquiry

- No infective symptoms.

Identifies key information from rest of history

- Establishes risk factors for venous thromboembolism
- Smoking
- Previous VTE
- Family history of VTE
- Oral contraceptive/hormone replacement
- Recent immobility
- Recent surgery
- Known active malignancy.

Relevant factors from employment, housing, social support

- Nil of note.

Completing the patient history

- Drug and allergy history: nil regular medications and no allergies
- Previous medical history: no personal history of DVT, PE or miscarriage
- Social and occupational history: part-time worker in a shop, smoker 15 per day, minimal alcohol intake, lives with husband and old pet cat
- Family history: sister possible DVT, no other known family history of DVT, PE.

Summarises important areas of the history back to the patient

Invites patient to ask questions and is able to deal with them appropriately

Establishes patient's ideas, concerns and expectations

- Establishes that patient believes that she has a chest infection and is expecting to have a chest X-ray and go home later today.

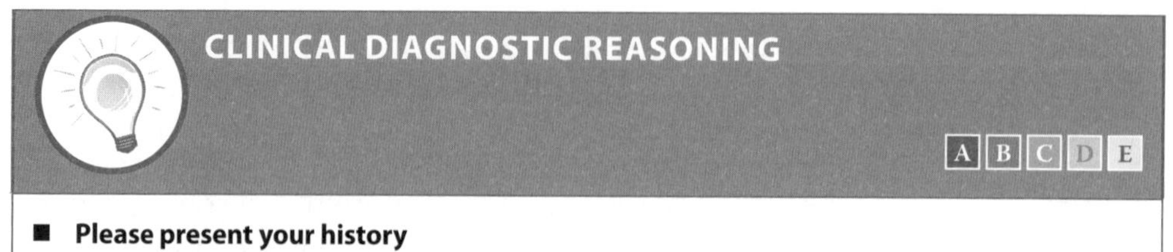

- **Please present your history**
  - Candidate offers a logical, well-structured account of the history
- **What is your diagnosis?**
  - Candidate offers the correct diagnosis and appropriate differentials
  - A sensible differential diagnosis would include infections such as tuberculosis as well as other causes of pleuritic chest pain, such as pneumothorax, although the history is very suggestive of venous thromboembolism.

GLOBAL HISTORY MARK

A B C D E

Station 2 – Examination

Patient script

If you are an actor/patient, read the patient history and physical signs fully – when the candidate comes to an abnormal site in their examination, act-out tenderness and/or volunteer the relevant physical sign.

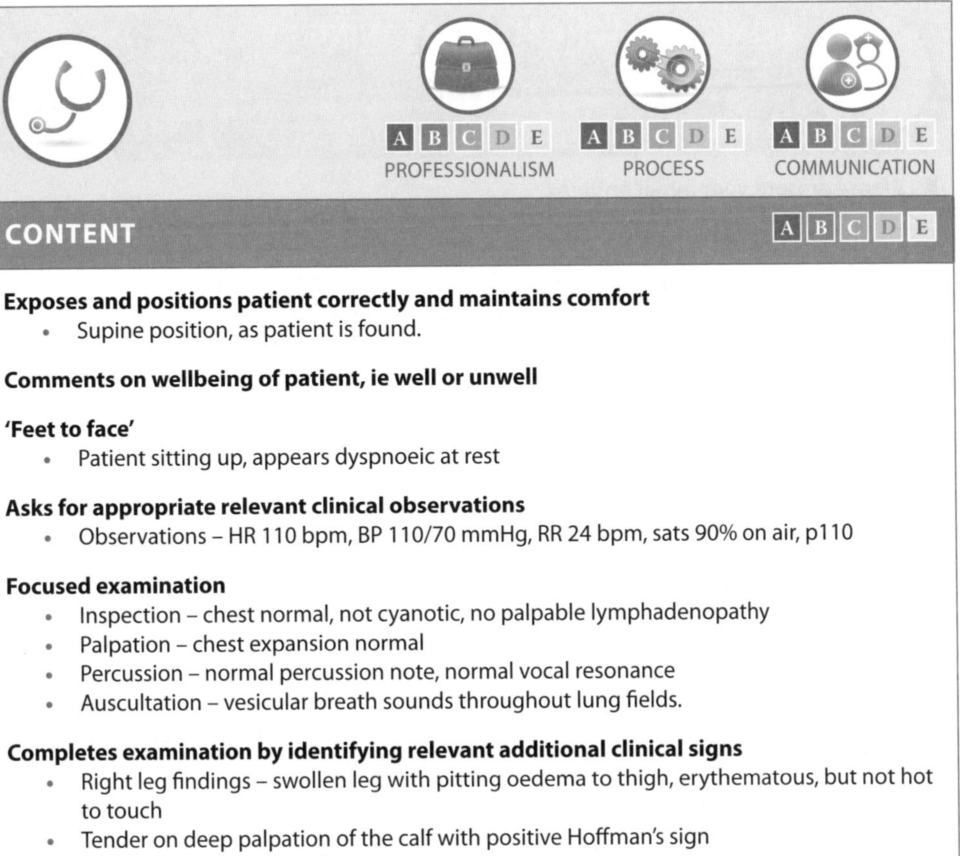

CONTENT

Exposes and positions patient correctly and maintains comfort
- Supine position, as patient is found.

Comments on wellbeing of patient, ie well or unwell

'Feet to face'
- Patient sitting up, appears dyspnoeic at rest

Asks for appropriate relevant clinical observations
- Observations – HR 110 bpm, BP 110/70 mmHg, RR 24 bpm, sats 90% on air, p110

Focused examination
- Inspection – chest normal, not cyanotic, no palpable lymphadenopathy
- Palpation – chest expansion normal
- Percussion – normal percussion note, normal vocal resonance
- Auscultation – vesicular breath sounds throughout lung fields.

Completes examination by identifying relevant additional clinical signs
- Right leg findings – swollen leg with pitting oedema to thigh, erythematous, but not hot to touch
- Tender on deep palpation of the calf with positive Hoffman's sign
- Auscultation of heart and JVP assessment.

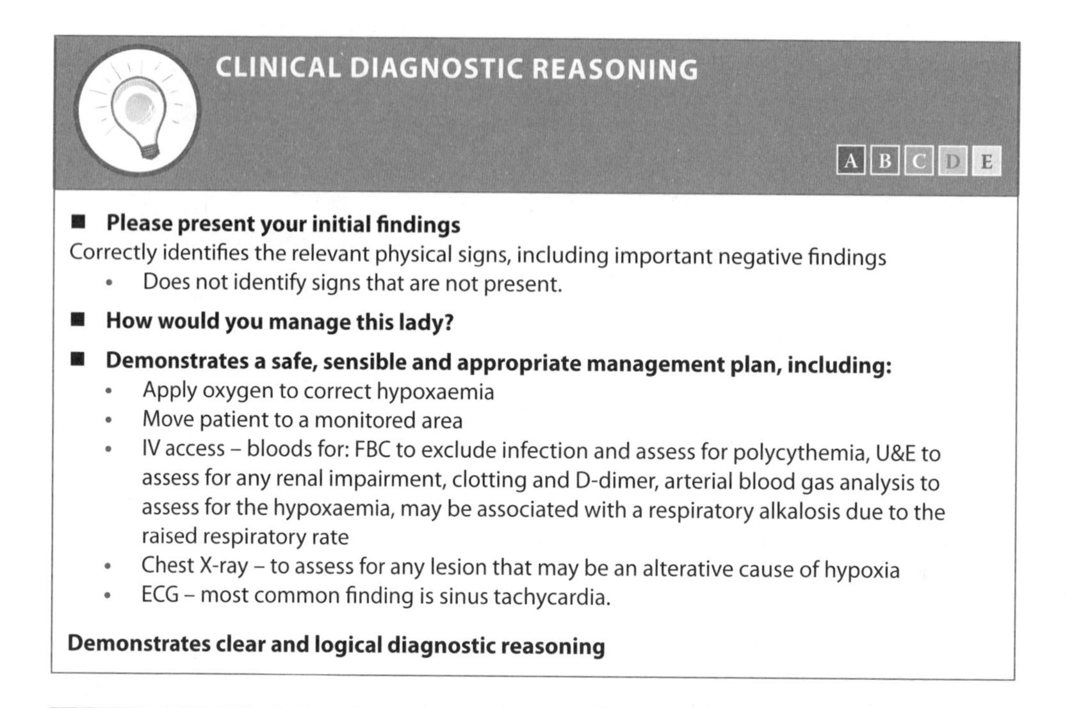

CLINICAL DIAGNOSTIC REASONING

A B C D E

- **Please present your initial findings**

Correctly identifies the relevant physical signs, including important negative findings
  - Does not identify signs that are not present.
- **How would you manage this lady?**
- **Demonstrates a safe, sensible and appropriate management plan, including:**
  - Apply oxygen to correct hypoxaemia
  - Move patient to a monitored area
  - IV access – bloods for: FBC to exclude infection and assess for polycythemia, U&E to assess for any renal impairment, clotting and D-dimer, arterial blood gas analysis to assess for the hypoxaemia, may be associated with a respiratory alkalosis due to the raised respiratory rate
  - Chest X-ray – to assess for any lesion that may be an alterative cause of hypoxia
  - ECG – most common finding is sinus tachycardia.

Demonstrates clear and logical diagnostic reasoning

GLOBAL EXAMINATION MARK

A B C D E

Station 3 – Data interpretation

Part 1 Wells' score = 8. This is a high Wells' score, making the diagnosis of PE a high probability.

Part 2

1 (C) (d)

This man has developed secondary polycythaemia due to his chronic airways disease with resultant pulmonary hypertension. The polycythaemia causes a procoagulant state, which in severe cases leads to thromboembolic disease. Treatment should include treatment of the underlying airways disease and regular venesection, with the aim of reducing the haematocrit (Hct) to 0.50 or less.

2 (E) (c)

This patient demonstrates a pancytopenia secondary to an aplastic anaemia. Thrombocytopenia of less than 10×10^9/l carries a significant risk of spontaneous bleeding, in this case a spontaneous intracranial haemorrhage. Causes of aplastic anaemia include:

Congenital; Fanconi's anaemia; Acquired; Idiopathic; Infection – TB, hepatitis A; Toxins – chemicals and insecticides; irradiation; Drugs – antibiotics, anti-epileptics, anti-inflammatories, antihistamines, antithyroid, oral hypoglycaemics, chemotherapeutic agents.

3 (D) (e)

Primary thrombocythaemia is a relatively uncommon haematological disorder, which presents with bleeding (due to abnormal platelet function), bruising and thromboembolic phenomena. It is intimately related to the myeloproliferative disorders – in particular polycythaemia rubra vera.

4 (A) (b)

Alcohol excess is shown in the peripheral blood film by macrocytosis and thrombocytopenia. Alcohol abusers are at increased risk of subdural haemorrhage because of increased falls, thrombocytopenia and coagulopathy (causing a raised INR and prolonged APTT) owing to the liver's inability to produce clotting factors.

5 (B) (a)

This patient has suffered an intracranial haemorrhage due to a grossly elevated INR. This has arisen due to the interaction of erythromycin with warfarin. Caution must be used when prescribing medications for patients on oral anticoagulants and the oral contraceptive pill.

GLOBAL DATA INTERPRETATION MARK A B C D E

Station 4 – Prescribing skills

Check: DRUG DRs Don't Forget Signing Off (page 373)

(a) Anticoagulation

Low molecular weight heparin – initial anticoagulation should be administered once the diagnosis of pulmonary embolus is suspected; previously infusions of unfractionated heparin were used, but these are complicated and require multiple blood tests; subcutaneous injections of low molecular weight heparin can be given once daily; there are various formulations, but enoxaparin (Clexane®) is often used in trusts across the NHS – 1.5 mg/kg once daily is a usual dose.

Warfarin – once the diagnosis of pulmonary embolus has been made, anticoagulation with warfarin should be initiated once a patient has been counselled and screened for any contraindications.

Warfarin should be loaded over a number of days, the first dose should be 10 mg for rapid anticoagulation. The subsequent days doses should be guided by the INR results. See further reading for information on the Fennerty regime for rapid antiocoagulation. Heparin should be continued until the warfarin is within the target range.

(b) Analgesia

Appropriate analgesia such as regular paracetamol and an NSAID such as ibuprofen 400 mg tds as required for breakthrough pain.

(c) Oxygen

Mrs Reilly has no history of respiratory disease, so target oxygen saturations should be above 94%.

Allergies, sensitivities and adverse drug reactions					Patient details/addressograph
No known allergies ✓		Initials SY 113	Gender M (F)		NHS/ Hospital No: 5672341
Not possible to ascertain ☐		Date 13.01	Weight (kg)	Date	
Medicine/substance	Reaction & Severity	Initials & Date	70		Surname: REILLY
			Height		First name: ELEANOR
			1.65m		
Alerts			Surface area (m²)		Date of birth: 01.12.49

IN-PATIENT MEDICATION PRESCRIPTION AND ADMINISTRATION RECORD

PasTest HOSPITAL

Consultant	Trainee Dr. Name and Bleep no.	Date of admission	Date chart reboarded	Estimated date of discharge
APPLEBY	SYED 113	13.01.12		
This chart is no. 1 of 1	Transcribing Check by Pharmacy Sign .... Date	Ward 1. MAU 2.		

Supplementary Medication charts in use: Other (please specify): 1 .... 2 ....

Epidural/PCA ☐ Syringe driver ☐ TPN ☐ Chemotherapy ☐ Insulin sliding scale ☐

Once only medications – loading doses, pre-medication, PGDs or surgical antibiotic propylaxis

Date	Time to be given	Medicine (approved name)	Dose	Route	Signature and bleep no.	Pharmacy	Time given	Given by	Checked by
13.01	11.30	ENOXAPARIN	105mg	SC	SY 113				
		[70 x 1.5 mg]							

Regular prescriptions continued

Regular medications

	Dose			Date 13	14	15	16	17									
Date	13.01			Medication ENOXAPARIN					Instructions (1.5mg kg x 70) = 105 mg				Signature and bleep no. SY 113			Pharmacy ☐	
Route	SC																
Signature	SY																
06																	
(09)	105mg			X													
12																	
18																	
22																	
24																	

Regular prescriptions continued																	
Regular medications																	
	Dose			Date 13	14	15	16	17									
Date	13.01			Medication PARACETAMOL					Instructions				Signature and bleep no. SY 113			Pharmacy ☐	
Route	PO																
Signature	SY																
06																	
(9)	1g																
(12)	1g																
(18)	1g																
(22)	1g																
02																	

Regular prescriptions continued																	
Regular medications																	
	Dose			Date 13	14	15	16	17									
Date	13.01			Medication CODEINE PHOSPHATE					Instructions				Signature and bleep no. SY 113			Pharmacy ☐	
Route	PO																
Signature	SY																
06																	
(9)	30mg																
(12)	30mg																
(18)	30mg																
(22)	30mg																
02																	

Oxygen			
Target Saturation	88-92% ☐	94/98% ☑	If oxygen saturation falls below target range on prescribed oxygen, patient needs urgent clinical review. If oxygen saturation is above targent range on prescribed oxygen, ask for review.
Other specify)		*Device: N= nasal cannula, SM = simple face mask, V = venturi, H = humidified, RM = reservoir mask, OTHER = other eg. NCPAP/NIPPV	Pharmacy
Target Saturation not applicable ☐			

	Date Started	Date Changed	Date Changed	Enter Time	Enter details below											
* Device	HUDSON															
% or L/min (Specify a range eg 1-12 L/min)	5L/M															
Signature and Bleep No.	SY 113															

GLOBAL PRESCRIPTION MARK

A B C D E

SCENARIO 16

Station 5 – Procedural skills

Procedure: subcutaneous injection

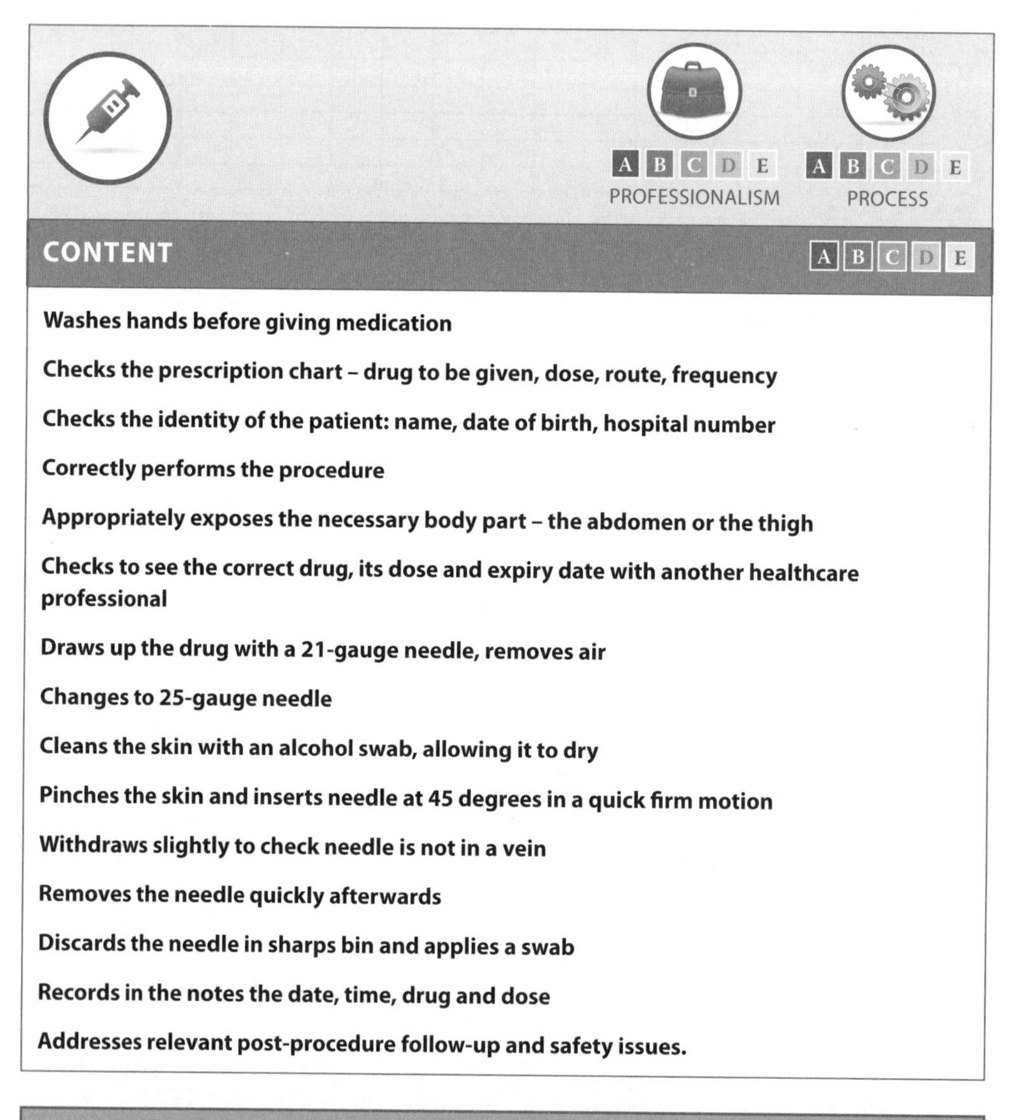

CONTENT A B C D E

Washes hands before giving medication

Checks the prescription chart – drug to be given, dose, route, frequency

Checks the identity of the patient: name, date of birth, hospital number

Correctly performs the procedure

Appropriately exposes the necessary body part – the abdomen or the thigh

Checks to see the correct drug, its dose and expiry date with another healthcare professional

Draws up the drug with a 21-gauge needle, removes air

Changes to 25-gauge needle

Cleans the skin with an alcohol swab, allowing it to dry

Pinches the skin and inserts needle at 45 degrees in a quick firm motion

Withdraws slightly to check needle is not in a vein

Removes the needle quickly afterwards

Discards the needle in sharps bin and applies a swab

Records in the notes the date, time, drug and dose

Addresses relevant post-procedure follow-up and safety issues.

GLOBAL PROCEDURE MARK A B C D E

Station 6 – Clinical communication skills

Patient script

You are a 62-year-old woman who has been in hospital for 5 days after been diagnosed with a clot in your leg and lung. You were both upset and shocked by this diagnosis. Your breathlessness and chest pain have improved and you are looking forward to going home.

You understand that the doctors have been looking for a reason that you have developed this problem and to this end you have had some blood tests and a scan of your abdomen. You are feeling quite concerned that there may be something else going on as you have been feeling slightly bloated and lethargic over recent months when you think about it. You would rather hear the information when your husband arrives and are keen to know the 'full story'.

When you are told that the likely diagnosis is a cancer of the ovary, you are very upset and have a number of questions, such as:

- Is it curable?
- Will I have to have chemotherapy?

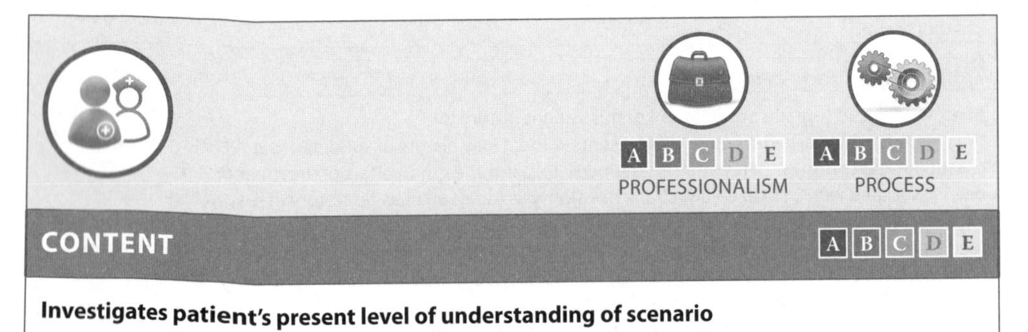

Investigates patient's present level of understanding of scenario

Summarises and confirms what has happened so far

- Establishes that a DVT and a PE has been diagnosed
- Establishes that treatment with anticoagulation has been initiated
- Establishes that an ultrasound scan has been performed.

Establishes patient's ideas, concerns and expectations

- Establishes that the patient is concerned that there is an underlying problem causing her to have these clots.

Explains the key, important information

- Gives warning that there is difficult information to be given
- Asks if any family members should be present
- Establishes how much the patient would like to know
- Explains news in clear chunks of information, checking understanding throughout – 'scan is abnormal', 'likely to be cancer', need further investigation with CT scan and biopsy
- Is empathetic and sensitive to patient throughout, with good use of silence.

Invites patient to ask questions as they proceed through the consultation and is able to deal with them appropriately

Summarises important areas of the consultation back to the patient

Formally ends the consultation and ensures appropriate follow-up has been discussed

- Arranges further meeting with consultant and further imaging.

GLOBAL COMMUNICATION MARK

A B C D E

Scenario 16: Reflection and consolidation

History

An example of an A-grade presentation of this patient history is:
"Mrs Reilly is a 62-year-old woman who presents with a 1-day history of sudden-onset left-sided pleuritic chest pain and shortness of breath. This has persisted, and she is now short of breath at rest. This has been associated with a small volume frank haemoptysis today. She has no history of respiratory disease or infective symptoms. She has clinical evidence of a likely DVT with a 1-week history of swelling of her calf and tenderness on walking. She is a current smoker but has no personal history of venous thromboembolism; however, her sister had post-operative DVT. She has not had recent immobility or surgery. She takes no regular medication, including hormonal therapy.
The most likely diagnosis is that of a pulmonary embolism and right leg deep vein thrombosis."

Examination

On examination, Mrs Reilly is tachypnoeic at rest, with a respiratory rate of 24 beats per minute. She is hypoxic with saturations of 90% on room air. She is tachycardic at 110 beats per minute, but she is not hypotensive. Her respiratory examination is unremarkable. On inspection of her legs there are signs suggestive of a right leg deep vein thrombosis with swelling, pitting oedema and dilated superficial veins.
The examination suggests a right leg deep vein thrombosis and associated pulmonary embolus.
The examination of the patient with a possible pulmonary embolus is usually normal. For the most part the purpose of the examination is to ensure that there is not another cause of chest pain/hypoxia, such as consolidation or pneumothorax.
The clinical suspicion for PE must remain high, as this is a diagnosis with a significant mortality if untreated (approximately 30%), and this is a condition that is often not confirmed until post-mortem.

Investigation

Once the clinical suspicion of pulmonary embolus has been raised, patients should be risk stratified by the Wells' score and investigated based on the result of this.

- **Low clinical probability**
- If negative D-dimer, PE is excluded
- If positive D-dimer, obtain CTPA and base treatment on results.
- **Moderate clinical probability**
- If negative D-dimer, PE is excluded
- If positive D-dimer, obtain CTPA and base treatment on results.
- **High clinical probability**
- Proceed to CTPA
- If positive, treat
- If negative, additional tests are needed to exclude PE.

The use of ventilation/perfusion scanning (nuclear medicine) is becoming less common. However, it is useful in particular situations – especially those with a normal chest X-ray.

Management

The management of pulmonary embolus is with anticoagulation. However, acute treatment with thrombolysis is indicated in patients with evidence of cardiovascular compromise as a result of pulmonary embolus – hypotension, cardiac arrest or massive PE with right heart strain on ECHO.
Surgical thrombectomy is an uncommon treatment because of poor outcomes but can be used in selected patients.
Inferior vena cava filter can be used when anticoagulation has not prevented further pulmonary emboli after a DVT or in those who cannot be anticoagulated owing to an active bleeding risk.

Further reading and web links
Warfarin loading guidance:
www.cks.nhs.uk/knowledgeplus/test_of_the_week/anticoagulant_monitoring/warfarin_monitoring
British Thoracic Society guidelines for management of suspected acute pulmonary embolism:
Wells PS et al. 2001 Ann Intern Med 17;135(2):98-107

Scenario 17: 'Couldn't get up'

Station 1

History *10-minute station*

You are a final year medical student on rotation in the Emergency Department. Your Consultant has asked you to take a history from an elderly patient who has been brought in by ambulance. Her name is Eileen Brierly.

- **Please take a focused history from Mrs Brierly. Once you have finished you should present your history to the Consultant and then answer any questions he may have.**

You will be assessed on the following areas, as well as the content and diagnostic reasoning of your history – take them into account in your presentation.

Professionalism

- Professional appearance (NHS dress code) – including general appearance, hair and jewellery
- Maintains patient and personal safety
- Polite introduction; identifies patient or interviewee correctly; confirms patient's date of birth from name band or other source
- Obtains informal consent; maintains patient's privacy
- Displays empathetic and caring attitudes and behaviours throughout.

Process

- Good organisation and structure; appropriate use of open and closed questions
- Appropriate fluency/rhythm/pace to the interview – this may change depending on environment and acute nature of the problem
- Appropriate time for the patient to respond/reply to questions
- Appropriate acknowledgement of difficult or emotional areas of the patient's history.

Communication skills

- Demonstrates caring and sympathetic attitude
- Asks open questions
- Invites patient to ask questions and answers them appropriately
- Addresses patient's ideas, concerns and expectations.

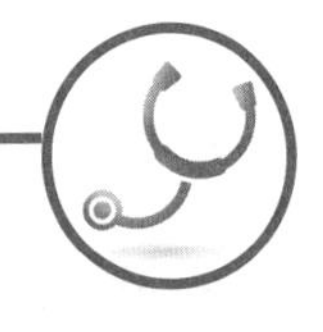

Station 2

Examination *10-minute station*

Now that you have taken a history from Mrs Brierly, you and your Consultant agree that a hip fracture seems likely. In anticipation of this diagnosis, your Consultant goes off to request an X-ray. He asks that you perform an examination that will aid the orthopaedic/anaesthetic team in expediting the patient's surgery should the presumed diagnosis be confirmed. A set of observations (which you may ask for) has been taken by the Emergency Department nurse.

- **Please complete your examination and then turn the page for a summary of the findings. You should then present your examination findings (from within the station) and answer the questions that your Consultant has for you.**

You will be assessed on the following areas, as well as the content and skills of your examination – take them into account in your presentation.

Professionalism

- Professional appearance; maintains infection control standards, including hand cleaning and appropriate use of gloves and aprons
- Maintains patient and personal safety
- Polite introduction; identifies patient and confirms date of birth from name band or other source
- Obtains informal consent; maintains patient privacy and dignity
- Displays empathetic and caring attitudes and behaviours throughout.

Process

- Appropriate fluency/rhythm/pace to the examination – this may change depending on environment and acute nature of problem
- Good organisation and structure of examination; sensitive and empathetic approach
- Uses appropriate clinical techniques throughout
- Maintains privacy and dignity throughout.

Clinical communication

- Explains proposed examination/procedure; explains examination/procedure as it proceeds
- Offers information in a clear, structured and fluent manner, avoiding jargon
- Listens to patient and responds appropriately
- Demonstrates appropriate body language.

Please read the information below and present your examination findings to the Consultant. ***[NB If you have a model do not read this section]***

Clinical findings

- o Frail elderly lady, slim build (estimated weight 65 kg)
- o Observations – HR 72 bpm, BP 101/67 mmHg, RR 14 bpm, O_2 sats 99% on air, temperature 36.9 °C
- o General examination – pulse irregularly irregular; no signs of anaemia, jaundice, cyanosis, pallor; warm and well perfused; not clinically dehydrated
- o Abdominal examination – soft, non-tender, bowel sounds present, no organomegaly
- o Cardiovascular examination – apex not displaced, HS I+II+0, no carotid bruits, no peripheral oedema
- o Respiratory examination – fine bibasal crepitations, otherwise good air entry and vesicular breath sounds
- o Orthopaedic examination – left leg is shortened and externally rotated; no swelling or bruising seen; marked tenderness at left hip especially on palpation anteriorly; no pain on palpation of the thigh or knee; unable to flex hip actively due to severe pain, not attempted passively because of pain; able to move ankle fully (dorsiflexion and plantarflexion); normal sensation at all dermatomes of left leg; distal pulses normal on palpation, and temperature of skin comparable to right leg.

Station 3

Data interpretation *10-minute station*

Mrs Brierly has now had her X-ray.

- Take a look at the following series of X-rays (all from different patients) and describe the fractures to your Consultant, in a concise and accurate manner as if making a referral to the Orthopaedic Registrar on the telephone.

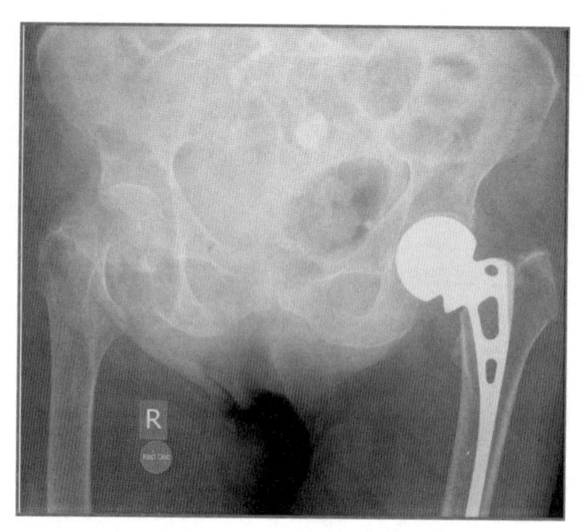

Figure 17.1

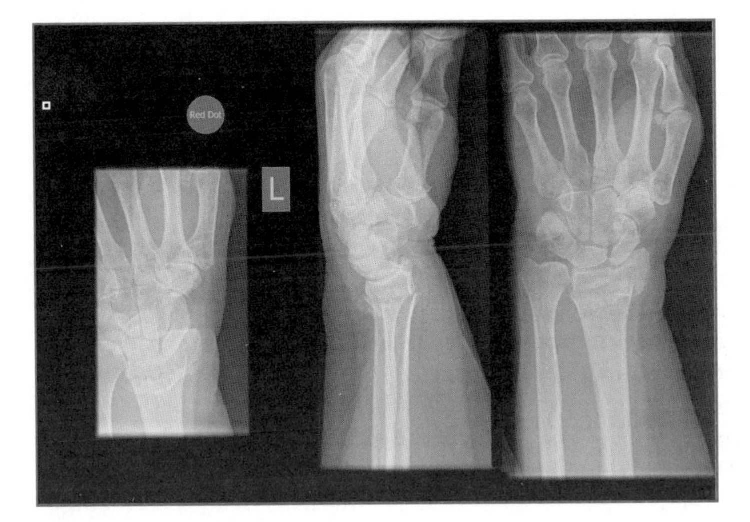

Figure 17.2

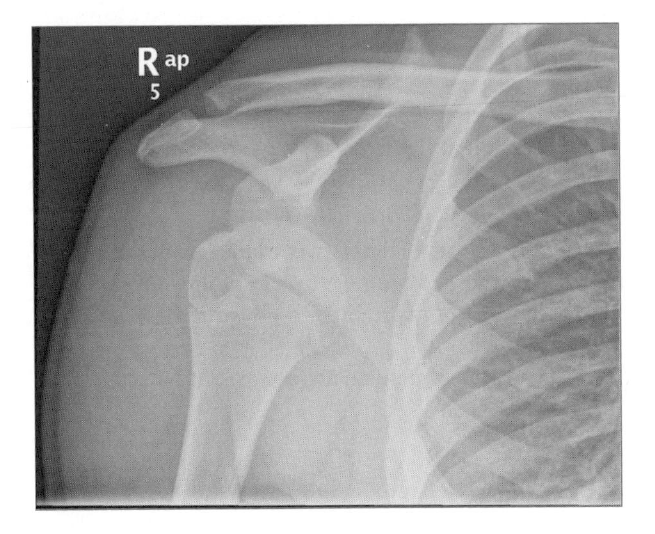

Figure 17.3

Station 4

Procedural skills *10-minute station*

Procedure

Mrs Brierly is going to be admitted to the Orthopaedic Ward to await surgery for her hip fracture. Your hospital has an infection control policy which mandates that all newly admitted patients must have swabs taken from the throat, nose and axilla in order to screen for meticillin-resistant *Staphylococcus aureus* (MRSA) colonisation. The Emergency Department Sister suggests that she observe you taking these swabs.

- **Using the following equipment, please perform the swab sampling and label the samples so that they can be sent to the Microbiology Laboratory.**

Equipment provided

- **Charcoal swab sticks × 3**
- **Sterile saline**
- **Gloves**
- **Apron**

Station 5

Clinical communication skills *10-minute station*

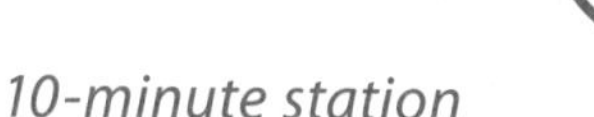

Mrs Brierly's daughter has arrived in the Emergency Department and has been informed by the Consultant that her mother has broken her hip and will require surgery. She seems to be concerned that her mother is being tested for MRSA and has some questions to ask.

- **The Consultant asks you to explain about the screening procedure and answer any questions that the patient's daughter has to ask.**

Answers

Station 1 – History

Patient script

Your name is Eileen Brierly, DOB 3 January 1934. You are 78 years old. You are reporting severe pain at your left hip since falling at home this morning. You slipped on the tiled floor in the kitchen after removing your lunch from the microwave and fell awkwardly onto your left side, landing heavily on the floor. You felt sudden pain at your hip that was so severe that you were unable to get up. You were thankfully able to reach your alarm cord, which alerted the warden at your accommodation, who came round straight away and called an ambulance.

The pain is sharp in nature and localized to your left hip and is excruciating when you try and move. When you lie still the pain is tolerable. The ambulance crew gave you an injection of some strong medicine, which helped, before putting you onto the stretcher and transporting you to hospital. You do not feel that the pain radiates anywhere else. You have not been able to bear weight at all since the fall. You do not report any numbness at the leg.

If asked about the fall, you suspect that you slipped on some tiles that had been cleaned by your carer this morning. You suffered no other injuries and do not recall feeling unwell before slipping. You have not had any chest pain, shortness of breath, palpitations, light-headedness, headache, cough or cold, urinary frequency or burning, or other symptoms prior to the event.

Your last meal was breakfast this morning (5 hours ago now). You had a cup of tea 3 hours ago.

Your previous medical problems include high blood pressure, tablet-controlled diabetes, an irregular heartbeat and a stroke 7 years ago. Since the stroke you have had some residual weakness of the right arm and leg.

The medications that you take are aspirin, bisoprolol, ramipril, metformin, gliclazide and simvastatin. You are not sure of the doses and have them dispensed from a dosset box. You are not aware of any allergies.

You were widowed 12 years ago and live alone in a warden-controlled ground-floor flat, having found your mobility restricted by the stroke 7 years ago. You are able to walk independently but only with the assistance of a zimmer frame. You have a carer once a day in the morning to help you with washing and getting dressed. Your daughter and grandchildren live nearby and come to visit you most days – they also help with your shopping and cleaning, and take you out regularly. You have never smoked. When you are with your family you will often have a sherry or small glass of wine, but no more.

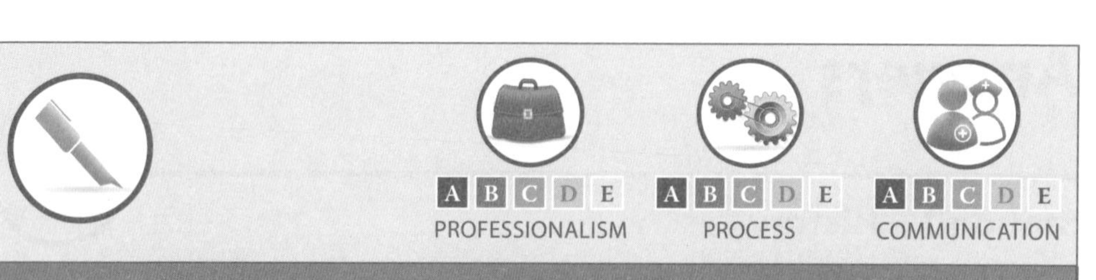

CONTENT

A B C D E

Identifies key information

- Pain after fall at home – unable to get up
- Left hip pain, sharp, no radiation, worse on movement, no numbness.

Includes important negatives, including systemic enquiry

- No other injuries
- No chest pain, no shortness of breath, no palpitations, no urinary symptoms, no recent cough or cold, no headache, no light-headedness, previous stroke but no new symptoms of weakness.

Identifies key information from rest of history

- Last ate meal five hours ago; last drank three hours ago.

Relevant factors from employment, housing, social support

- Lives alone in warden-controlled ground-floor accommodation
- Once daily carer, supportive family
- Mobilises with Zimmer frame.

Completing the patient history

- Drug and allergy history: aspirin, metformin, gliclazide, ramipril, simvastatin, bisoprolol; no known allergies
- Previous medical history: stroke 7 years ago, leading to residual right-sided weakness; tablet-controlled diabetes; hypertension; atrial fibrillation
- Social and occupational history: non-smoker, occasional alcohol.

Summarises important areas of the history back to the patient

Invites patient to ask questions and is able to deal with them appropriately

Establishes patient's ideas, concerns and expectations

CLINICAL DIAGNOSTIC REASONING

A B C D E

- **Please present your history**
  - Candidate offers a logical, well-structured account of the history
- **What is your diagnosis?**
  - Candidate offers the correct diagnosis and appropriate differentials
  - Diagnosis: fractured neck of femur
  - Differentials could include: other fractures such as pubic ramus fracture, acetabular fracture or femoral shaft fracture; muscular injuries such as adductor tear; bruising and soft tissue contusion.

GLOBAL HISTORY MARK

A B C D E

Station 2 – Examination

Patient script

If you are an actor/patient, read the patient history and physical signs fully – when the candidate comes to an abnormal site in their examination, act-out tenderness and/or volunteer the relevant physical sign.

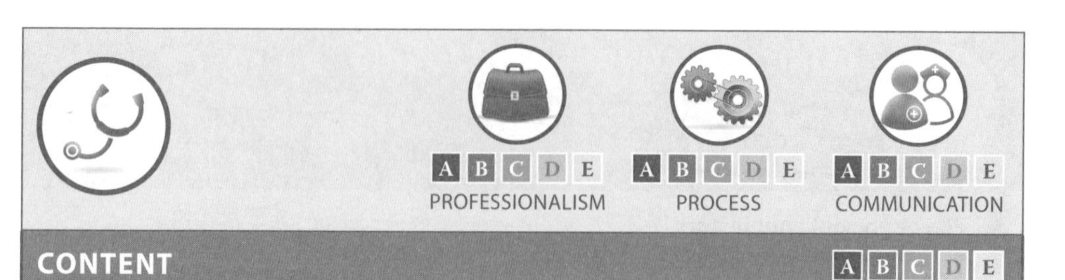

CONTENT

A B C D E

Exposes and positions patient correctly and maintains comfort

- Supine position, as patient is found.

Comments on wellbeing of patient, ie well or unwell

'Feet to face'

- Frail, elderly patient
- Slim build (estimated weight 65 kg).

Asks for appropriate clinical observations

- HR 72 bpm, BP 101/67 mmHg, RR 14 bpm, O_2 sats 99% on air, temperature 36.9 °C.

General/systematic examination

- Hands – pulse irregularly irregular
- Face and neck – no signs of anaemia, jaundice, cyanosis or pallor; warm and well perfused, euvolaemic
- Cardiovascular examination – apex beat not displaced, HS I+II+0, no carotid bruits, no peripheral oedema
- Respiratory examination – fine bibasal crepitations, otherwise vesicular breath sounds, good air entry
- Abdominal examination – soft, non-tender, bowel sounds present.

Focused orthopaedic examination of left hip

- LOOKS for deformity – left leg 'appears' shortened and externally rotated, no bruising seen
- FEELS for tenderness – tenderness on palpation of hip joint, especially anteriorly, no tenderness at thigh or knee
- MOVES: unable to flex hip actively owing to pain, and not attempted passively owing to patient discomfort; able to move leg distally (full range of ankle movement)
- Examines for neurological or vascular involvement – normal sensation and presence of pedal pulses, capillary refill time.

Thanks patient, offers assistance, maintains patient's dignity and privacy until they are dressed

CLINICAL DIAGNOSTIC REASONING

A B C D E

- **Please present your examinations**

Correctly identifies the relevant physical signs, including important negative findings

- Does not identify signs that are not present.

- **What investigations should be arranged before anaesthetic prior to surgery for a fractured hip**
  - Bloods – FBC, U&E, glucose, bone profile, clotting screen, group and crossmatch (2–4 units)
  - Chest X-ray
  - Electroc.

- **What measures would you take to minimise the risk of venous thromboembolism**
  - Early surgery followed by early mobilisation after surgery
  - Anti-embolic compression stockings (eg TED) and use of intermittent pneumatic compression boots
  - Pharmacological prophylaxis with low molecular weight heparin, eg tinzaparin.

GLOBAL EXAMINATION MARK

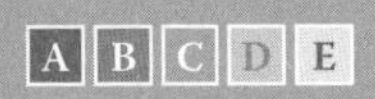

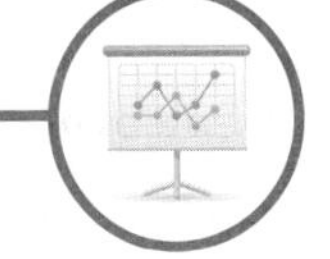

Station 3 – Data interpretation

X-ray 17.1

There is a subcapital fracture of the right femoral neck – the trabecular pattern is normal, indicating that this fracture is undisplaced. It can be classified as a Garden Type II fracture. The patient has had a previous left hip fracture treated with an Austin Moore prosthesis.

X-ray 17.2

This fracture of the distal radius is a typical Colles fracture, with dorsal angulation and radial deviation of the distal fragment, together with impaction. There may be an associated fracture of the ulnar styloid process, and, with fragmentation of the distal radius, the fracture may extend into the wrist joint.'

X-ray 17.3

There is anterior dislocation of the right glenohumeral joint; no fracture is seen.

GLOBAL DATA INTERPRETATION MARK

A B C D E

Station 4 – Procedural skills

Procedure

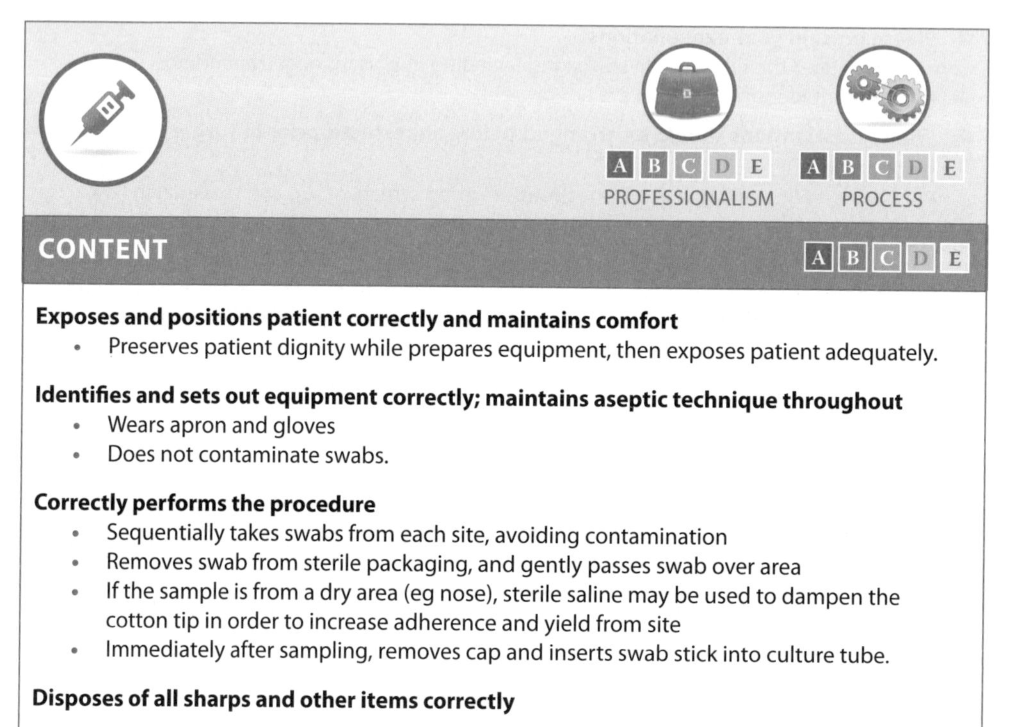

CONTENT A B C D E

Exposes and positions patient correctly and maintains comfort

- Preserves patient dignity while prepares equipment, then exposes patient adequately.

Identifies and sets out equipment correctly; maintains aseptic technique throughout

- Wears apron and gloves
- Does not contaminate swabs.

Correctly performs the procedure

- Sequentially takes swabs from each site, avoiding contamination
- Removes swab from sterile packaging, and gently passes swab over area
- If the sample is from a dry area (eg nose), sterile saline may be used to dampen the cotton tip in order to increase adherence and yield from site
- Immediately after sampling, removes cap and inserts swab stick into culture tube.

Disposes of all sharps and other items correctly

Addresses relevant post-procedure follow-up and safety issues

- Labels samples appropriately, and clearly identifies site of sample without mixing up sites.

GLOBAL PROCEDURE MARK A B C D E

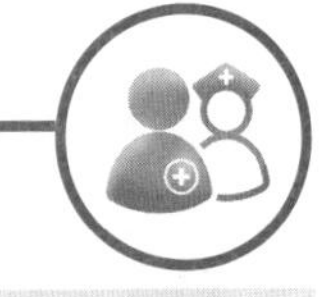

Station 6 – Clinical communication skills

Patient script

You are Catherine, the daughter of Mrs Brierly. You have just arrived in the Emergency Department after receiving a call from the warden at your mother's accommodation. You have spoken with the Emergency Medicine Consultant and have been told that your mother has broken her hip and will be admitted to the Orthopaedic Ward for surgery to fix the fracture. You are grateful to the team for the care that they have provided so far, but are a little confused and concerned that your mother is being screened for MRSA.

Beliefs – you understand that MRSA is a superbug and you've read that it can kill people from horrible infections. You thought people caught it in hospital and you are worried that your mother is being tested for it. You are not aware of any screening protocol for MRSA until it is explained to you.

Expectations – you are worried about what it would mean if your mother's MRSA screening was positive.

You have several specific questions:

- Why would my mother have MRSA? How would she have got it if she does have it?
- What would it mean if the screening test shows MRSA? Will she die of a nasty infection like those that have been all over the news?
- What is the treatment if she does test positive?

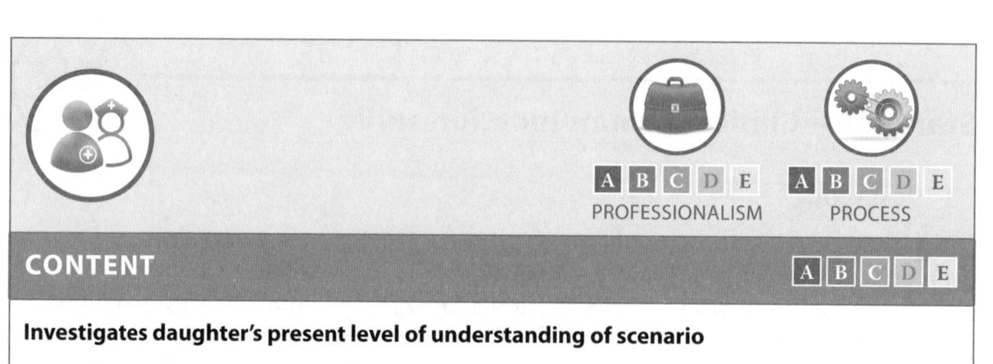

CONTENT

A B C D E

Investigates daughter's present level of understanding of scenario

Summarises and confirms what has happened so far

- Mrs Brierly has fractured her hip and will require admission for surgery.

Establishes daughter's ideas, concerns and expectations

- Daughter is concerned about why her mother is being screened for MRSA
- Believes that MRSA is a superbug that can kill people by causing horrible infections.

Explains the key, important information

- Explains that MRSA is a common bacterium that lives on many people's skin/throat/nose normally – explains meaning of colonisation
- Explains that MRSA can cause serious infections, but this is different to colonisation
- Explains that elderly people are more at risk from hospital-acquired infections, as they may have weakened immune systems when they are unwell
- Reassures that all patients that are admitted have routine MRSA screening
- Explains results of screening swabs will normally take 2–3 days
- Explains that if test is positive it means colonisation, not infection, and treatment with specific soap, mouthwash and nasal spray for several days is normally sufficient.

Invites daughter to ask questions as they proceed through the consultation and is able to deal with them appropriately

Summarises important areas of the consultation back to the daughter

Formally ends the consultation and ensures appropriate follow-up has been discussed

GLOBAL COMMUNICATION MARK

A B C D E

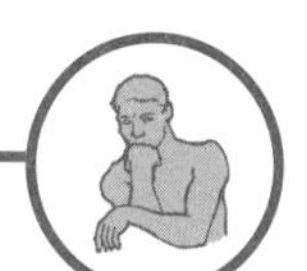

Scenario 17: Reflection and consolidation

History

Mrs Brierly is a 78-year-old lady who presented by ambulance after she slipped at home in her kitchen. She fell onto her left side and hurt her left hip, preventing her from being able to get up. She thinks that she slipped on the tiles, and denies any precipitating symptoms such as chest pain, shortness of breath, headache or dizziness, or the feeling of another stroke.

Her previous medical history includes a stroke, which has left her with a right-sided with motor deficit, tablet-controlled diabetes, hypertension and atrial fibrillation. Her regular medications are aspirin, bisoprolol, ramipril, metformin, gliclazide and simvastatin. She has no allergies. She lives alone in a ground-floor warden-controlled flat, and has a carer once daily to assist her with washing and dressing. She also has a supportive family, who help her with her shopping and cleaning. She mobilises independently with a Zimmer frame.

Examination

When examining orthopaedic injuries such as this, a patient must never be subjected to the pain of unnecessary movement of the injured limb, especially when the diagnosis is self-evident from the deformity that may be visible from the foot of the bed. Early X-ray of the relevant bone or joint will demonstrate the fracture, and if radiographic imaging is unrevealing, and the patient has received adequate analgesia, mobilization of the injured limb may then be undertaken to identify other pathologies such as ligamentous, tendinous or muscular injuries. In all orthopaedic injuries, examination of the limb distal to the injury is essential to assess for any neurological or vascular compromise that may have resulted from the injury.
In this context, where a patient is almost certainly going to require surgical intervention, the initial examination should help identify other comorbidity (particularly respiratory or cardiovascular) that will help inform the anaesthetist, and assist in ongoing management of the patient's care.

Management of hip fractures

Hip fractures are common, especially in the elderly, and are associated with high mortality and morbidity. Many hospitals have dedicated 'hip fracture pathways' to help facilitate early analgesia, expedient X-ray, and surgery at the earliest opportunity. Patients should be mobilised early post-operatively in order to help reduce common complications such as infection, thromboembolism and pressure sores form prolonged bed rest.
Surgical intervention includes dynamic hip screw, hemiarthroplasty and total hip replacement.

Describing fractures on X-ray

There are many ways to describe fractures and various features that an orthopaedic surgeon will need to know when taking a referral.
In general, the following should all be considered and commented on (where present):

- Open or closed
- Spiral, greenstick, transverse, comminuted
- Displacement
- Angulation
- Rotation
- Shortening.

There are many classification systems that help to describe fractures in more specific situations, eg Salter-Harris classification of epiphyseal fractures, Garden classification of femoral neck fractures, Weber classification of ankle fractures.

MRSA

Hospital-acquired infection has been in the glare of the media spotlight over the past few years, particularly regarding MRSA and *Clostridium difficile*. MRSA is now screened for in all elective and emergency admissions, so that infection control measures such as eradication therapy and isolation can be undertaken in those that are colonised. If requiring surgery such as in this case, specific antibiotics (such as vancomycin) will be given if identified preoperatively this is upon induction of anaesthesia to reduce the risk of surgical site infection.

Further reading and web links
Management of fracture neck of femur:
www.sign.ac.uk/pdf/sign111.pdf
MRSA:
www.patient.co.uk/health/MRSA.htm

Scenario 18: 'Heart's a flutter'

Station 1

History *10-minute station*

You are an FY1 doctor on call for general medicine in the Emergency Department. A patient, Mrs Eleanor Cooper, has been referred by her GP with a history of shortness of breath and palpitations since last night.

- **Please take a history from Mrs Cooper and present it to the Medical Registrar on call.**

You will be assessed on the following areas, as well as the content and diagnostic reasoning of your history – take them into account in your presentation.

Professionalism

- Professional appearance (NHS dress code) – including general appearance, hair and jewellery
- Maintains patient and personal safety
- Polite introduction; identifies patient or interviewee correctly; confirms patient's date of birth from name band or other source
- Obtains informal consent; maintains patient's privacy
- Displays empathetic and caring attitudes and behaviours throughout.

Process

- Good organisation and structure; appropriate use of open and closed questions
- Appropriate fluency/rhythm/pace to the interview – this may change depending on environment and acute nature of the problem
- Appropriate time for the patient to respond/reply to questions
- Appropriate acknowledgement of difficult or emotional areas of the patient's history.

Communication skills

- Demonstrates caring and sympathetic attitude
- Asks open questions
- Invites patient to ask questions and answers them appropriately
- Addresses patient's ideas, concerns and expectations.

Station 2

Examination *10-minute station*

Your Registrar has asked you to examine the cardiorespiratory system of Mrs Cooper and make a global assessment of her cardiovascular status.

- **Please present your examination (from information within the station) and give your differential diagnosis.**
- **Your Registrar agrees with your likely differential diagnosis and asked you to order the required basic investigations. Please list your investigations and a reason for each request.**

You will be assessed on the following areas, as well as the content and skills of your examination – take them into account in your presentation.

Professionalism

- Professional appearance; maintains infection control standards, including hand cleaning and appropriate use of gloves and aprons
- Maintains patient and personal safety
- Polite introduction; identifies patient and confirms date of birth from name band or other source
- Obtains informal consent; maintains patient privacy and dignity
- Displays empathetic and caring attitudes and behaviours throughout.

Process

- Appropriate fluency/rhythm/pace to the examination – this may change depending on environment and acute nature of problem
- Good organisation and structure of examination; sensitive and empathetic approach
- Uses appropriate clinical techniques throughout
- Maintains privacy and dignity throughout.

Clinical communication

- Explains proposed examination/procedure; explains examination/procedure as it proceeds
- Offers information in a clear, structured and fluent manner, avoiding jargon
- Listens to patient and responds appropriately
- Demonstrates appropriate body language.

Please read the information below and present this case to the ST4 Medical Registrar as if you were on a busy medical take.
[NB If you have a model do not read this section]

Clinical findings

- o **Patient appears comfortable at rest; not sweaty or dyspnoeic, able to complete sentences**
- o **Observations – HR 140 bpm, BP 105/75 mmHg, RR 18 bpm, sats 96% on air, temperature 36.6 °C**
- o **General examination – peripheral capillary refill time <2 s, pulse irregularly irregular in rhythm, carotid pulse normal in volume, JVP not elevated, apex beat not displaced, no evidence of thyrotoxicosis, no pedal or sacral oedema**
- o **CV examination – heart sounds easily heard, no rubs, no third heart sound**
- o **RS examination – no signs of pulmonary oedema, no effusions**

Station 3

Procedural skills *10-minute station*

Procedure
Your Registrar has asked you to perform an ECG on this patient and then interpret your findings.

- **In Fig 18.1 below please indicate the positions of the following leads: aVR, aVL, aVF, V1, V2, V3, V4, V5, V6.**

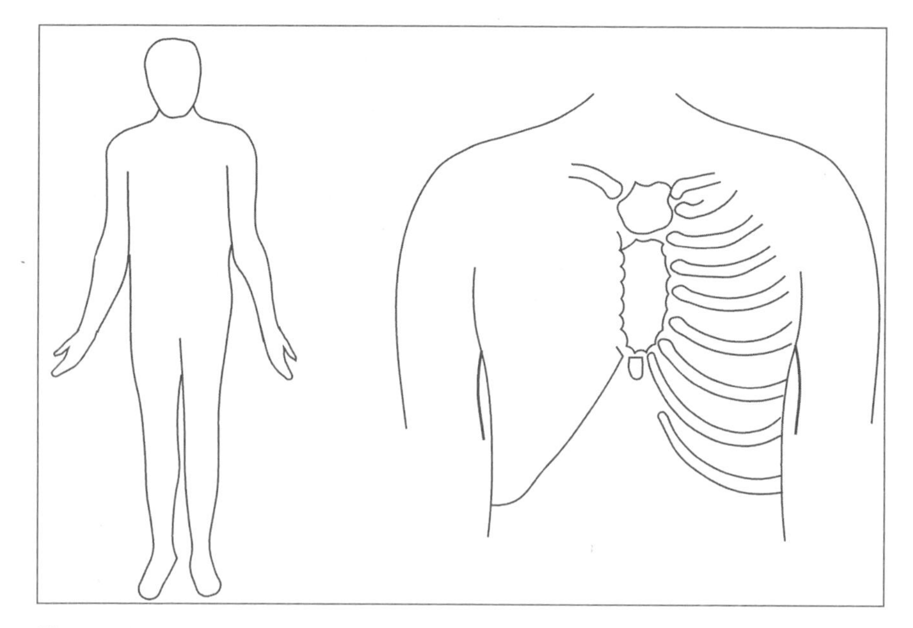

Figure 18.1

Station 4

Data interpretation *10-minute station*

Part 1:

Mrs Cooper is being monitored in Resus and you now have her 12-lead ECG.

- **Please comment on the abnormalities seen in Mrs Cooper's ECG, below.**

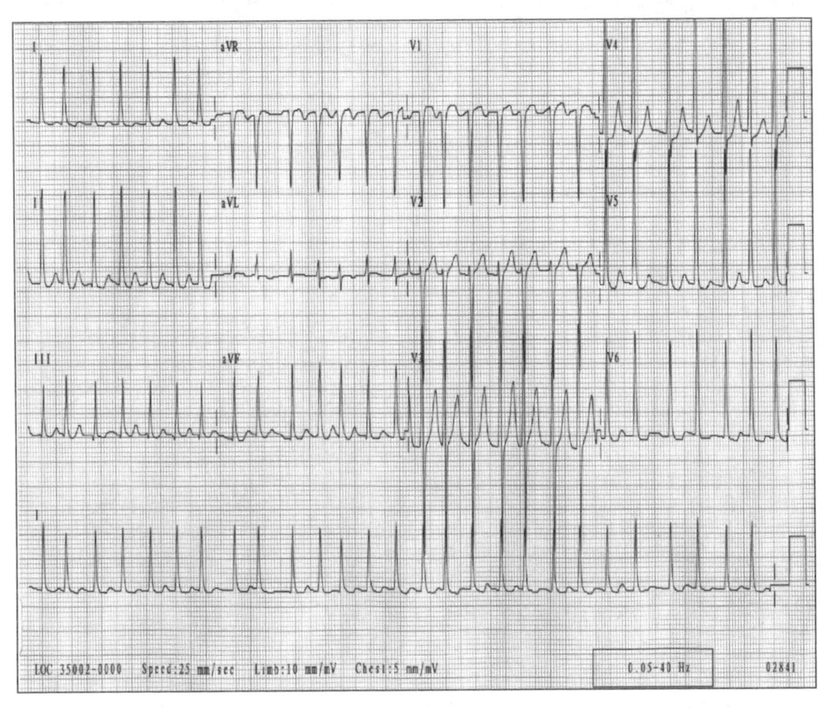

Figure 18.2

- **Please identify an abnormality in Mrs Cooper's blood results, which may have contributed to her arryhthmia.**

  FBC: Hb 12.4 g/dl, MCV 92 fl, WCC 7.6 × 10^9/l, neutrophils 5.3 × 10^9/l, platelets 167 × 10^9/l

  U&Es: Na^+ 131 mmol/l, K^+ 3.2 mmol/l, urea 6.7 mmol/l, creatinine 86 μmol/l

  RBG: 4.7 mmol/l

  Coagulation: INR 1.1, APTT 28 s

  CCa^{2+} 2.23 mol/l, PO_4^- 0.78 mmol/l, Mg 1.02 mmol/l

  TFTs awaited

Mrs Cooper's chest X-ray shows cardiomegaly but no evidence of pulmonary oedema.

Part 2:

- **Your Registrar shows you three further ECGs of patients admitted to the Medical Admissions Unit in the last week. For each one, please describe the abnormalities present on the ECGs and recommend a treatment for each patient.**

Figure 18.3: ECG of a 65-year-old patient with chest pain

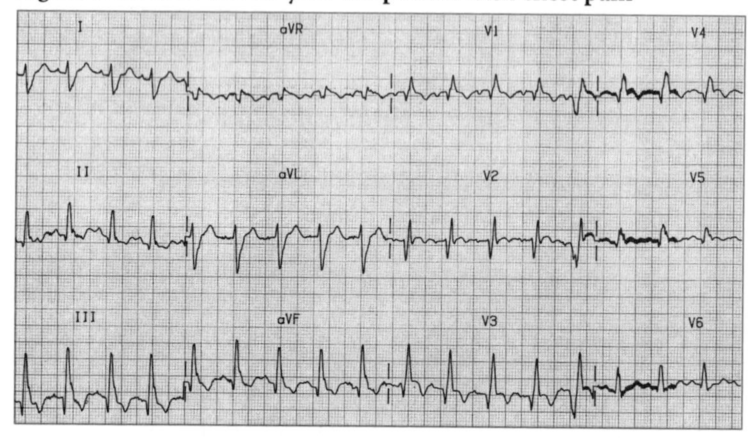

Figure 18.4: ECG of a 57-year-old man with chest pain

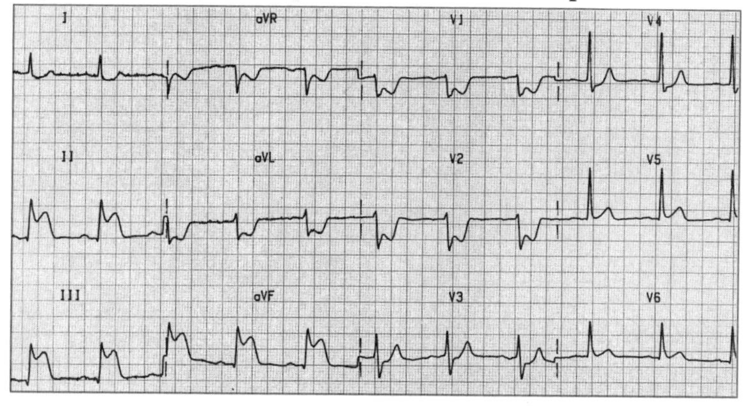

Figure 18.5: ECG of a 65-year-old obese man with hypertension and hypercholesterolaemia, who presented to the Emergency Department with left leg cellulitis

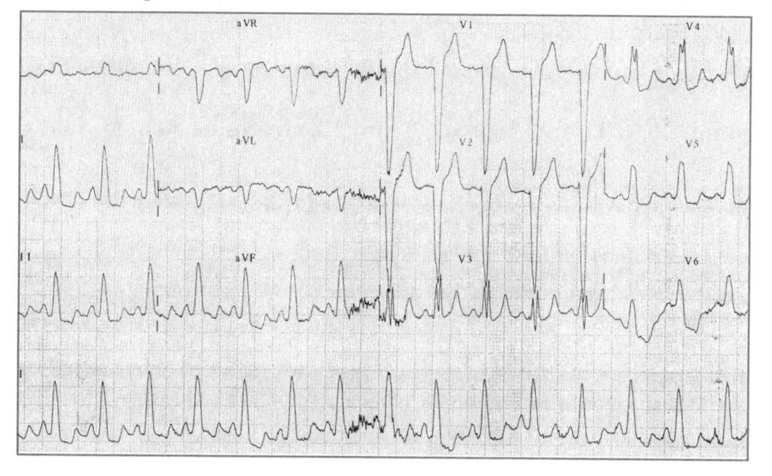

Station 5

Prescribing skills *10-minute station*

Your Registrar has asked you to prescribe the appropriate medication for the initial treatment of Mrs Cooper's episode of atrial fibrillation. Your Registrar wants to chemically cardiovert Mrs Cooper and has decided to use amiodarone as well as supplementing her potassium.

- **Using the BNF and the drug chart provided, write up Mrs Cooper's required medications. Please ensure you prescribe the correct fluid dilutant for her amiodarone infusion.**

Details

Mrs Eleanor Cooper; Hospital No. 50160282; DOB: 10/07/1934;
Drug allergies: β blocker; Weight: approx. 72 kg; Ward: MAU;
Consultant: Dr Burrage; Stat side: amiodarone 300 mg IV STAT;
Infusions: amiodarone 600 mg to run over 24 hours after initial stat infusion of amiodarone via a central line

Remember: DRUG DRs **D**on't **F**orget **S**igning **O**ff (page 373)

Station 6

Clinical communication skills *10-minute station*

Mrs Cooper's heart rate reverts to sinus rhythm after her initial treatment; however, she then develops AF once more 36 hours later on the ward. Her ECHO shows mild MR and a moderately impaired left ventricular function. After the Cardiology Team reviews her, the decision is made to aim to control the rate of AF showing NICE guidelines. As Mrs Cooper is over 75 with hypertension and impaired LV function, the recommendation is that she receive oral anticoagulation with warfarin.

- **Your Consultant has asked you to explain long-term anticoagulation therapy to Mrs Thomas. You should make sure you explain the rationale behind the therapy and that there are no contraindications to the therapy. Also ensure you mention both common and important side-effects of warfarin and any interactions you feel are relevant. Your Consultant has already established that there are no contraindications to anticoagulation with warfarin, so you do not need to spend time on that area of the consultation.**

You should mention the following:
(A) Adherence: important to take dose prescribed as this will keep patient's blood at the correct dilution; stress importance of not missing doses
(B) Effect: stops blood clotting so easily, decreasing the risk of clots forming due to the irregular heartbeat and causing strokes
(C) Side-effects:
- **(a) Haemorrhage – if there are any problems with ongoing bleeding the patient should seek medical attention immediately**
- **(b) Easy bruising**
- **(c) Others (rare) – nausea, rashes.**

(D) Warfarin/anticoagulant clinic: visit once a fortnight; the warfarin book will explain treatment
(E) Interactions with other drugs, eg antibiotics.
You should also attempt to answer any questions Mrs Cooper may have.

Answers

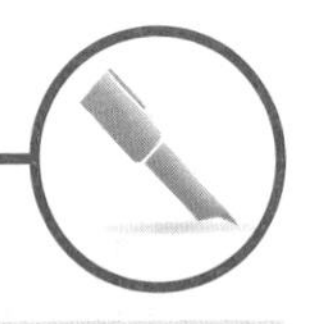

Station 1 – History

Patient script

You are a 78-year-old woman (DOB 10 July 1933) who attended your GP today having developed palpitations last night when doing the washing-up after your evening meal. You are very aware that your heart is racing very quickly. You have been feeling light-headed since it started. You have no chest pain but do feel slightly short of breath. You did not get any sleep last night.

You have never had this sensation before, although you are often very aware of your heartbeat and feel that it 'skips a beat'. You have high blood pressure, for which you have been taking bendroflumethiazide for many years. You were previously given β-blocker medication for your high blood pressure but you developed wheeze so stopped it.

You have previously been treated for depression and anxiety. You have no history of heart attacks, kidney problems, diabetes or thyroid problems. You have been quite well recently. You do not smoke, you drink three to four glasses of wine per week. You drink one or two cups of tea a day. You live alone as your husband died last year. You are a retired teacher.

On direct questioning, the palpations are irregular and if asked you will admit to having had rheumatic fever as a child.

You think that your heart is racing because you are very anxious and that it will sort itself out if you could calm down. You do not like being in hospital and are scared that you will have to stay in the hospital.

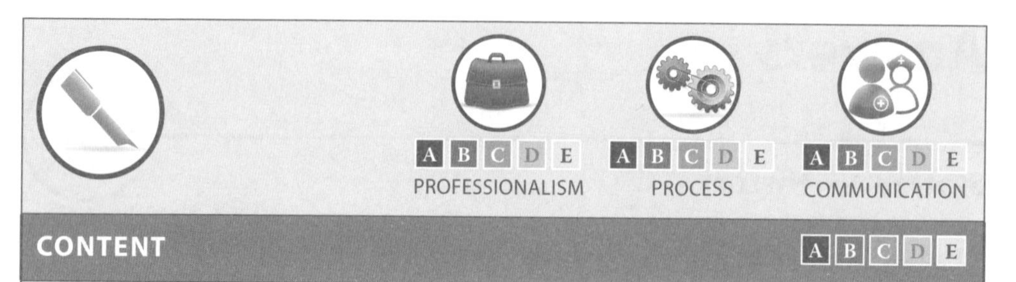

CONTENT

A B C D E

Identifies key information

- Establishes duration of illness – less than 24 hours
- Establishes nature of palpations – rapid and irregular
- Establishes presence of shortness of breath and light-headedness and absence of chest pain.

Includes important negatives, including systemic enquiry

- No previous episodes of significant palpitations
- No precipitating factors – alcohol, caffeine, illicit substances, thyrotoxicosis.

Completing the patient history

- Drug and allergy history: bendroflumethiazide, previously been given a β blocker and developed wheeze
- Previous medical history: hypertension, depression and anxiety, rheumatic fever as child
- Social and occupational history: retired teacher, lives alone, non-smoker, drinks 6–8 units of alcohol per week
- No relevant family history.

Summarises important areas of the history back to the patient

Invites patient to ask questions and is able to deal with them appropriately

Establishes patient's ideas, concerns and expectations

- Establishes that Mrs Cooper believes that her symptoms are related to anxiety and is not keen to stay in hospital.

CLINICAL DIAGNOSTIC REASONING

A B C D E

- **Please present your history**
  - Candidate offers a logical, well-structured account of the history.
- **What is your diagnosis?**
  - Candidate offers the correct diagnosis and appropriate differentials
  - The most likely diagnosis is that of atrial fibrillation
  - The differential diagnosis should include other tachyarrhythmias such as: supraventricular tachycardia, atrial flutter, pulsed VT, anxiety.
- **What are the common precipitants of new-onset atrial fibrillation?**
  - Intercurrent illness such as PE or pneumonia
  - Alcohol excess
  - Caffeine
  - Thyrotoxicosis
  - Mitral valve disease and ischaemic heart disease.

GLOBAL HISTORY MARK

A B C D E

Station 2 – Examination

Patient script

If you are an actor/patient, read the patient history and physical signs fully – when the candidate comes to an abnormal site in their examination, act-out tenderness and/or volunteer the relevant physical sign.

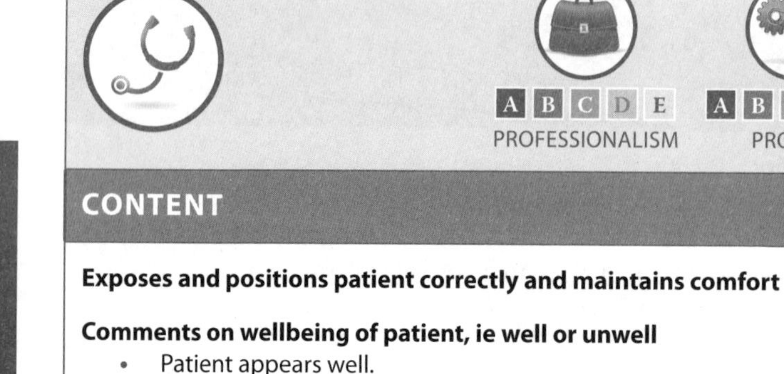

CONTENT

A B C D E

Exposes and positions patient correctly and maintains comfort

Comments on wellbeing of patient, ie well or unwell

- Patient appears well.

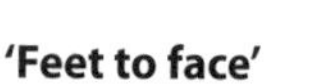

'Feet to face'

- Patient sitting comfortably on trolley
- Patient not sweaty or breathless.

Focused examination

- Inspection – hands: warm and well perfused, no clubbing or evidence of subacute bacterial endocarditis; pulse at wrist irregularly irregular, rate 140, carotid pulse irregular, normal volume and character, JVP not elevated; face: patient not cyanotic, not anaemic; chest: no scars
- Palpation – no palpable heaves or thrills, apex beat not displaced
- Percussion – normal percussion note
- Auscultation – precordium, listens in all areas, including axillae and carotids, normal heart sounds heard; vesicular breath sounds throughout both lung fields.

Asks for appropriate relevant clinical observations

- HR 140 bpm, BP 105/75 mmHg, RR 18 bpm, sats 96% on air, temperature 36.6 °C.

Completes examination by identifying relevant additional clinical signs

- No pedal or sacral oedema.

CLINICAL DIAGNOSTIC REASONING

A B C D E

Correctly identifies the relevant physical signs, including important negative findings

- Does not identify signs that are not present.

Correctly identifies the necessary investigations and gives a valid reason for each

- 12-lead ECG to assess and confirm atrial fibrillation
- IV access and blood tests: U&Es – electrolyte imbalance may precipitate arrhythmia; TFTs – to look for thyrotoxicosis; calcium and magnesium – electrolyte imbalance may precipitate arrhythmia; FBC – to assess for anaemia
- CXR – to assess for evidence of pulmonary oedema.

GLOBAL EXAMINATION MARK

A B C D E

Station 3 – Procedural skills

Procedure: performing an ECG

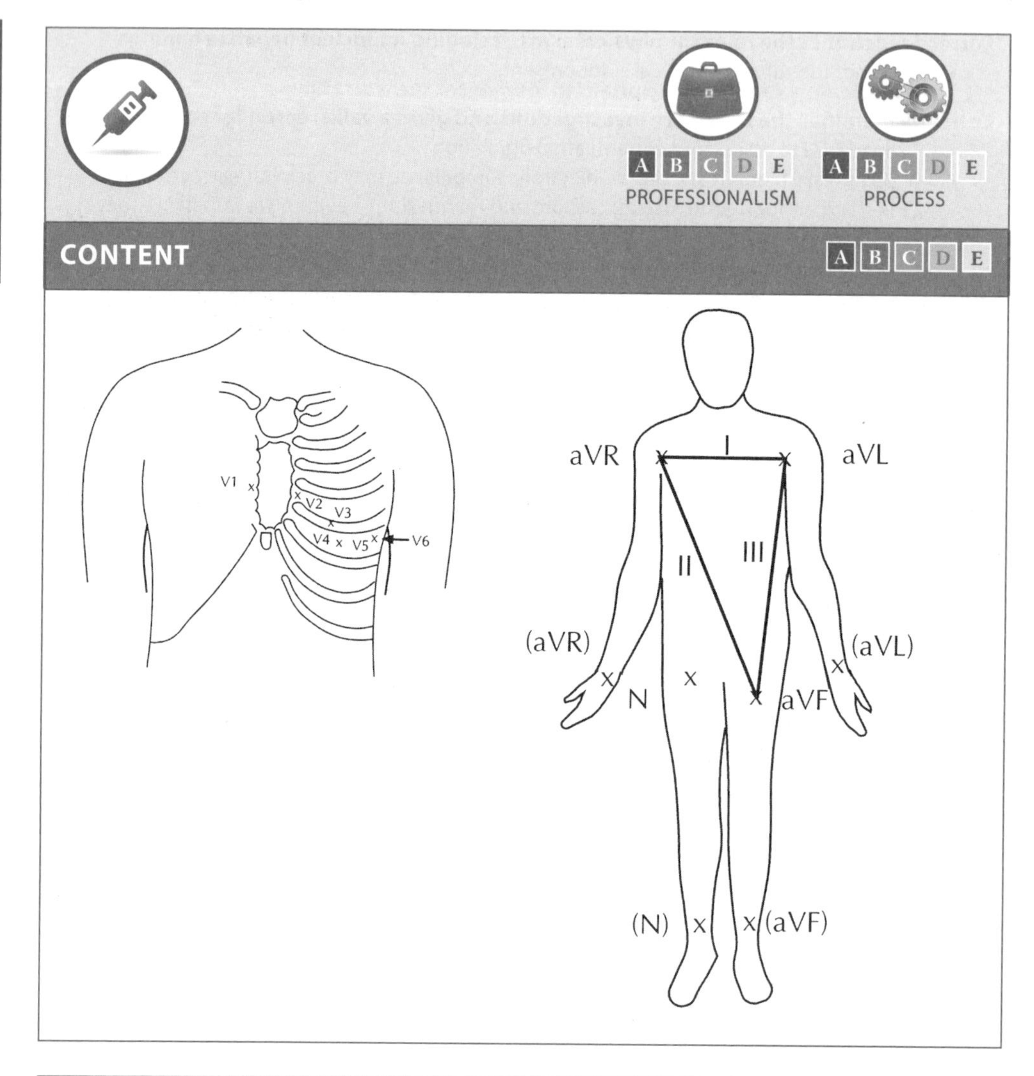

GLOBAL PROCEDURE MARK

A B C D E

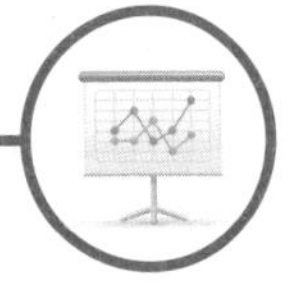

Station 4 – Data interpretation

Part 1:

1. **Absence of P waves, rapid ventricular rate 160, left ventricular hypertrophy**
2. **Hypokalaemia can be a precipitant to new onset tachyarrythmias**

Part 2:

ECG 1 (Figure 18.3)

- Abnormalities – sinus tachycardia, RBBB, S1Q3T3 (S wave prominent in lead I, Q waves and T wave inversion in lead III)
- Diagnosis – pulmonary embolus
- Treatment – treatment dose low molecular weight heparin, if evidence of haemodynamic compromise then for thrombolysis.

ECG 2 (Figure 18.4)

- Abnormalities – inferior ST elevation with ST depression in anterior leads, first-degree heart block
- Diagnosis – inferoposterior acute myocardial infarction
- Treatment – aspirin, clopidogrel and percutaneous coronary intervention in nearest unit (if not available then thrombolysis is second line).

ECG3 (Figure 18.5)

- Abnormalities – LBBB
- Diagnosis – incidental finding of LBBB
- Treatment – LBBB is always a pathological finding, and if it is a new finding associated with a clinical picture suggestive of acute myocardial infarction, it is an indication for PCI/thrombolysis; however, as patient has known ischaemic heart disease and this is an incidental finding, then the most appropriate treatment is not to review old ECGs and to give no specific treatment.

GLOBAL DATA INTERPRETATION MARK A B C D E

SCENARIO 18

Station 5 – Prescribing skills

Check: DRUG DRs Don't Forget Signing Off (page 373)

Allergies, sensitivities and adverse drug reactions					Patient details/addressograph
No known allergies ✓		Initials JAC 312	Gender M (F)		NHS/ Hospital No: 50160282
Not possible to ascertain ☐		Date 13.01	Weight (kg)	Date	
Medicine/substance	Reaction & Severity	Initials & Date			Surname: COOPER
BETABLOCKER	WHEEZE				
			Height		First name: ELEANOR
Alerts			Surface area (m²)		Date of birth: 10.07.33

IN-PATIENT MEDICATION PRESCRIPTION AND ADMINISTRATION RECORD

PasTest HOSPITAL

Consultant	Trainee Dr. Name and Bleep no.	Date of admission	Date chart reboarded	Estimated date of discharge
BURRAGE	JACKSON 312	13.01.12		
This chart is no. 1 of 1	Transcribing Check by Pharmacy Sign .... Date	Ward MAU 1. .... 2.		

Supplementary Medication charts in use: Other (please specify): 1 .... 2 ....

Epidural/PCA ☐ Syringe driver ☐ TPN ☐ Chemotherapy ☐ Insulin sliding scale ☐

Once only medications – loading doses, pre-medication, PGDs or surgical antibiotic propylaxis

Date	Time to be given	Medicine (approved name)	Dose	Route	Signature and bleep no.	Pharmacy	Time given	Given by	Checked by
13.01	18.00	AMIODARONE	300mg	CVL	JAC 312				
		[see infusion chart]							
13.01	18.00	SANDO-K	ṫṫ	PO	JAC 312				

Thromboprophylaxis please prescribe treatment regimens in the regular medications section

Choice of mechanical prophylaxis and leg(s) to be applied to							Enter Time	Enter details below
Graduated elastic compression stockings ☐		Intermittend pneumatic compression device (IPC) ☐	Leg					
			Left	Right	Both			
13.01 Start Date:	End Date:	Signature and Bleep No.	☐	☐	✓			
Start Date:	End Date:	Signature and Bleep No.						

Medication		Dose	Dose Change	Enter Time	Enter details below
CLEXANE		40mg			
Please ensure you have completed the VTE risk assessment form	Date	13.01.12			
	Route	SC			
	Signature	JAC		Instructions	Pharmacy
	Bleep no.	312			

Regular prescriptions continued

Regular medications

	Dose			Medication	Instructions	Signature and bleep no.	Pharmacy
Date	13.01			SANDO-K	UNTIL K+ 7 4.0	JAC 312	
Route	PO						
Signature	SY						

Time		Dose			13	14	15											
06																		
(09)		ii																
12																		
(18)		ii																
22																		
24																		

Regular prescriptions continued

Regular medications

	Dose			Medication	Instructions	Signature and bleep no.	Pharmacy
Date	13.01			AMIODARONE	SEE INFUSION CHART	JAC 312	
Route	OVL						
Signature	SY						

Time		Dose			13	14	15											
06																		
10																		
14																		
18																		
22																		
02																		

Regular prescriptions continued

Regular medications

	Dose			Medication	Instructions	Signature and bleep no.	Pharmacy
Date	13.01			BENDROFLUMETHIAZIDE		JAC 312	
Route	PO						
Signature	SY						

Time		Dose			13	14	15											
06																		
(10)		2.5mg	X	X	X													
14																		
18																		
22																		
02																		

SCENARIO 18

Infusion prescriptions continued										SC = subcutaneous		IVC = intravenous central IVP = intravenous peripheral		
Date & time	Route	Infusion Fluid		Medication		Duration	Rate	Prescriber's signature & bleep no.	Date given	Given by / Added by	Check by	Start time	Finish time	Pharmacy
		Name & strength	Volume	Approved name with expiry / unit number	Dose									
13/01	CVL	5% DEXTROSE Exp: Batch/unit no:	200ml 1.5mg	AMIODARONE run @ 15mg/MIN	300 mg		20 mins	JAC 312						
13/01	CVL	5% DEXTROSE Exp: Batch/unit no:	500ml 1.5mg	AMIODARONE run @ 0.42mg/MIN	600 mg		24 hours	JAC 312						

As required prescriptions			Date	Time	Dose	Route	Date	Time	Dose	Route	Date	Time	Dose	Route	Date	Time	Dose	Route
Drug PARACETAMOL	Allergies Checked	Dose 1g																
Frequency	Max Dose/24 hrs 6 HR	Route PO																
Indication																		
Signature JAC	Pharmacy	Start 13.01																

NOTES

Thromboprophylaxsis – prophylaxsis at usual dose is appropriate, although there is some argument for full dose anti-coagulation as patient is likely to be warfarinised if she remains in atrial fibrillation.

Bendroflumethizide should be withheld in view of electrolyte abnormalities.

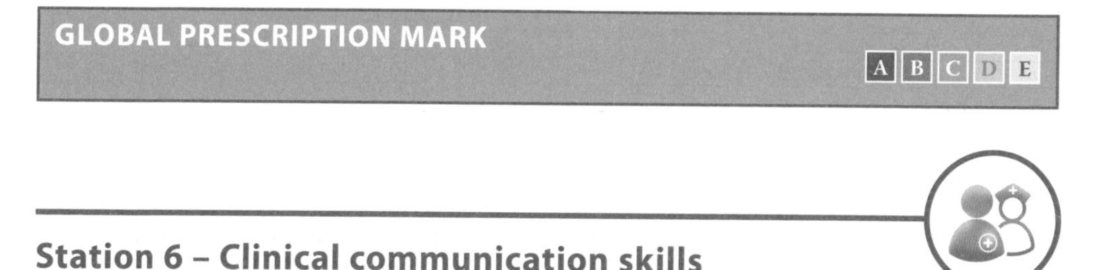

Station 6 – Clinical communication skills

Patient script

You have heard of warfarin, as your neighbour was on it after a 'clot in the leg'. You are unclear why you need this for your irregular heartbeat and are concerned that you have been diagnosed with a blood clot already if you have to take this medication.

You know that your neighbour had to attend for blood tests 'all the time' and you are not keen because of this.

After appropriate explanation of the therapy and its importance you are willing to start therapy.

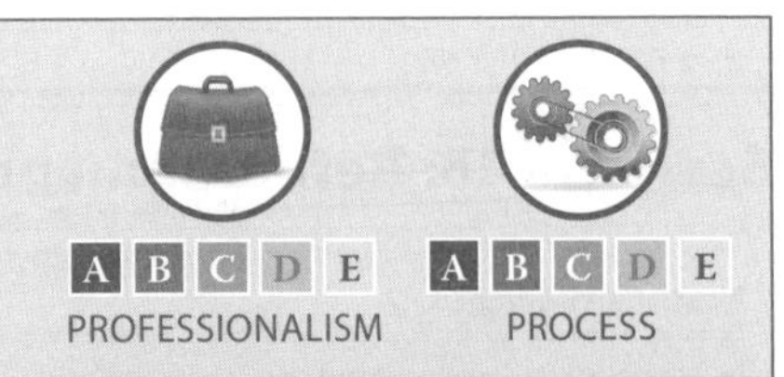

CONTENT

A B C D E

Investigates patient's present level of understanding of scenario

Summarises and confirms what has happened so far

- Explains clearly the link between AF and stroke
- Explains what warfarin is and how it will decrease the risk of future stroke.

Asks what, and how much information the patient would like to be told

Establishes patient's ideas, concerns and expectations

Explains the key, important information

- Why patient is taking treatment – in order to decrease chance of TIA and stroke
- Duration of therapy
- Importance of adherence to therapy
- Side-effects – principally haemorrhage and bruising
- What to do in case of bleeding
- Need for blood monitoring in anticoagulation clinic
- Need to carry anticoagulation book
- Interaction with other medications/alcohol
- Need to tell dentist or other doctors about treatment.

Invites patient to ask questions as they proceed through the consultation and is able to deal with them appropriately

Summarises important areas of the consultation back to the patient

Formally ends the consultation and ensures appropriate follow-up has been discussed

- Explains that anticoagulation clinic will contact patient with an appointment for her first blood test.

GLOBAL COMMUNICATION MARK

A B C D E

Scenario 18: Reflection and consolidation

History

Mrs Cooper is a 78-year-old woman who presents with a less than 24-hour history of sudden onset rapid irregular palpitations. This is associated with shortness of breath and light-headedness but no chest pain. She has not had rapid palpitations before this episode. She has a past medical history of treated hypertension, depression and rheumatic fever as a child. She takes 2.5 mg bendroflumethiazide once daily and is intolerant of β blockers. She is non-smoker, does not take excessive alcohol, illicit substances or excessive caffeine. She does not have symptoms suggestive of thyrotoxicosis. The most likely diagnosis is that of a new tachyarrhthymia, probably new-onset atrial fibrillation.

The history of AF will allow you to categorise AF and help guide ongoing management

- Paroxysmal AF – episodes of AF that terminate spontaneously within 7 days (most episodes last less than 24 hours)
- Persistent AF – episodes of AF that last more than 7 days and may require either pharmacologic or electrical intervention to terminate
- Permanent AF – AF that has persisted for more than 1 year, either because cardioversion has failed or because cardioversion has not been attempted.

Examination

On examination of Mrs Cooper's cardiorespiratory system she appears to be comfortable at rest. She is clinically in atrial fibrillation with an irregularly irregular pulse of 140 beats per minute. She has no evidence of cardiovascular compromise due to her arrhythmia, as evidenced by the adequate BP (105/75) and lack of clinical evidence of cardiac failure. On auscultation of her heart, both heart sounds are normal with no added sounds. Her apex beat is non-displaced. There are no crackles at the bases of the lungs and the JVP is not elevated.

Overall this examination is suggestive of atrial fibrillation or atrial flutter with a variable block. Mrs Cooper is not compromised by this, as there is no evidence of heart failure or hypotension.

The examination of a patient with tachyarrhthymia is focused on whether there is evidence of cardiovascular compromise. If the patient is compromised by her arrhythmia, urgent DC cardioversion is required. The signs of compromise are:

- Shock – hypotension (systolic blood pressure <90 mmHg), pallor, sweating, cold, clammy extremities, confusion or impaired consciousness
- Syncope – transient loss of consciousness due to global reduction in blood flow to the brain
- Myocardial ischaemia – typical ischaemic chest pain and/or evidence of myocardial ischaemia on 12-lead ECG
- Heart failure – pulmonary oedema and/or raised jugular venous pressure (with or without peripheral oedema and liver enlargement).

Investigations and management

The management of chronic AF aims to decrease the chance of thromboembolic events (stroke and TIAs) due to the stagnant blood in the fibrillating atria. This can either be by converting the heart back to sinus rhythm (rhythm control) or rate control and anticoagulation.
The approach of rhythm control is most appropriate in those who:

- Have recent-onset AF
- Are younger than 65
- Have a precipitant that has been successfully treated
- Have a structurally normal heart
- Are very symptomatic from their AF.

The approach of rate control and anticoagulation is most appropriate in those who are in permanent AF with structurally abnormal hearts. Rate control can be achieved with a number of agents that work by increasing the degree of block at the level of the AV node, effectively decreasing the number of atrial impulses that conduct into the ventricles.

- Beta blockers (preferably the 'cardioselective' beta blockers such as metoprolol or bisoprolol)
- Calcium-channel blockers (ie diltiazem or verapamil)
- Digoxin has limited use, apart from in the sedentary elderly patient.

The decision regarding the agent for anticoagulation depends on each patient's co-morbidities and risk factors. The CHADS2-Vasc score takes into account age and co-morbidities such as hypertension, heart failure, diabetes, stroke/TIA, vascular disease and both age and gender. In low-risk patients aspirin can be used for anticoagulation but in higher risk patients anticoagulation with warfarin or new agents such as dabigatran.

Further reading and web links

ALS guidelines on treatment of tachyarrhythmia:
www.resus.org.uk/pages/periarst.pdf
NICE guidelines on treatment of atrial fibrillation:
www.nice.org.uk/CG36
CHA2DS2-VASc score for stroke risk in atrial fibrillation:
www.gpnotebook.co.uk/simplepage.cfm?ID=x20110126111707933383

Scenario 19: 'Don't sweat it'

Station 1

History *10-minute station*

You are a final year medical student attached to the Respiratory Team. You are in clinic and your Consultant has asked you to take a history from Mr Yan Nowak, a 27-year-old man who has been referred by his GP with a fever, night sweats and productive cough.

- **Please take a history and present this, along with your differential diagnosis, to your Consultant.**

You will be assessed on the following areas, as well as the content and diagnostic reasoning of your history – take them into account in your presentation.

Professionalism

- Professional appearance (NHS dress code) – including general appearance, hair and jewellery
- Maintains patient and personal safety
- Polite introduction; identifies patient or interviewee correctly; confirms patient's date of birth from name band or other source
- Obtains informal consent; maintains patient's privacy
- Displays empathetic and caring attitudes and behaviours throughout.

Process

- Good organisation and structure; appropriate use of open and closed questions
- Appropriate fluency/rhythm/pace to the interview – this may change depending on environment and acute nature of the problem
- Appropriate time for the patient to respond/reply to questions
- Appropriate acknowledgement of difficult or emotional areas of the patient's history.

Communication skills

- Demonstrates caring and sympathetic attitude
- Asks open questions
- Invites patient to ask questions and answers them appropriately
- Addresses patient's ideas, concerns and expectations.

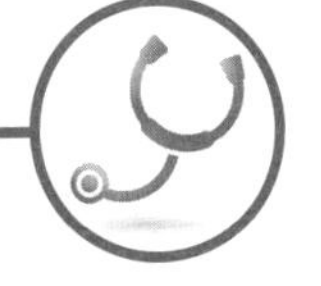

Station 2

Examination *10-minute station*

After presenting your history, you have been asked to complete a formal respiratory system examination in front of your Consultant in order to aid your preparation for your upcoming final year examinations.

- **You have 10 minutes to perform your examination (using the information within the station) and will be expected to present your positive findings once you have finished.**

You will be assessed on the following areas, as well as the content and skills of your examination – take them into account in your presentation.

Professionalism

- Professional appearance; maintains infection control standards, including hand cleaning and appropriate use of gloves and aprons
- Maintains patient and personal safety
- Polite introduction; identifies patient and confirms date of birth from name band or other source
- Obtains informal consent; maintains patient privacy and dignity
- Displays empathetic and caring attitudes and behaviours throughout.

Process

- Appropriate fluency/rhythm/pace to the examination – this may change depending on environment and acute nature of problem
- Good organisation and structure of examination; sensitive and empathetic approach
- Uses appropriate clinical techniques throughout
- Maintains privacy and dignity throughout.

Clinical communication

- Explains proposed examination/procedure; explains examination/procedure as it proceeds
- Offers information in a clear, structured and fluent manner, avoiding jargon
- Listens to patient and responds appropriately
- Demonstrates appropriate body language.

Please read the information below before presenting this case to the Respiratory Consultant in the clinic.
[NB If you have a model do not read this section]

Clinical findings

- Patient appears comfortable at rest, is not sweaty or dyspnoeic, able to complete sentences
- Observations – HR 92 bpm, BP 110/65 mmHg, RR 14 bpm, O_2 sats 95% on air, temperature 37.7 °C
- General examination – thin but not cachectic, smoothly enlarged lymph nodes in the right supra-clavicular fossa, not cyanosed, in hands normal capillary refill, no flap of CO_2 retention, no clubbing
- Chest examination – trachea central, decreased right side chest expansion, stony dull percussion note at right base but normal in other zones, reduced breath sounds at right base but vesicular in all other zones, reduced vocal resonance at right base
- Additional signs – no hepatomegaly or peripheral oedema, heart signs audible and normal

Station 3

Data interpretation *10-minute station*

You have requested a chest X-ray for Mr Nowak. Whilst in clinic your conultant has also asked you to review three chest X-rays of other patients in the Respiratory clinic, as well as that of Mr Nowak.

- Please state whether the following statements regarding the chest X-rays are true or false

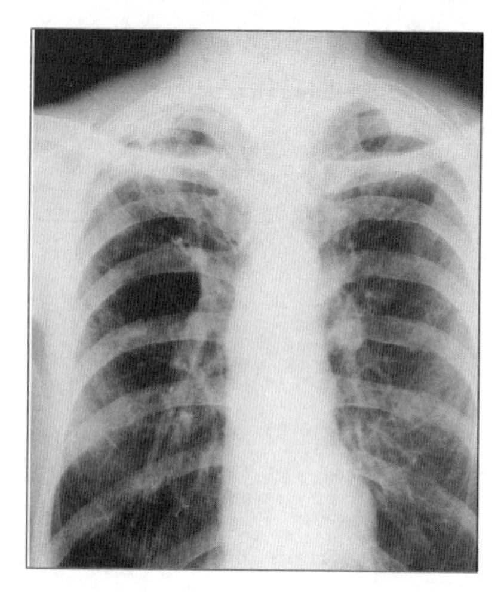

Figure 19.1 CXR 1

1. This is a PA CXR.
2. The hilar are enlarged.
3. There is pulmonary pruning.
4. There is hyperexpansion of the lung.
5. This patient has evidence of apical fibrosis.

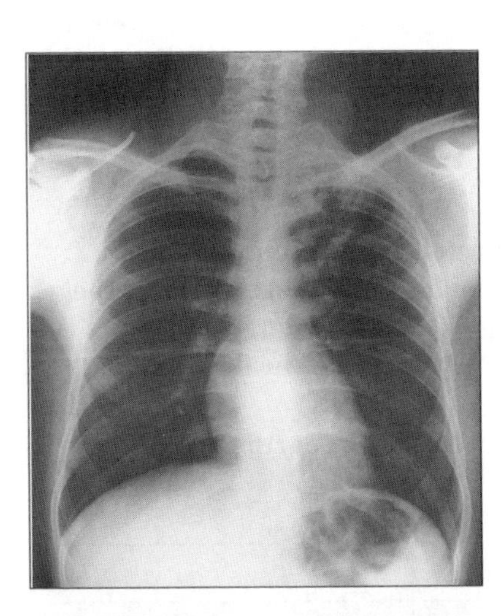

Figure 19.2 CXR 2

1. This CXR is poorly penetrated.
2. The radiograph is rotated.
3. There is cavitation in the left upper lobe.
4. One cause of this appearance is tuberculosis.
5. The patient requires a bronchoscopy.

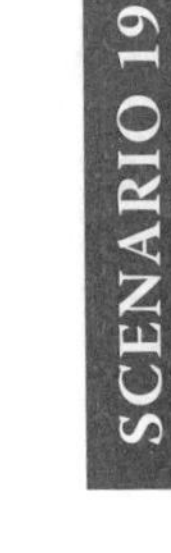

Figure 19.3 CXR 3

1. This CXR shows a left-sided pleural plaque.
2. This CXR shows left lower lobe collapse.
3. This CXR shows a haemothorax.
4. There is evidence of chronic lung disease on this CXR.
5. There is a large left-side pleural effusion.

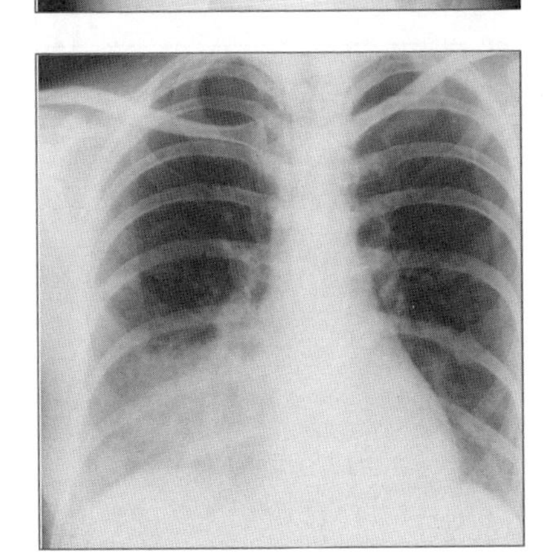

Figure 19.4 CXR 4

1. This is a well-penetrated CXR.
2. The cardiothoracic ratio is normal.
3. There is a right-sided pneumothorax.
4. There is a right-sided pleural effusion.
5. The lung fields are hyperexpanded.

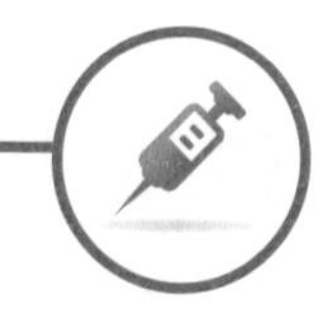

Station 4

Procedural skills *10-minute station*

The ST5 Registrar in respiratory medicine has performed an ultrasound-guided aspiration of pleural fluid for diagnostic purposes. You have been asked to label the samples of fluid and request the appropriate tests.

- **Please complete the request forms for the tests you require on the fluid that has been aspirated.**

Mr Yan Nowak; Hospital No. 98734561; DOB: 16/11/1984; Department: Outpatients; Consultant: Dr Malir

Hospital		Patient details	
Laboratory department		Name	
Date		DOB	
		Hospital No.	
Clinical details		Consultant	
Tests required			
Person requesting tests			
Contact details		Signature	

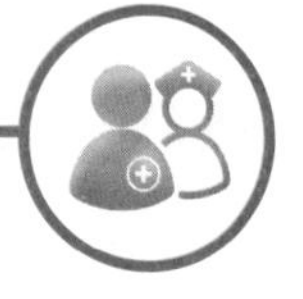

Station 5

Clinical communication skills *10-minute station*

Mr Nowak has been diagnosed with fully sensitive pulmonary TB. This has been explained to him by the Respiratory Specialist Nurse; however, Mr Nowak is about to start on his therapy and still has some questions.

- **Please explain the basic outline of Mr Nowak's therapy for the next 6 months and answer any concerns/questions that may arise. Include the following information in your explanation:**
    1. **Therapy will last 6 months**
    2. **He will be on four medications in a combination pill; please explain the common side-effects of these medications and when he should contact the specialist TB team:**
       Isoniazid – 6 months
       Rifampicin – 6 months
       Ethambutol – first 2 months only
       Pyrazinamide – first 2 months only
    3. **Any monitoring that will need to occur**
    4. **Importance of completing therapy for patient and those around him.**

Answers

Station 1 – History

Patient script

You are Mr Yan Nowak, a 27-year-old builder originally from Poland (DOB 16 November 1984). You have been living in the UK for 6 months.

You have felt unwell for approximately 2 months but have continued to work. Initially you noticed that you had a dry cough, but this has become productive over the last 2 weeks. Your sputum is greenish and increasing in quantity and you have noticed that there is some fresh blood streaked within it, which is worrying you. You attended your GP as you had become increasingly short of breath on exertion over the last 2 weeks.

You have no chest pain or coryzal symptoms. You are having fevers and episodes of sweating every night, to the point that you are changing your bedclothes daily. You have also noticed that you have lost some weight, as your trousers are much looser than they were, despite a stable appetite. You have no headaches, visual disturbances, rashes or gastrointestinal upset. You have noticed some lumps on the side of your neck over the last few months.

You live in a very cramped flat with five other men. One of your flatmates had similar symptoms, but he left for a job in Manchester 2 weeks ago. You drink heavily on the weekends (approximately 30–40 units) and you have smoked 15–20 cigarettes per day for 12 years. You admit to having a poor diet. You have no medical history of note, and no regular medication or allergies. You know of no significant illnesses in your family. You never had TB as a child. You do not recall having the BCG vaccination. You have never had an HIV test, and you have never travelled outside Europe.

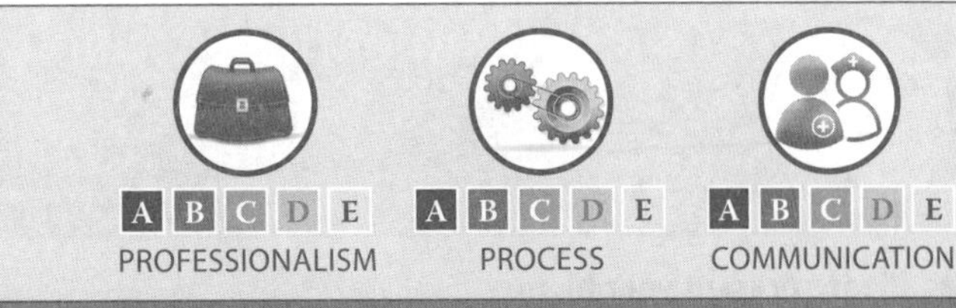

CONTENT

A B C D E

Identifies key information

- Duration of illness
- Presence of productive cough – including characteristics of sputum and haemoptysis
- Presence of night sweats and fever
- Presence of systemic upset – weight loss
- Presence of shortness of breath and decreased exercise tolerance.

Includes important negatives, including systemic enquiry

- Full and systematic review of systems to ascertain absence of headaches, visual disturbances, rashes or gastrointestinal upset
- No lymphadenopathy.

Identifies key information from rest of history

Relevant factors from employment, housing, social support

- Overcrowding
- Exposure in household to possible TB contacts
- Immunosuppression – assess for possible HIV
- Poor diet and excess alcohol intake
- Lack of vaccination.

Completing the patient history

- Drug and allergy history: nil regular and no allergies
- Previous medical history: nil of note, no childhood TB
- Social and occupational history: alcohol intake 30–40 units per week, cigarette smoking 15–20 per day
- No relevant family history.

Summarises important areas of the history back to the patient

Invites patient to ask questions and is able to deal with them appropriately

Establishes patient's ideas, concerns and expectations

- Mr Nowak does not believe he is very unwell and is keen to just 'get back to work'.

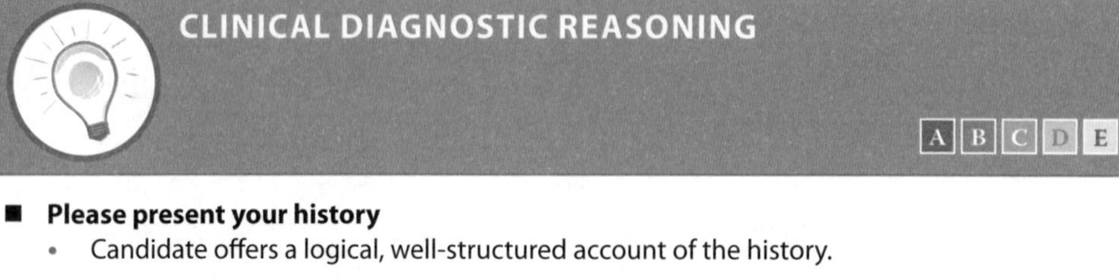

- **Please present your history**
  - Candidate offers a logical, well-structured account of the history.
- **What is your diagnosis?**
  - The combination of night sweats, fever and haemoptysis makes a diagnosis of pulmonary tuberculosis most likely, although other respiratory infections such as atypical pneumonia should be considered along with possible lymphoma.
- **What is your initial management plan?**
  - Examination of patient
  - Likely to require CXR
  - Sputum examination for MC&S as well as acid-fast bacilli
  - Basic blood tests – FBC, LFTs, clotting profile.

Demonstrates clear and logical diagnostic reasoning

GLOBAL HISTORY MARK

A B C D E

Station 2 – Examination

Patient script

If you are an actor/patient, read the patient history and physical signs fully – when the candidate comes to an abnormal site in their examination, act-out tenderness and/or volunteer the relevant physical sign.

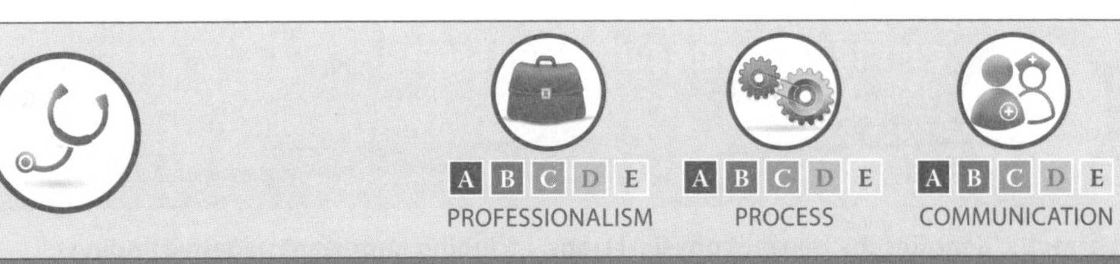

CONTENT

A B C D E

Exposes and positions patient correctly and maintains comfort

- Patient should be exposed to the waist and sitting at 45 degrees.

Comments on wellbeing of patient, ie well or unwell

'Feet to face'

- Observes and comments on patient and surroundings from foot of bed.

Asks for appropriate relevant clinical observations

- BP 110/65 mmHg, HR 92 bpm, RR 14 bpm, O_2 sats 95% on air, temperature 37.7 °C

Focused examination

- Inspection – assesses for hand and nails for signs such as clubbing, palmar erythema; assesses neck for lymphadenopathy in all regions, supra-clavicular, cervical, sub-mental, pre- and post-auricular and occipital, right supra-clavicular lymph nodes; assesses trachea
- Palpation – assesses chest expansion anteriorly and posteriorly
- Percussion – in all zones, including apices; examines for any change in tactile vocal resonance
- Auscultation – auscultates in all areas, no breath sounds audible at right base.

Completes examination

- Listens to heart and assesses for apex beat and JVP (signs of pericardial tamponade/ pericardial effusion)
- Palpates for hepatosplenomegaly
- Asks to examine for systemic lymphadenopathy.

Thanks patient, offers assistance, maintains patient's dignity and privacy until they are dressed

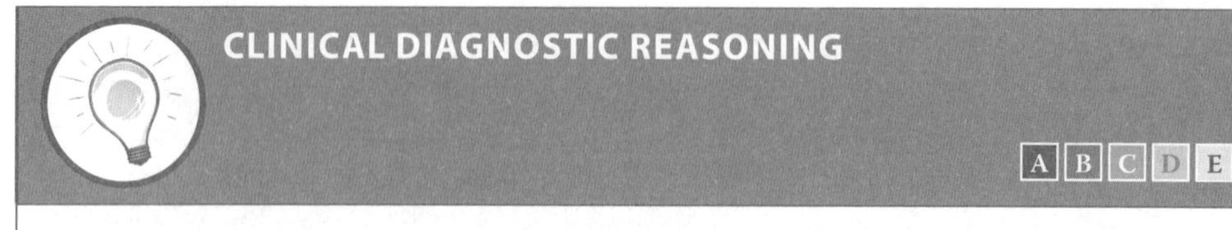

Correctly identifies the relevant physical signs, including important negative findings

- Does not identify signs that are not present.

Correctly identifies the appropriate tests that should be requested on the sputum that Mr Nowak is producing

- Sputum MC&S
- Sputum for acid-fast bacilli and TB culture.

GLOBAL EXAMINATION MARK

A B C D E

Station 3 – Data interpretation

CXR 1

1 True 2 False 3 False 4 True 5 True

This is a PA poorly penetrated CXR showing hyperexpanded lung fields and flattened diaphragms. There is marked pulmonary apical fibrosis resulting in the hilar being pulled upwards towards the apices. The fibrosis was secondary to TB in this patient; other causes include pneumoconiosis, ankylosing spondylitis, rheumatoid arthritis and malignancy.

CXR 2

1 False 2 False 3 True 4 True 5 False

This is a well-penetrated, well-centred PA chest radiograph showing a cavitating area in the left apex. The commonest cause of this appearance is tuberculosis. Other causes of cavitation include *Staphylococcus, Klebsiella, Pseudomonas,* fungal infection and malignancy.

CXR 3

1 False 2 False 3 False 4 False 5 True

This chest X-ray shows a left side pleural effusion. Causes of pleural effusions should be divided by their protein content, into transudates (<30 g/l) and exudates (>30 g/l). However, these criteria can misidentify up to a quarter of transudates as exudates, especially in those with a low serum albumin. Hence the Lights criteria for pleural effusion are used to compare the levels of LDH and protein in the pleural fluid to the serum levels. Exudative pleural effusions meet at least one of the following criteria, where as transudative pleural effusions meet none:

- pleural fluid protein/serum protein >0.5
- pleural fluid LDH/serum LDH >0.6
- pleural fluid LDH more than two-thirds normal upper limit for serum.

CXR 4

1 True 2 False 3 False 4 False 5 False

This is a well-penetrated, slightly rotated chest radiograph showing a right middle lobe pneumonia, with loss of definition of the right heart border. A lateral view would show the consolidated lobe. The heart and left lung are normal.

GLOBAL DATA INTERPRETATION MARK A B C D E

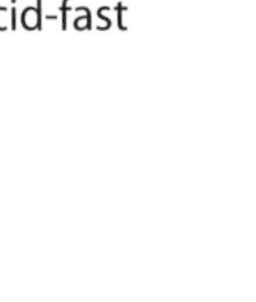

Station 4 – Procedural skills

Requests the correct tests

- Biochemistry – glucose, protein, LDH, amylase
- Cytology – to exclude a malignant cause of effusion
- Microbiology – samples for microscopy, culture and sensitivity (MC&S) and for acid-fast bacilli (microscopy and culture).

Includes the correct information on each request form

- Patient's name
- Patient's DOB
- Patient's medical record no.
- Date of request
- Concise clinical details – right-side pleural effusion ?TB
- Signature and contact details of person requesting test.

GLOBAL PROCEDURE MARK A B C D E

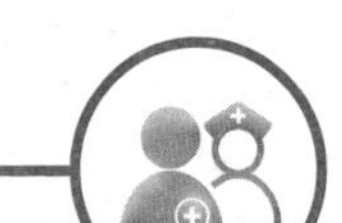

Station 5 – Clinical communication skills

Patient script

You are a 27-year-old man with a recent diagnosis of pulmonary TB. You understand that you will need to take some medications, but you are unsure if this is all necessary as you are feeling quite well. You are concerned with side-effects of medications and just want to get back to work as soon as possible. You are unaware of how you caught TB and how contagious it is. If this is explained clearly to you, you agree to undertake the therapy and attend for follow-up.

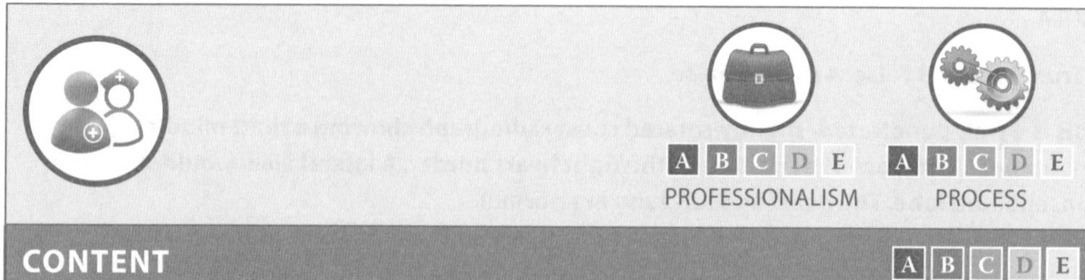

CONTENT

A B C D E

Investigates patient's present level of understanding of scenario

Summarises and confirms what has happened so far

- Establishes understanding of TB and emphasises that it is a transmissible disease
- Establishes that TB treatment is curative but treatment must be completed
- Raises issue of contact tracing and confirms this has taken place.

Establishes patient's ideas, concerns and expectations

- Need for full 6 months of therapy.

Explains the key, important information

- Duration of therapy
- Blood tests that occur at start, after 2 weeks and throughout treatment
- Common side-effects of medications – isoniazid (hepatitis and peripheral neuropathy 'tingling in fingers and toes'); rifampicin (hepatitis and turning all secretions orange-pink); ethambutol (retro-bulbar neuritis – loss of colour vision is first sign); pyrazinamide (hepatitis)
- Explains if any of the above side-effects occur to call TB team.

Invites patient to ask questions as they proceed through the consultation and is able to deal with them appropriately

Summarises important areas of the consultation back to the patient

Formally ends the consultation and ensures appropriate follow-up has been discussed

- Follow-up with Respiratory Specialist Nurse
- Ensure baseline LFTs/FBC/U&E have been scheduled.

GLOBAL COMMUNICATION MARK

A B C D E

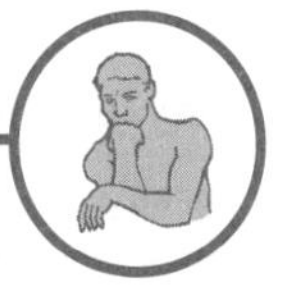

Scenario 19: Reflection and consolidation

History

Mr Nowak is a 27-year-old builder who presents with a 2-month history of intermittent fever, night sweats and a cough productive of sputum. He describes some fresh haemoptysis mixed in with the green sputum he is expectorating. He has also had weight loss despite a stable food intake. He describes no lymphadenopathy, headache or gastrointestinal symptoms. He denies any previous medical history, including previous TB. He has not had a BCG vaccination against TB.

He lives in cramped conditions and is a heavy smoker (12 pack year history) and binges on alcohol most weekends. His flatmate had similar symptoms but he has now left and his diagnosis is not clear.

The most likely diagnosis is that of pulmonary tuberculosis, but a sensible differential diagnosis would include atypical pulmonary infections, bronchiectasis or lung malignancy.

Examination

On examination of the respiratory system of Mr Nowak, he is comfortable at rest, with a respiratory rate of 14, and saturations of 95% on room air. He appears thin but not cachectic. On inspection of his hands he is has no evidence of clubbing and no stigmata of respiratory disease. His trachea is central and he has palpable lymph nodes in the right supra-clavicular fossa. He has reduced chest expansion on the right with associated stony dull percussion note, absent breath sounds and reduced tactile vocal resonance. He has no hepatomegaly. These signs are suggestive of a right-sided pleural effusion.

Tuberculosis is a caused by the organism *Mycobacterium tuberculosis*. The primary infection is usually when alveolar macrophages ingest the organism. The mycobacterium then multiplies at a slow rate and then spreads via the lymphatic vessels and regional lymph nodes. This infection, 'the primary complex', should then be controlled by an immune-competent patient, leaving a calcified inactive lesion seen on chest X-ray. However, this complex can cause local symptoms, such as persistent cough or bronchial obstruction. It may also lead to primary progressive TB when the duplication of the mycobacterium is not controlled and can spread (via the lymphatics and bloodstream). This leads to both many pulmonary and extrapulmonary manifestations of TB.

The extrapulmomary manifestations are wide and varied. They include:

- Pericarditis and pericardial effusion
- Osteomyelitis and septic arthritis, even leading to spinal cord compression
- TB meningitis or a tuberculoma
- Skin manifestations such as lupus vulgaris and erythema nodosum.

Close examination and a high clinical suspicion of occult TB is needed in order not to miss this very treatable infection.

Investigations

The investigation of pleural effusions is a common problem on the acute medical take. The key to identify the aetiology of the effusions and classify whether or it is an exudate or a transudate.

Transudates tend to be bilateral and are caused by the 'failures':

- Congestive cardiac failure
- Renal failure with associated fluid overload
- End-stage liver failure
- Thyroid 'failure' in myoedema coma.

Exudates are more likely to be unilateral and caused by local disease processes:

- Parapneumonic effusion
- Empyema
- TB
- Malignancy – lung, pleural and metastatic disease.

Management

TB is a notifiable disease and its incidence in the UK is increasing owing to factors such as increased immigration from areas where TB is endemic and increased numbers of immunocompromised patients with HIV-AIDS. Only patients with open pulmonary TB are able to transmit the disease. Also the disease is only transmissible to those who have close contact with those with TB. Therefore contact tracing is limited to those who have had close contact with a patient diagnosed with TB.

Further reading and web links
NICE guidelines TB treatment:
www.nice.org.uk/CG033
TB alert – national TB charity:
www.tbalert.org

Scenario 20: 'Unsteady on my feet'

Station 1

History *10-minute station*

You are an FY1 doctor attached to the General Neurology Team. You are in the Outpatients Clinic and your Consultant has asked you to take a history from Mr Brian Kemp, who has been referred by his GP with a history of movement difficulty and unsteady gait over the last 9 months.

- **Please take a history from Mr Kemp and then be prepared to present your history and differential diagnosis to your Consultant.**

You will be assessed on the following areas, as well as the content and diagnostic reasoning of your history – take them into account in your presentation.

Professionalism

- Professional appearance (NHS dress code) – including general appearance, hair and jewellery
- Maintains patient and personal safety
- Polite introduction; identifies patient or interviewee correctly; confirms patient's date of birth from name band or other source
- Obtains informal consent; maintains patient's privacy
- Displays empathetic and caring attitudes and behaviours throughout.

Process

- Good organisation and structure; appropriate use of open and closed questions
- Appropriate fluency/rhythm/pace to the interview – this may change depending on environment and acute nature of the problem
- Appropriate time for the patient to respond/reply to questions
- Appropriate acknowledgement of difficult or emotional areas of the patient's history.

Communication skills

- Demonstrates caring and sympathetic attitude
- Asks open questions
- Invites patient to ask questions and answers them appropriately
- Addresses patient's ideas, concerns and expectations.

Station 2

Examination *10-minute station*

Your Consultant has asked you to perform a neurological examination of the upper and lower limbs of Mr Kemp.

- **Please only assess the motor system. You can perform any further examinations (using information from within the station) you think are indicated.**

You will be assessed on the following areas, as well as the content and skills of your examination – take them into account in your presentation.

Professionalism

- Professional appearance; maintains infection control standards, including hand cleaning and appropriate use of gloves and aprons
- Maintains patient and personal safety
- Polite introduction; identifies patient and confirms date of birth from name band or other source
- Obtains informal consent; maintains patient privacy and dignity
- Displays empathetic and caring attitudes and behaviours throughout.

Process

- Appropriate fluency/rhythm/pace to the examination – this may change depending on environment and acute nature of problem
- Good organisation and structure of examination; sensitive and empathetic approach
- Uses appropriate clinical techniques throughout
- Maintains privacy and dignity throughout.

Clinical communication

- Explains proposed examination/procedure; explains examination/procedure as it proceeds
- Offers information in a clear, structured and fluent manner, avoiding jargon
- Listens to patient and responds appropriately
- Demonstrates appropriate body language.

Please read the information below before presenting this case to the Consultant Neurologist. ***[NB If you have a model do not read this section]***

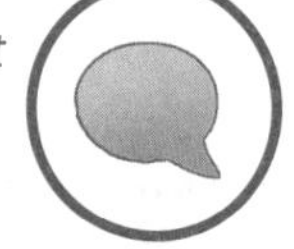

Clinical findings

- Patient appears comfortable at rest; not sweaty or dyspnoeic, able to complete sentences
- Observations – HR 75 bpm, BP 140/70 mmHg, RR 18 bpm, O_2 sats 97% on air, temperature 36.6 °C
- General examination – asymmetrical resting tremor affecting the right hand, no wasting or fasciculations, face has reduced expression
- Motor examination of upper limbs – tone of left arm normal, right arm increased tone with 'cogwheel' rigidity; power normal bilaterally; co-ordination: no pastpointing, dysdiadochokinesis, tremor improves on movement
- Motor examination of lower limbs – tone normal; power normal; co-ordination normal; difficulty initiating movement, hesitant gait with reduced arm swing
- Romberg's test negative
- Handwriting small and illegible when tested.

Station 3

Data interpretation *10-minute station*

Part 1:

Your Consultant is happy with your assessment of Mr Kemp and agrees that the diagnosis is likely to be idiopathic Parkinson's disease. However, the triad of symptoms that define parkinsonism (bradykinesia, rigidity and tremor) are seen in a number of other clinical situations.

A MPTP poisoning
B Multiple system atrophy
C Idiopathic Parkinson's disease
D Drug-induced parkinsonism
E Progressive supra-nuclear palsy
F Cortico-basilar degeneration
G Vascular parkinsonism
H Diffuse Lewy body disease
I Normal pressure hydrocephalus
J Wilson's disease

- Please match each of the clinical scenarios with the most likely diagnosis (A–J) below.

1. A 73-year-old man with cognitive decline, vivid hallucinations and bradykinesia.
2. A 62-year-old man with balance problems, erectile dysfunction and urinary incontinence.
3. An 83-year-old man with falls, symmetrical rigidity, pronounced gait dysfunction with a history of AF, hypertension and a previous TIA.
4. A 28-year-old man with rigidity, tremor, mood alteration and deranged LFTs.
5. A 45-year-old man with a history of schizophrenia with uncontrollable facial movement, rigidity and falls.

SCENARIO 20

Part 2:
Mr Kemp is to be started on a trial of levodopa, one of the treatments for Parkinson's disease. Your Consultant has explained to you about the different pharmacological treatments for Parkinson's disease.

- **Please match the following treatments for Parkinson's and their common side-effects.**

Treatment	Mechanism of action	Side-effect
1 Levodopa	(a) Reduces dopamine breakdown	(A) Postural hypotension and 'on–off' dyskinesia
2 Dopamine agonist (cabergoline, bromocriptine)	(b) Provides background dopamine concentration	(B) Pulmonary fibrosis
3 Catechol-*O*-methyltransferase inhibitors (entacapone)	(c) Increases cerebral dopamine concentration	(C) Risk of hepatic failure
4 Procyclidine	(d) Anticholinergic agent decreases tremor	(D) Confusion, dry mouth and blurred vision

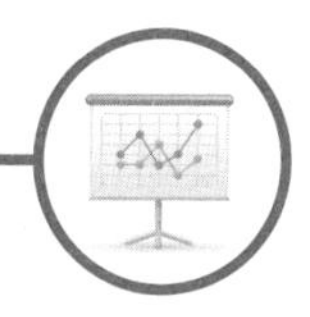

Station 4

Prescribing skills *10-minute station*

- **Using a BNF and the FP10 prescription provided, please prescribe the medication for Mr Kemp's trial of medication on this outpatient script. Please select and prescribe a combination therapy of levodopa and dopa decarboxylase inhibitor three times per day for 1 month.**

Details

Mr Brian Kemp; DOB: 10/05/1958; Address: 8 Winchester Road, London; No known drug allergies; NHS No. 789456213; FBC, U&Es and LFTs normal

Remember: DRUG DRs Don't Forget Signing Off (page 373)

Station 5

Clinical communication skills *10-minute station*

- **Mr Kemp is to begin a trial of pharmacological therapy for his Parkinson's disease. His diagnosis has been explained to him, but your Consultant would like you to explain his new medications to him, including any important side-effects. Please address any questions or concerns that Mr Kemp raises.**

Medications

Sinemet® CR (50–200) – levodopa and dopa decarboxylase inhibitor

Two tablets at 0600 h, 1200 h and 1600 h

Benefits – increased dopamine in the brain, leading to decreased disability and increased functional ability; they do not stop disease progression or outcome.

Side-effects

Common – postural hypotension, gastrointestinal upset, mood lability

Important – impulsivity can be a problem

Over years on–off dyskinesia can occur

This is a trial of therapy and alterations will be made depending on initial response; the response will be monitored in a movement disorder clinic.

Answers

Station 1 – History

Patient script

You are Mr Brian Kemp, a 53-year-old accountant (DOB 10 May 1958), who attended your GP with increasingly difficult movement over the last 9 months. You initially noticed that you found it difficult to 'get going' when you got out of bed in the morning. This has become more noticeable in recent months. It feels as though you are stiff but once you start moving there is less resistance. However, you do feel that you are not as steady on walking and have fallen twice when you have had to make an abrupt turn. You have recently noticed that you have some shaking of your hands, mostly on the right, which is most obvious when you are sitting still, eg watching television. It disappears as soon as you are doing anything purposeful. Doing some day-to-day activities, such as chopping food, has become difficult, as you notice that you get less co-ordinated and are tired with repetitive movement.

You have no weakness in your arms or legs; you have no abnormal sensation in your arms or legs; you have had no headaches/problems with bladder or bowel. You have no episodes of freezing.

If you are questioned directly:

You wife does describe that you appear 'bored' all the time and your face is less expressive.

Your concentration has suffered and you are finding it more difficult to complete paperwork at home.

Your handwriting has changed and become very small and nearly illegible.

You are an otherwise well man with no significant medical history. You have never had a stroke or heart attack. You take no regular medication and have never smoked, You do enjoy a glass of red wine most evenings. You have no drug allergies. You live with your wife and two children and your only family history is that your mother had a 'clot on the lung' in her 50s.

You are very worried about your symptoms as they have affected your ability to do your work and they seem to getting worse month on month. You believe that you are going to end up in a wheelchair and unable to provide for your family.

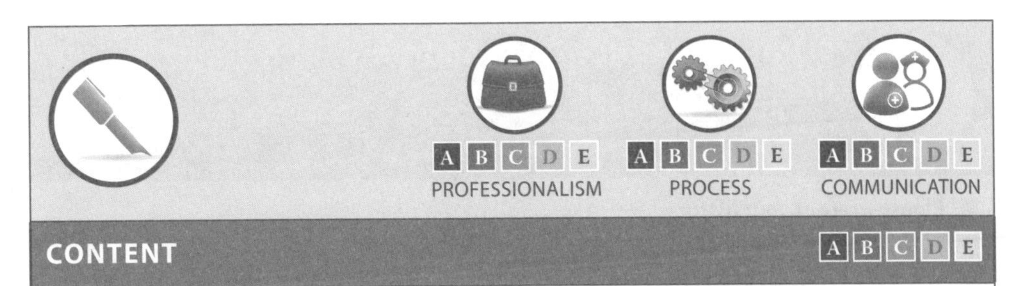

CONTENT

A B C D E

Identifies key information

- Presence of progressive bradykinesia – difficulty initiating movement, rigidity, loss of spontaneous movement, reduced facial expression
- Presence of resting tremor
- Presence of postural instability – affecting balance and posture with unsteady gait and falls
- Asymmetry of onset
- Cognitive dysfunction with poor concentration.

Excludes important negatives, including systemic enquiry

- No sensory symptoms, bladder or bowel dysfunction
- No bulbar dysfunction
- No vascular risk factors.

Relevant factors from employment, housing, social support

- Assess functional impact of symptoms.

Completing the patient history

- Drug and allergy history: nil regular medications, no allergies
- Previous medical history: nil of note
- Social and occupational history: accountant, non-smoker, moderate alcohol intake, lives with wife and 2 children
- Family history: no history of neurological disorders.

Summarises important areas of the history back to the patient

Invites patient to ask questions and is able to deal with them appropriately

Establishes patient's ideas, concerns and expectations

- Identifies that the patient is extremely concerned that he will require a wheelchair.

CLINICAL DIAGNOSTIC REASONING

A B C D E

- **Please present your history**
  - Candidate offers a logical, well-structured account of the history.
- **What is your diagnosis?**
  - Candidate offers the correct diagnosis and appropriate differentials
  - Parkinsonism – most likely idiopathic Parkinson's disease
  - Other possibilities are the Parkinson plus syndromes such as multiple system atrophy or progressive supra-nuclear palsy
  - Considers Wilson's disease or drug toxicity, but no risk factors.

Demonstrates a safe and sensible initial management plan

- Full neurological examination including gait assessment
- Cognitive assessment including handwriting
- Parkinson's disease is a clinical diagnosis, so routine biochemical investigations are unlikely to give any further information.

Demonstrates clear and logical diagnostic reasoning

GLOBAL HISTORY MARK

A B C D E

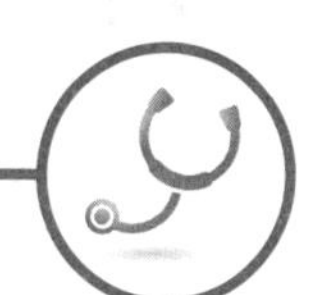

Station 2 – Examination

Patient script

If you are an actor/patient, read the patient history and physical signs fully – when the candidate comes to an abnormal site in their examination, act-out tenderness and/or volunteer the relevant physical sign.

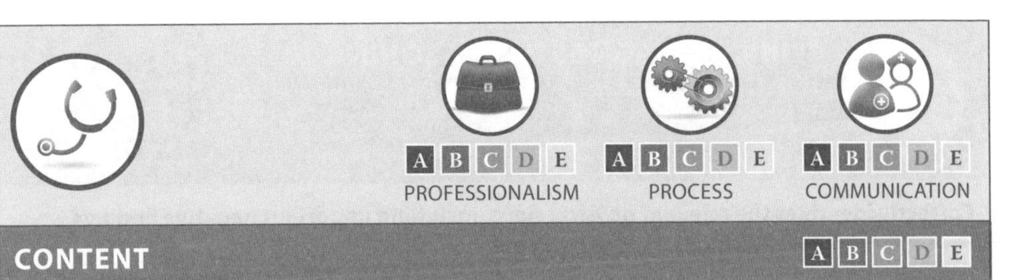

CONTENT

A B C D E

Exposes and positions patient correctly and maintains comfort

- Patient has exposed arms and legs.

Comments on wellbeing of patient, ie well or unwell

- Comments on any obvious wasting or weakness
- Notices 'pill rolling' asymmetrical low-frequency tremor at rest.

'Feet to face'

- Observes and comments on patient and surroundings from foot of bed
- Comments on absence of any aids to walking.

General and systematic examination

- Upper limb assessment: tone (including assessment for 'cog wheel' rigidity); power in shoulder (ab- and adduction), elbow (flex and extend), wrist (flex and extend, supinate and pronate) and fingers (ab- and adduction); reflexes (biceps, triceps and supinator); co-ordination (past pointing and assessment for dysdiadochokinesis)
- Lower limb assessment: tone (assessment for movement of foot with leg rolling and clonus); power in hip (flex and extend, ab- and adduction), knee (flex and extend), ankle (inversion, eversion, plantar and dorsiflexion); reflexes (knee jerk, ankle jerk and plantars – ensure safe approach); co-ordination (heel shin co-ordination).

Completes examination

- Gait: asks patient to walk across the room and turn and then return; difficulty initiating, festinant shuffling gait with small steps, reduced arm swing, difficulty on turning
- Postural instability: asks patient to stand with feet together and close their eyes; ensures patient safety and reassurance that they will not fall
- Can ask to assess handwriting and comment on facial paucity of movement.

Thanks patient and offers assistance

CLINICAL DIAGNOSTIC REASONING

A B C D E

Correctly identifies the relevant physical signs, including important negative findings

- Does not identify signs that are not present.

Correctly identifies other information that should be looked for when assessing for Parkinson plus syndromes

- Progressive supra-nuclear palsy – gaze abnormalities
- Multiple system atrophy – postural BP
- Dementia with Lewy bodies – dementia, visual hallucinations.

GLOBAL EXAMINATION MARK

A B C D E

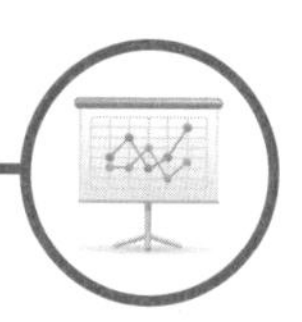

Station 3 – Data interpretation

Part 1:

1. H

2. I

3. G

4. J

5. D

Part 2:

1 (d) (D)

2 (b) (A)

3 (a) (C)

4 (d) (B)

Complications of drug therapy in Parkinson's disease

- 'Wearing off' phenomenon – increase in symptoms prior to next dose: this can be modified with prolonged release preparation, and adding in catechol-O-methyltransferase (COMT) inhibitors
- 'On-off' fluctuations (patients may switch from severe dyskinesia to immobility in a few minutes): this can be modified by combining levodopa with a dopamine agonist such as cabergoline
- Dyskinesias (may occur either at the beginning or end of a dose, or sometimes at its peak).

GLOBAL DATA INTERPRETATION MARK

A B C D E

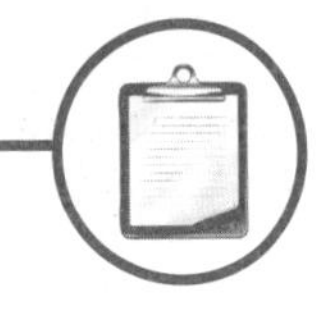

Station 4 – Prescribing skills

Sinemet® CR (50–200) two tablets at 0600 h, 1200 h and 1600 h with meals

For an outpatient prescription to be valid, it needs to include:

- Patient's date of birth
- Patient's name
- Patient's title, eg Mr
- Quantity of the product to be supplied
- Prescriber's qualifications
- Date prescription was signed
- Instructions to the patient on how to use the product
- Prescriber's signature.

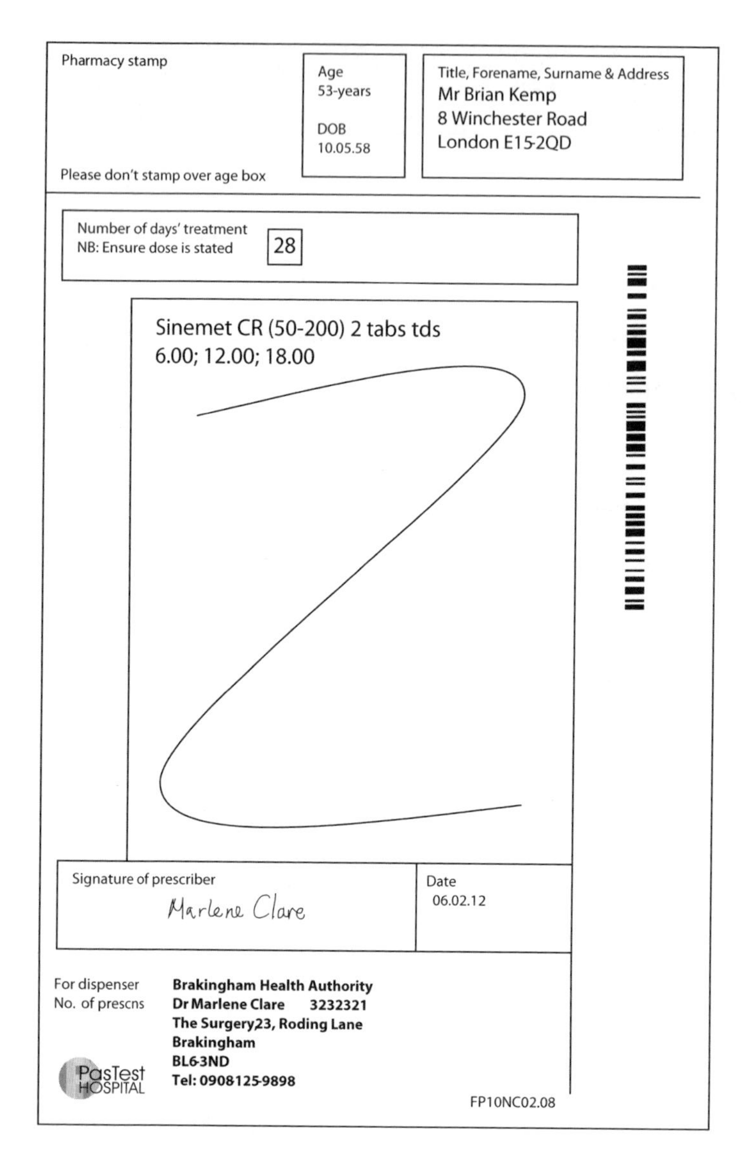
Pharmacy stamp

Please don't stamp over age box

Age
53-years

DOB
10.05.58

Title, Forename, Surname & Address
Mr Brian Kemp
8 Winchester Road
London E15-2QD

Number of days' treatment
NB: Ensure dose is stated
28

Sinemet CR (50-200) 2 tabs tds
6.00; 12.00; 18.00

Signature of prescriber
Marlene Clare

Date
06.02.12

For dispenser
No. of prescns

Brakingham Health Authority
Dr Marlene Clare 3232321
The Surgery, 23, Roding Lane
Brakingham
BL6-3ND
Tel: 0908125-9898

PasTest HOSPITAL

FP10NC02.08

Note: Patients who are suspected of having idiopathic Parkinson's disease are often trialled on smaller doses of L-dopa and a peripheral decarboxylase inhibitor, such as Madopar. If they demonstrate clinical improvements this low dose is rapidly increased and converted to a modified or slow release preparation. As 'on/off' periods and reduced response occur, doses are often split and spread over the full waking hours. Other medications including dopamine receptor agonists (carbegoline, pergolide and ropinrole), MAO-B inhibitor (selegiline) and Catechol-*O*-Methyltransferase (COMT) inhibitors (Entacapone and Tolcapone) and apomorphine are used in addition. All PD patients should be cared for by an expert MDT.

GLOBAL PRESCRIPTION MARK

A B C D E

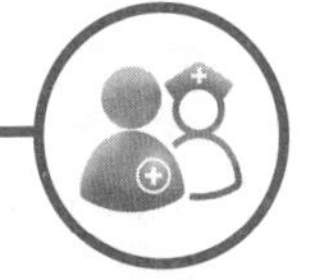

Station 6 – Clinical communication skills

Patient script

You are extremely upset about your diagnosis of Parkinson's disease. You know it cannot be cured and feel as though there is no point getting treatment if you have no chance of a cure.

You are not keen on any tablets, as you are 'just about' managing as you are and your wife is able to do the more complicated tasks at home.
After appropriate explanation and reassurance that your symptoms can be improved, you are willing to try the new medication.

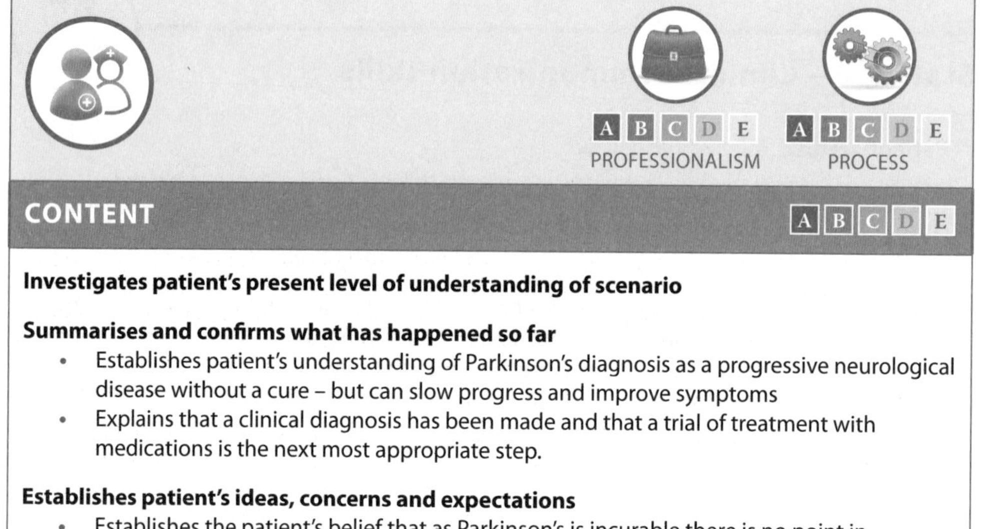

CONTENT

A B C D E

Investigates patient's present level of understanding of scenario

Summarises and confirms what has happened so far

- Establishes patient's understanding of Parkinson's diagnosis as a progressive neurological disease without a cure – but can slow progress and improve symptoms
- Explains that a clinical diagnosis has been made and that a trial of treatment with medications is the next most appropriate step.

Establishes patient's ideas, concerns and expectations

- Establishes the patient's belief that as Parkinson's is incurable there is no point in embarking on treatment
- Sensitively explains that symptom control with medication can be effective and improve quality of life.

Explains the key, important information

- Medications increase the amount of dopamine in the brain to improve ability to start movement, decrease rigidity and speed of movement
- Tablets taken three times per day with meals
- Take some weeks to monitor response and will be titrated up and down
- Common side-effects – postural hypotension 'dizziness', GI upset, labile mood.

Invites patient to ask questions as they proceed through the consultation and is able to deal with them appropriately

Summarises important areas of the consultation back to the patient

Formally ends the consultation and ensures appropriate follow-up has been discussed

- Gives prescription, informs patient they will need to see GP in next 2 weeks and will be seen in movement disorder clinic.

GLOBAL COMMUNICATION MARK

A B C D E

Scenario 20: Reflection and consolidation

History

Mr Kemp is a 52-year-old man who presents with a progressive of bradykinesia, resting tremor and unsteadiness of gait. His bradykinesia has been a problem for at least 9 months and is characterised by a long-standing history of loss of facial expression and increasing difficulty initiating movement, but he is able to complete movements without significant difficulty. He has unsteadiness of gait and has fallen twice. He has a history of resting tremor, which was initially unilateral. He also describes poor concentration and micrographia. He has no significant medical history and is a non-smoker. He has no bulbar dysfunction and no sensory symptoms. The likely diagnosis is of idiopathic Parkinson's disease.

Investigations

On examination of this man's neurological system, he has no obvious wasting or fasciculation. He has a blank expression and reduced expressiveness. He has a resting tremor, more noticeable on the right side. This improves on movement. He has an increase in tone with cog wheeling more noticeable on the right. His power is normal throughout. He has no pastpointing, dysdidochokinesis or impaired lower limb co-ordination.

He has difficulty initiating movement and his gait is hesitant and shuffling with reduced arm swing.

The triad of bradykinesia, rigidity and resting tremor suggests a diagnosis of parkinsonism, most likely due to idiopathic Parkinson's disease.

The diagnosis is clinical and based on typical history and examination. Any investigations are based on excluding other causes of parkinsonism.

- CT or MRI brain can be needed to exclude rare secondary causes (eg supratentorial tumours and normal pressure hydrocephalus) and extensive subcortical vascular pathology
- Positron emission tomography (PET) scans can localise dopamine deficiency in the basal ganglia, while autonomic tests can confirm a diagnosis of multiple system atrophy
- Further investigations for young-onset disease may include measurement of ceruloplasmin levels (Wilson's disease), tests for the Huntington gene and syphilis serology.

Management

Multidisciplinary management is essential

- Nurses with a special interest in Parkinson's disease who can monitor the clinical condition and adjust medication
- Physiotherapy – to help improve gait, balance and flexibility, increase independence and provide advice regarding fall prevention and other safety information
- Occupational therapy – give advice and help on maintaining all aspects relating to activities of daily living
- Speech and language therapy – improving loudness and intelligibility of speech where possible, ensuring methods of communication are available as the disease progresses, and to help with swallowing.

Further reading and web links

Parkinson's disease: diagnosis and management in primary and secondary care:
www.nice.org.uk/guidance/index.jsp?action=byID&r=true&o=10984

Parkinson's UK: up-to-date patient and clinician information:
www.parkinsons.org.uk

Prescription charts

Allergies, sensitivities and adverse drug reactions					Patient details/addressograph
No known allergies ☐		Initials	Gender M / F		NHS/ Hospital No:
Not possible to ascertain ☐		Date	Weight (kg)	Date	
Medicine/substance	Reaction & Severity	Initials & Date			Surname:
			Height		First name:
Alerts			Surface area (m²)		Date of birth:

IN-PATIENT MEDICATION PRESCRIPTION
AND ADMINISTRATION RECORD

PasTest HOSPITAL

Consultant	Trainee Dr. Name and Bleep no.	Date of admission	Date chart reboarded	Estimated date of discharge
This chart is no. .... of	Transcribing Check by Pharmacy Sign .... Date	Ward 1. .... 2.		

Supplementary Medication charts in use: Other (please specify): 1 .... 2 ....

Epidural/PCA ☐ Syringe driver ☐ TPN ☐ Chemotherapy ☐ Insulin sliding scale ☐

Once only medications – loading doses, pre-medication, PGDs or surgical antibiotic propylaxis

Date	Time to be given	Medicine (approved name)	Dose	Route	Signature and bleep no.	Pharmacy	Time given	Given by	Checked by

Regular prescriptions						
Oral anticoagulation follow the anticoagulation guidelines available on the intranet						
Indication	Target INR	Baseline INR (if applicable)	Duration of therapy Date therapy started	Date of anticoagulation follow-up appointment (clinic or other)*	Anticoagulant record book given or updated. Sign and date	Date patient counselled and sign
* A follow-up appointment must be booked with the anti-coagulant clinic or enhanced provider of primary care services. If not, the TTA will not be dispensed						

Initiating warfarin	Perform baseline coagulation screen, LFTs, U&Es and FBC	Prescribe initiation dose as per guidelines	CHECK INR ON DAY 3	FOLLOW DOSING ALGORITHM IN GUIDELINE
Continuing warfarin	Maintenance therapy	FOLLOW MAINTENANCE DOSING ALGORITHM IN GUIDELINE		
Do not use the initiation protocol for patients already on warfarin. More frequent INR monitoring may be required for patients on interacting drug(s)				

Medication				Date													
1				INR													
Route	Frequency OD	Time 18.00	Start	Dose													
			Stop	Dr sign													
Signature		Bleep no.	Pharmacy	Given													

Initiating warfarin – Reduced dosing regimen in red. Refer to anticoagulation policy																		
Day	One	Two	Three							Four and above								
INR	<1.4	No test	<2.0	2.0-2.1	2.2-2.5	2.6-2.9	3.0-3.3	3.4-4.0	>4.0	<1.4	1.4-1.5	1.6-1.7	1.8-1.9	2.0-2.3	2.4-3.0	3.1-4.0	4.1-4.5	>4.5
Dose mg	10 5	10 5	10	5	4	3	2	1	0	9	8	7	6	5	4	3	Miss 1 day	Miss 2 day

Thromboprophylaxis please prescribe treatment regimens in the regular medications section									
Choice of mechanical prophylaxis and leg(s) to be applied to							Enter Time	Enter details below	
Graduated elastic compression stockings		Intermittend pneumatic compression device (IPC)	Leg						
			Left	Right	Both				
Start Date: ☐	End Date: ☐	Signature and Bleep No.	☐	☐	☐				
Start Date: ☐	End Date: ☐	Signature and Bleep No.	☐	☐	☐				

Medication		Dose	Dose Change	Enter Time	Enter details below
Please ensure you have completed the VTE risk assessment form	Date				
	Route				
	Signature			Instructions	Pharmacy ☐
	Bleep no.				

Oxygen		☐	☐	
Target Saturation		88-92%	94/98%	If oxygen saturation falls below target range on prescribed oxygen, patient needs urgent clinical review. If oxygen saturation is above targent range on prescribed oxygen, ask for review.
Other specify)				*Device: N= nasal cannula, SM = simple face mask, V = venturi, H = humidified, RM = reservoir mask, OTHER = other eg. NCPAP/NIPPV — Pharmacy ☐
Target Saturation not applicable ☐				

	Date Changed	Date Changed	Enter Time	Enter details below
Device				
% or L/min (specify a range eg 1-21 L/min)				
Signature and Bleep no.				

Regular prescriptions continued																		
Regular medications																		
		Dose			Date													
Date					Medication					Instructions				Signature and bleep no.			Pharmacy	
Route																		
Signature																		
06																		
09																		
12																		
18																		
22																		
24																		

Regular prescriptions continued																		
Regular medications																		
		Dose			Date													
Date					Medication					Instructions				Signature and bleep no.			Pharmacy	
Route																		
Signature																		
06																		
09																		
12																		
18																		
22																		
24																		

Infusion prescriptions continued										SC = subcutane-ous		IVC = intravenous central IVP = intravenous peripheral		
Date & time	Route	Infusion Fluid		Medication		Duration	Rate	Prescriber's signature & bleep no.	Date given	Given by / Added by	Check by	Start time	Finish time	Pharmacy
		Name & strength	Volume	Approved name with expiry / unit number	Dose									
		Exp: Batch/unit no:												
		Exp: Batch/unit no:												
		Exp: Batch/unit no:												
		Exp: Batch/unit no:												
		Exp: Batch/unit no:												
		Exp: Batch/unit no:												
		Exp: Batch/unit no:												
		Exp: Batch/unit no:												
		Exp: Batch/unit no:												

As required medications																									
Medication				Date																					
Indication				Time																					
Dose	Route	Maximum frequency / dose	Start date	Dose																					
			Stop date	Route																					
Signature			Bleep no.	Given																					
Additional instructions:																	Pharmacy								

As required medications																									
Medication				Date																					
Indication				Time																					
Dose	Route	Maximum frequency / dose	Start date	Dose																					
			Stop date	Route																					
Signature			Bleep no.	Given																					
Additional instructions:																	Pharmacy								

FP10

Pharmacy stamp

Please don't stamp over age box

Age

DOB

Title, Forename, Surname & Address

Number of days' treatment
NB: Ensure dose is stated

Signature of prescriber

Date

For dispenser
No. of prescns

FP10NC02.08

Drug chart

PRESCRIBING PROFORMA

Generic Prescribing: The following details were completed and correct:

- Patient's name, DOB, age, weight, height
- The ward, consultant, responsible junior doctor and bleep number.

The drug chart is legible
For each of the drugs prescribed the following details are correctly completed:

(**DRUG DR**s **D**on't **F**orget **S**igning **O**ff)

DRUG - name (generic)
Dose
Route of administration
Signature
Dose
Frequency
Signature
Others – duration, gated, maximum dose per 24 hours, levels

As it is written – the drug can be dispensed

Station Index

communication skills x, xix, xxi
- alcohol abuse 241, 250–2
- aortic stenosis 224, 236–7
- asthma 5, 16–17
- atrial fibrillation 323–4, 334–5
- cancer diagnosis 291, 301–2
- cancer has spread 267, 283–4
- consent for surgery 43, 52–4
- diabetes 185, 199–201
- DNAR orders 77, 92–4
- epilepsy 58, 68–9
- hypothyroidism 101, 109–11
- MRSA screening 308, 315–16
- multiple sclerosis 167, 175–6
- Parkinson's disease 357, 365–6
- peripheral vascular disease 134, 143–4
- pneumonia 119, 129–30
- tuberculosis 343, 349–50
- unstable angina 24, 35–6

data interpretation x, xx–xxi
- angiography (anatomy) 137–8, 147
- arterial blood gases 182–3, 191, 206, 212–13
- blood tests
  - alcohol abuse 241–2, 252–3
  - coagulopathy screens 289, 296–7
  - diabetes 181–2, 190–1
  - gastroenteritis 75, 85, 96
  - metastatic breast cancer 264–5, 274
  - pulmonary lesions 118, 126–7
- CT abdomen (anatomy) 41, 48
- ECGs 221–3, 231, 321–2, 331
  - unstable angina 21–2, 29–30, 37
- hepatitis screening 242–3, 253
- lumbar punctures 166, 174–5
- lung function tests 4, 11
- microbiology (gastroenteritis) 75–6, 85
- MRI of spine 265, 274
- multiple sclerosis therapy 167, 175
- Parkinson's disease 355–6, 362
- thyroid function tests 100–1, 109, 114
- upper GI bleeding 151–2, 159
- Wells' score for PE 288, 296
- X-rays
  - fractures 306–7, 313, 317
  - pulmonary disease 340–1, 348–9
  - unstable angina 22–3, 37

examination x, xii, xviii, xix
- acute cord syndrome 263–4, 271–3, 285
- alcohol abuse 240–1, 248–50, 260
- aortic stenosis 220–1, 228–30, 238
- appendicitis 40–1, 46–7, 54
- asthma 2–3, 9–10, 17
- atrial fibrillation 319–20, 327–9, 336
- COPD 204–5, 210–11, 217
- diabetes 180–1, 188–90, 202
- epilepsy 56–7, 62–4, 70
- gastroenteritis 73–4, 83–4, 96
- hip fracture 305–6, 311–13, 317
- hypothyroidism 99–100, 106–8, 114
- multiple sclerosis 164–5, 170–2, 177
- Parkinson's disease 354–5, 360–2, 367
- peripheral vascular disease 133–4, 142–3, 148
- pneumonia 116–17, 122–4, 130
- pulmonary embolism 287–8, 294–6, 303
- tuberculosis 339–40, 346–8, 351
- unstable angina 20–1, 27–9, 37
- upper GI bleeding 150–1, 156–8, 162

history ix, xii, xviii, xix
- acute cord syndrome 262, 268–71, 284
- alcohol abuse 239, 245–8, 260
- aortic stenosis 219, 225–8, 238
- appendicitis 39, 44–5, 54
- asthma 1, 6–8, 17

atrial fibrillation 318, 325–7, 336
COPD 203, 208–10, 217
diabetes 179, 186–8, 201
epilepsy 55, 59–62, 70
gastroenteritis 72, 79–82, 96
hip fracture 304, 309–11, 316–17
hypothyroidism 98, 103–6, 113
multiple sclerosis 163, 168–70, 177
Parkinson's disease 353, 358–60, 367
peripheral vascular disease 132, 139–41, 147
pneumonia 115, 120–2, 130
pulmonary embolism 286, 292–4, 302
tuberculosis 338, 344–6, 351
unstable angina 19, 25–7, 37
upper GI bleeding 149, 154–6, 162

prescribing skills x, xxi
acute cord syndrome 266–7, 278–82
alcohol abuse 244, 256–9
aortic stenosis 224, 232–5
appendicitis 42, 48–51
asthma 5, 12–15
atrial fibrillation 323, 332–4
COPD 207, 213–17
diabetes 184, 195–8
epilepsy 58, 66–7, 69
gastroenteritis 76, 86–91, 97
hypothyroidism 101–2, 111–13
Parkinson's disease 356, 363–4
peripheral vascular disease 134–6, 145, 148
pneumonia 118–19, 127–8, 131
pulmonary embolism 290, 297–9
unstable angina 23–4, 30–4, 37
upper GI bleeding 153, 159–61

procedural skills x, xxi
arterial blood sampling 183–4, 192–3, 205, 212
blood glucose testing 166, 174
cannulation 117, 126
confirmation of death 77–8, 94–5
ECGs 320, 330
emergency blood transfusion 244, 255
in epileptic seizures 57, 65–6
infusion pumps 137, 146, 148
intramuscular injections 43, 51–2
nasogastric tube insertion 184, 193–4
nebuliser administration 3, 10
pleural effusion testing 342, 349
subcutaneous injection 290, 300
swabbing for MRSA 308, 314
urinary catheterization 153, 161, 266, 275–7
venepuncture 165, 173
for blood cultures 117, 125
for crossmatching 243–4, 254

Subject Index

abdominal CT scans 41, 48
abdominal examination 41, 46–7
ABGs *see* arterial blood gases
ACE inhibitors 237
acid–base balance 182–3, 191, 206, 212–13
ACTH (adrenocorticotrophic hormone), ectopic 118, 127
acute cord syndrome *see* spinal cord compression, acute
AF *see* atrial fibrillation
airway management 57, 65
alcohol abuse 239–61
  counselling 241, 250–2
  examination 240–1, 248–50, 260
  history 239, 245–8, 260
  investigations 241–2, 252–3, 289, 297
  management 243–4, 252, 254–9, 260
amiodarone 102, 113, 323, 332–4
anaemia, aplastic 289, 296–7
anaesthesia, risks 52
angina *see* unstable angina
angiograms 137–8, 147
antibiotics
  in gastroenteritis 76, 86–8
  interactions with anti-epileptics 69
anticoagulants
  heparin 134–6, 145, 148, 297
  warfarin 297, 323–4, 334–5
anti-epileptic drugs 58, 66–7, 69
  with thyroxine 102, 113
aortic stenosis 219–38
  communication 224, 236–7
  examination 220–1, 228–30, 238
  history 219, 225–8, 238
  management 224, 232–5, 238
appendicitis 39–54
  consenting for surgery 43, 52–4
  examination 40–1, 46–7, 54
  history 39, 44–5, 54
  management 42–3, 48–52, 54
APTT ratio, heparin and 136, 145
arterial blood gases (ABGs)
  differential diagnosis 182–3, 191, 206, 212–13
  sampling procedure 183–4, 192–3, 205, 212
asthma 1–18
  communication 5, 16–17
  examination 2–3, 9–10, 17
  history 1, 6–8, 17
  investigations 4, 11, 18, 183, 191
  management 3, 5, 10, 12–15, 18
atrial fibrillation (AF) 318–37
  communication (re warfarin) 323–4, 334–5
  examination 319–20, 327–9, 336
  history 318, 325–7, 336
  investigations 320–1, 330–1
  management 323, 332–4, 337
autoimmune thyroid disease 108

Barrett's oesophagus 151, 159
blood tests
  ABGs *see* arterial blood gases
  alcohol abuse 241–2, 252–3
  diabetes 181–2, 190–1
  gastroenteritis 75, 85, 96
  for glucose 166, 174
  hepatitis screen 242–3, 253
  metastatic breast cancer 264–5, 274
  thyroid function 100–1, 109, 114
  venous sampling 117, 125, 165, 173, 243–4, 254
blood transfusions 153, 159–61
  emergency 244, 255
breaking bad news
  cancer diagnosis 291, 301–2
  cancer has spread 267, 283–4
  discussing DNAR orders 77, 92–4

multiple sclerosis 167, 175–6
breast cancer, metastatic *see* spinal cord compression
bronchitis 217

CAGE questionnaire 246
calcium abnormalities 118, 126–7, 264–5, 274
cannulation 117, 126
carbimazole 102, 112
carcinoid syndrome 118, 126
cardiovascular disorders
aortic stenosis 219–38
atrial fibrillation 318–37
differential diagnosis on ECG 221–3, 231, 321–2, 331
unstable angina 19–38
cerebellar system examination 63
cerebral angiograms 137–8, 147
chest X-rays
NG tube insertion 194
pulmonary infections 340–1, 348–9
unstable angina 22–3
clinical communication (domain) xix
clinical diagnostic reasoning (domain) xx
coagulation screens
DIC 181–2, 191
differential diagnosis 289, 296–7
liver disease 241–2, 252–3
consent for surgery 43, 52–4
content (domain) xix
continuous positive airway pressure (CPAP) 119, 129–30, 131
COPD (chronic obstructive lung disease) 203–18
examination 204–5, 210–11, 217
history 203, 208–10, 217
investigations 182, 191, 206, 213, 218
management 207, 213–17, 218
cranial nerve examination 63
Crohn's disease 152, 159
CT (computed tomography) scans
abdominal 41, 48
pulmonary embolism 289

death, confirmation/certification 77–8, 94–5
dehydration 74, 84, 90, 97
diabetes mellitus type 1, new-onset 179–202
communication 185, 199–201
examination 180–1, 188–90, 202
history 179, 186–8, 201
investigations 181–2, 190–1, 202
management 184, 195–8, 202
diagnostic clinical assessment xii–xiii
diarrhoea and vomiting *see* gastroenteritis
disseminated intravascular coagulopathy (DIC) 181–2, 191
do not resuscitate (DNAR) orders 77, 92–4
domains xiv, xvi–xx
driving 69
drugs
acute cord syndrome 266–7, 278–82
acute coronary syndrome 23–4, 30–4, 35, 37
alcohol abuse 244, 252, 256–9
aortic stenosis 224, 232–5
appendicitis 42, 48–51
asthma 5, 12–15
atrial fibrillation 323–4, 332–5
COPD 207, 213–17
diabetes 184, 195–8
epilepsy 58, 66–7, 69
gastroenteritis 76, 86–91, 97
hypothyroidism 101–2, 111–13
multiple sclerosis 167, 175, 178
Parkinson's disease 356–7, 362–6
peripheral vascular disease 134–6, 145, 148
pneumonia 118–19, 127–8
pulmonary embolism 290, 297–9
upper GI bleeding 153, 159–61
duodenal ulcers 151, 159

electrocardiograms (ECG)

acute coronary syndrome 21–2, 29–30
atrial fibrillation 321, 331
differential diagnosis 221–3, 231, 321–2, 331
procedures 320, 330
electrolytes
diabetes 181–2, 190–1
gastroenteritis 75, 85
emphysema 4, 11, 217
epilepsy 55–71
communication 58, 68–9
examination 56–7, 62–4, 70
history 55, 59–62, 70
management 57–8, 65–7, 69, 71
euthyroidism 100–1, 109
exercise tolerance tests 36

fibrosing alveolitis 4, 11
fluids
in diabetes 197
in gastroenteritis 90, 97
fractures
hip *see* hip fracture
upper limb 307, 313

gastric carcinoma 151, 159, 182, 191
gastroenteritis 72–97
examination 73–4, 83–4, 96
history 72, 79–82, 96
investigations 75–6, 85, 96
management 76, 86–91, 97
gastrointestinal bleeding (upper) 149–62
examination 150–1, 156–8
history 149, 154–6, 162
investigations 151–2, 159, 162, 241–2, 252–3
management 153, 159–61, 162
gastro-oesophageal reflux disease 152, 159
glucose testing 166, 174
Guillain–Barré syndrome 206, 212

H_2 antagonists 102, 113
haematemesis *see* gastrointestinal bleeding (upper)
heart block 222, 231, 322, 331
heparin 134–6, 145, 148, 297
hepatic disease *see* liver disease
hepatitis, viral 242–3, 253
hip fracture 304–17
examination 305–6, 311–13, 317
history 304, 309–11, 316–17
investigations 306, 313, 317
MRSA screening 308, 314–16, 317
hyperthyroidism 100–1, 102, 108, 109, 112
hyperventilation 206, 213
hypothyroidism 98–114
communication 101, 109–11
examination 99–100, 106–8, 114
history 98, 103–6, 113
investigations 100–1, 109, 114
management 101–2, 111–13, 114

infusion pumps 137, 146, 148
injections
intramuscular 43, 51–2
subcutaneous 290, 300
insulin therapy 200
intermittent claudication *see* peripheral vascular disease
intramuscular injections 43, 51–2
intubation 57, 65
irritable bowel syndrome 152, 159

kidney disease 74, 84, 264–5, 274

left bundle branch block (LBBB) 322, 331
left ventricular hypertrophy (LVH) 221, 231
Legionella pneumophila 122
lithium 102, 113
liver disease
alcoholic
blood tests 241–2, 252–3
examination 241, 249
management 152, 159

metastatic 118, 127
viral hepatitis 242–3, 253
lower limb
hip fracture 304–17
neurological assessment 165, 171, 264, 272
vascular disease 132–48
lumbar punctures 166, 174–5
lung disease
asthma 1–18, 183, 191
COPD 203–18
differential diagnosis 4, 11, 118, 126–7, 206, 212–13
pneumonia 115–31, 341, 349
tuberculosis 338–52
see also pulmonary embolism
lung function tests 4, 11

Mallory–Weiss syndrome 151, 159
marking of OSCEs xxii–xxiii
meningitis 166, 175
microbiology
gastroenteritis 75–6, 85
MRSA screening 308, 314–16, 317
pneumonia 122, 130
taking a blood sample 117, 125
MRI (magnetic resonance imaging)
contraindications 36
spinal cord compression 265, 274
MRSA (meticillin-resistant *Staphylococcus aureus*) screening 308, 314–16, 317
multiple sclerosis 163–78
communication 167, 175–6
examination 164–5, 170–2, 177
history 163, 168–70, 177
lumbar puncture 166, 174
management 167, 175, 178
myasthenia gravis 4, 11
myocardial infarction 222, 231, 322, 331

nasogastric (NG) tube insertion 184, 193–4
nebuliser administration 3, 10
neck examination 107
neurological disorders
acute cord syndrome 262–85
epilepsy 55–71
multiple sclerosis 163–78
Parkinson's disease 353–67
non-invasive positive pressure ventilation (NIPPV) 119, 129–30, 131

obturator sign 47
oesophageal varices 151, 158, 159
oesophagogastroduodenoscopy (OGD) 152, 159, 162
oligoclonal bands 166, 174
OSCE examinations xi–xii, xiii–xiv
marking xxii–xxiii
ovarian cancer 291, 301–2

parathyroid hormone, ectopic 118, 126–7
Parkinson's disease 353–67
diagnosis 355, 362, 367
examination 354–5, 360–2, 367
history 353, 358–60, 367
management 356–7, 362–6, 367
PE *see* pulmonary embolism
pelvic CT scans 41, 48
pericarditis, acute 223, 231
peripheral vascular disease 132–48
communication 134, 143–4
examination 133–4, 142–3, 148
history 132, 139–41, 147
investigations 137–8, 147
management 134–7, 145–6, 148
peritonism 152, 159
phenytoin 58, 66–7, 69
with thyroxine 102, 113
phlebotomy *see* venepuncture
platelet abnormalities 289, 296–7
pleural effusions 341, 342, 348, 349, 351
pneumonia 115–31
examination 116–17, 122–4, 130
history 115, 120–2, 130

management 117, 118–19, 125–6, 127–8, 131
microbiology 122, 130
X-rays 341, 349
presentation skills xv–xvi
process (domain) xviii
professionalism (domain) xvii
propylthiouracil 102, 112
psoas sign 47
pulmonary embolism (PE) 286–303
communication 291, 301–2
examination 287–8, 294–6, 303
history 286, 292–4, 302
investigations 288–9, 296, 303
ABGs 183, 191, 206, 213
ECG 322, 331
management 290, 297–300, 303
pulmonary oedema, acute 206, 213

radiography *see* X-rays
radiotherapy 284
renal artery stenosis 237
renal disease 74, 84, 264–5, 274
respiratory arrest 57, 66
respiratory disease
asthma 1–18, 183, 191
COPD 203–18
differential diagnosis 4, 11, 118, 126–7, 206, 212–13
pneumonia 115–31, 341, 349
tuberculosis 338–52
see also pulmonary embolism
resuscitation, DNAR orders 77, 92–4

scenario design xv–xvi
seizures *see* epilepsy
shoulder, dislocated 307, 313
SIADH (syndrome of inappropriate ADH secretion) 118, 127
spinal cord compression, acute 262–85
communication 267, 283–4
examination 263–4, 271–3, 285
history 262, 268–71, 284
investigations 264–5, 274, 285
management 266–7, 275–82, 285
spirometry 4, 11
station design ix–x, xx–xxi
stomach carcinoma 151, 159, 182, 191
subarachnoid haemorrhage 166, 175
subcutaneous injections 290, 300
subdural haemorrhage 166, 175
syphilis 166, 175

T_3 (triiodothyronine) 100–1, 109
T_4 (thyroxine)
replacement therapy 101, 111–12
test results 100–1, 109
thromboembolism *see* pulmonary embolism
thyroid disorders 98–114
communication 101, 109–11
examination 99–100, 106–8, 114
history 98, 103–6, 113
management 101–2, 111–13, 114
thyroid function tests 100–1, 109, 114
transfusions *see* blood transfusions
TSH (thyroid stimulating hormone) 100–1, 109
tuberculosis 338–52
examination 339–40, 346–8, 351
history 338, 344–6, 351
investigations 340–2, 348–9, 351
management 343, 349–50, 352

unstable angina 19–38
communication 24, 35–6
examination 20–1, 27–9, 37
history 19, 25–7, 37
investigations 21–3, 29–30, 37
management 23–4, 30–4, 37
upper limb
neurological assessment 165, 171
X-rays 307, 313
uraemia 74, 84
urinary catheterization 153, 161, 266, 275–7

vascular disease *see* peripheral vascular disease; unstable angina
venepuncture 165, 173
  for crossmatching 243–4, 254
  for culturing 117, 125
venous thromboembolism *see* pulmonary embolism
ventilation
  intubation 57, 65
  in pneumonia 119, 129–30, 131
vomiting *see* gastroenteritis

warfarin 297, 323–4, 334–5
Wells' score 288, 296
wrist, fracture 307, 313

X-rays
  fractures 306–7, 313, 317
  NG tube insertion 194
  pulmonary infections 340–1, 348–9
  unstable angina 22–3